Case-Based Pathology and Laboratory Medicine

Nagy H. Mikhail, MD, FCAP

Associate Professor of Pathology and Laboratory Medicine,
Robert Wood Johnson Medical School, NJ
Laboratory Director, Southern Ocean County Hospital, NJ

Jana Raskova, MD

Professor of Pathology and Laboratory Medicine and
Chief, Division of Pathology Educational Programs, Robert Wood Johnson Medical School, NJ
Visiting Professor, 3rd Faculty of Medicine, Charles University, Prague

Stephen M. Shea, MD, FRCPath

Professor of Pathology and Laboratory Medicine,
Robert Wood Johnson Medical School, NJ

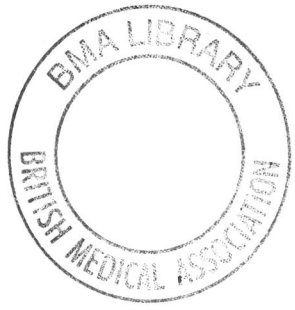
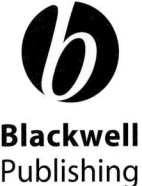
Blackwell
Publishing

Published by Blackwell Publishing Ltd
Blackwell Publishing, Inc., 350 Main Street, Malden, Massachusetts 02148-5020, USA
Blackwell Publishing Ltd, 9600 Garsington Road, Oxford OX4 2DQ, UK
Blackwell Publishing Asia Pty Ltd, 550 Swanston Street, Carlton, Victoria 3053, Australia

First published 2005

Library of Congress Cataloging-in-Publication Data
Mikhail, Nagy H.
    Case-based pathology and laboratory medicine / Nagy H. Mikhail, Jana Raskova, Stephen M. Shea.
        p. ; cm.
    Includes index.
    ISBN 1-4051-2056-8 (alk. paper)
    1. Pathology—Case studies. 2. Diagnosis, Laboratory—Case studies.
    I. Raskova, Jana. II. Shea, Stephen M. III. Title.
    [DNLM: 1. Clinical Medicine—methods—Case Reports. 2. Clinical Medicine—
methods—Problems and Exercises. 3. Clinical Laboratory Techniques—Case Reports.
4. Clinical Laboratory Techniques—Problems and Exercises.   WB 18.2 M636c 2004]
    RB112.M535 2004
    616.07'5—dc22

    2004018341

ISBN 1-4051-2056-8

A catalogue record for this title is available from the British Library

Set in 10/12 pt Minion by Sparks, Oxford – www.sparks.co.uk
Printed and bound in India by Replika Press Pvt. Ltd

Commissioning Editor: Vicki Noyes
Development Editor: Geraldine Jeffers
Editorial Assistant: Nic Ulyatt
Production Controller: Kate Charman

For further information on Blackwell Publishing, visit our website:
http://www.blackwellpublishing.com

The publisher's policy is to use permanent paper from mills that operate a sustainable forestry policy, and which has been manufactured from pulp processed using acid-free and elementary chlorine-free practices. Furthermore, the publisher ensures that the text paper and cover board used have met acceptable environmental accreditation standards.

Contents

Preface

In pre-clinical courses students acquire a large amount of scientific knowledge, aimed at the understanding of biological events or processes that ultimately lead to disorder and disease. There is no better way to test one's knowledge than to face exposure to the specific problem, or better, to the combination of problems that a patient usually presents when seeking medical help. Suddenly, facts learned must be conceptually integrated with clinical data, and new information and data must be sought and assimilated, until a diagnosis is finally reached. This process is described as diagnostic reasoning. With this in mind, we present a series of clinical cases arranged into chapters which cover a variety of major diseases.

Our clinical cases are divided into specific sections. The first part of each chapter is an exploratory component of the case. It consists of "Clinical history and presentation," including radiological and laboratory data, followed by probing multiple choice questions, "Clinical course," with additional laboratory and other findings, and more questions. These questions may vary in difficulty, since their primary purpose is to explore the clinical and scientific aspects of the case, rather than to assess mastery of material. Accordingly they are individually labeled by difficulty as Basic, Intermediate, or Advanced. Through this stage the reader is guided, but left to his or her own resources to arrive at a conclusion. The second part of the chapter is explanatory and didactic. It is composed of the following sections: "Figure descriptions," "Answers," "Final diagnosis and synopsis of the case," and in some cases a section on "Lab tips" is included. We recommend that the reader complete part one first without consulting part two. This approach would not only provide feedback on the reader's understanding of the problem, but also sharpen his or her skill in diagnostic reasoning.

At the end of this book we have compiled Appendices of information we consider to be useful for the reader's orientation and learning. These consist of a "SI Units Conversion Table," a listing of "Topics Explored," which is divided into "Pathology" and "Laboratory Medicine" sections, a list of "Lab Tips," and a list of "Final Diagnoses" for review of specific problems in any of the chapters.

The purpose of this book is not to provide the reader with more facts, but rather to teach him or her how best to make use of facts already known, and to develop skill in using them rationally. At the same time the book will serve as a review of many major diseases, and as a stimulus to consult reference texts.

The Authors
New Jersey

Acknowledgements

The authors first wish to acknowledge their enduring friendship, which survived the preparation and completion of this manuscript. Many thanks also belong to our long-time colleague, Frederick C. Skvara, MD, for his many contributions to the development of the clinical cases.

We also wish to express our appreciation to the following institutions, which were of great assistance to us: the Department of Pathology and Laboratory Medicine, Robert Wood Johnson Medical School, Piscataway, NJ; the Department of Pathology and Molecular Diagnostics, St Peter's University Hospital, New Brunswick, NJ; and the Departments of Pathology and Laboratory Medicine and of Radiology, Southern Ocean County Hospital, Manahawkin, NJ.

Finally, our profound thanks belong to our spouses, Mrs Cherine Mikhail, for her tireless proofreading of the many numbers we have generated, and to Karel Raska, MD, PhD, for his many comments, good and bad, and to our friend, Mrs Margee Chapin, for her invaluable administrative support.

Abbreviations

AAT Alpha1 antitrypsin
AB Antibody
ACE Angiotensin-converting enzyme
AG Antigen
AHG Antihuman globulin
ADH (AVP) Antidiuretic hormone (arginine vasopressin)
AFB Acid-fast bacilli
AFP Alpha fetoprotein
AIDS Acquired immune deficiency syndrome
Alk Phos (ALP) Alkaline phosphatase
ALL Acute lymphoblastic leukemia
ALT (SGPT) Alanine aminotransferase (glutamic-pyruvic transaminase)
ANA Antinuclear antibodies
A-P view Antero-posterior view
APTT (aPTT) Activated partial thromboplastin time
AST (SGOT) Aspartate aminotransferase (glutamic-oxaloacetic transaminase)
ATN Acute tubular necrosis
AVP Arginine vasopressin
B CLL Chronic lympocytic leukemia of B-lymphocytes
Baso Basophil
BNP B-type natriuretic peptide
BRAT Bananas, rice, apple-sauce, tea-toast diet
BUN Blood urea nitrogen
C3b Complement component, fragment C3b
C3d Complement component, fragment C3d
CA-125 Tumor marker
CALLA Common acute lymphoblastic leukemia antigen
CAT; CT scan Computerized axial tomography scan
CBC Complete blood count
CD Cluster designation
CEA Carcinoembryonic antigen
CFU Colony-forming units
CGD Chronic granulomatous disease
CHF Congestive heart failure
CK MB Creatine kinase, MB fraction
CK (CPK) Creatine kinase
CK 903 Cytokeratin 903
Cl Chloride

CO$_2$ Carbon dioxide
CSF Colony-stimulating factor
DNA Deoxyribonucleic acid
RNA Ribonucleic acid
EBV Epstein–Barr virus
EKG (ECG) Electrocardiogram
Eos Eosinophil
ESR Erythrocyte sedimentation rate
ET Essential thrombocytosis (Essential thrombocythemia)
Fig. Figure
FBC Full blood count
fL Femtoliter
GGTP (GGT) Gamma glutamyl transpeptidase (transferase)
GM-CSF Granulocyte-macrophage colony-stimulating factor
GI Gastrointestinal
H High (in tables)
H & E Hematoxylin and eosin stain
HCO$_3^-$ Bicarbonate
HCl Hydrochloric acid
HCT Hematocrit
HD Hodgkin's disease
Hg Mercury
HGB Hemoglobin
Hgb F Fetal hemoglobin
Hgb A$_{1c}$ Glycosylated hemoglobin
Hgb A$_2$ Hemoglobin A2
Hgb C Hemoglobin C
HLA-DR Class II major histocompatibility gene complex product
HPF High-power field
HPV Human papillomavirus
HTLV-1 Human T-cell lymphotropic virus type I
IgA Immunoglobulin A
IgD Immunoglobulin D
IgE Immunoglobulin E
IgG Immunoglobulin G
IgM Immunoglobulin M
IL-1 Interleukin-1

IL-2 Interleukin-2
IL-4 Interleukin-4
IL-6 Interleukin-6
INF-γ Interferon-γ
INR International normalized ratio
K Potassium
L Liter
L Low (in tables)
LCA Leukocyte common antigen (CD45)
LDH Lactate dehydrogenase
LDL Low-density lipoproteins
Lyme AB Antibodies to *Borrelia burgdorferi* (ELISA)
Lymph Lymphocyte
MALT Mucosa-associated lymphoid tissue
MCH Mean corpuscular hemoglobin
MCHC Mean corpuscular hemoglobin concentration
MCV Mean corpuscular volume
mEq Milliequivalent
mill Million
min Minute
mL Milliliter
mono Monocyte
MRI Magnetic resonance imaging
μL Microliter
μm Micrometer
Na Sodium
Neut; poly Neutrophil
ng Nanogram
NBT Nitroblue tetrazolium
O₂ Oxygen
O₂ sat. Oxygen saturation

PA Pernicious anemia
PAS Periodic acid-Schiff stain
PDW Platelet distribution width
PCO₂ Carbon dioxide partial pressure
pg Picogram
Plts Platelets
PO₂ Oxygen partial pressure
Poly; neut Neutrophil
PRBC Packed red blood cells
PRV Polycythemia rubra vera
PSA Prostate-specific antigen
PSAP Prostate-specific acid phosphatase
PT Prothrombin time
PTH Parathyroid hormone
RA Rheumatoid arthritis
RBC Red blood cell
RDW Red cell distribution width
Retic Reticulocyte
RPR Rapid plasma reagin
RS Reed–Sternberg cell
SAM *S*-adenosylmethionine
SPE Serum protein electrophoresis
TCR T-cell receptor
thou Thousand
TIBC Total iron-binding capacity
TNF Tumor necrosis factor
Transferrin sat. Transferrin saturation
U Unit
UTI Urinary tract infection
VLDL Very-low-density lipoproteins
WBC White blood cells

A 64-year-old woman with recurrent fever and cough

CASE AND MCQS

Clinical history and presentation

A 64-year-old woman was admitted to the hospital because of extreme weakness, cough, and fever of 4 days' duration. During the last 3 months the patient was twice hospitalized with pneumonia and had lost 6 pounds (2.8 kg). During her last admission a hilar lymphadenopathy was noted on chest X-ray. Currently she is on no medications. Her past medical history includes frequent episodes of bronchitis. She has a 40-year-long history of smoking one to two packs of cigarettes a day and admits to occasional drinking. Her mother died of lung cancer, her father is living and well.

Physical examination revealed a weak, lethargic, and pale woman. Her temperature was 102.8°F (39.3°C), blood pressure was 105/65 mmHg, pulse was 98/min and regular, and respiratory rate 28/min. Pertinent physical findings included dullness to percussion, decreased breath sounds, and rales on the right side of the chest. The rest of the physical examination was within normal limits. Sputum was obtained for Gram stain (Fig. 1.1) and cultures, and a chest X-ray (Fig. 1.3) was performed. Blood cultures were obtained.

Admission data

Table 1.1 Hematology

			SI Units	
WBC	13.47 H	(3.3–11.0 thou/µL)	13.47 H	(3.3–11.0 × 10⁹/L)
Neut	69	(44–88%)	69	(44–88%)
Band	10	(0–10%)	10	(0–10%)
Lymph	9 L	(12–43%)	9 L	(12–43%)
Mono	9	(2–11%)	9	(2–11%)
Eos	1	(0–5%)	1	(0–5%)
Baso	1	(0–2%)	1	(0–2%)
RBC	2.62 L	(3.9–5.0 mill/µL)	2.62 L	(3.9–5.0 × 10¹²/L)
HGB	7.9 L	(11.6–15.6 g/dL)	79 L	(116–156 g/L)
HCT	23.6 L	(37.0–47.0%)	0.236 L	(0.37–0.47)
MCV	89.9	(79.0–99.0 fL)	89.9	(79.0–99.0 fL)
MCH	30.3	(26.0–32.6 pg)	30.3	(26.0–32.6 pg)
MCHC	33.7	(31.0–36.0 g/dL)	337	(310–360 g/L)
Plts	154	(130–400 thou/µL)	154	(130–400 × 10⁹/L)

Table 1.2 Chemistry

			SI Units	
Glucose	97	(65–110 mg/dL)	5.38	(3.6–6.11 mmol/L)
BUN	21	(7–24 mg/dL)	7.5	(2.50–8.57 mmol/L)
Creatinine	1.0	(0.7–1.4 mg/dL)	88.4	(62.0–124.0 µmol/L)
Uric acid	8	(3.0–8.5 mg/dL)	0.47	(0.18–0.51 mmol/L)
Cholesterol	155	(150–200 mg/dL)	4.0	(3.88–5.17 mmol/L)
Calcium	10.6 H	(8.5–10.5 mg/dL)	2.65 H	(2.13–2.63 mmol/L)
Protein	4.8	(6–8 g/dL)	48	(60–80 g/L)
Albumin	2.7 L	(3.7–5.0 g/dL)	27 L	(37–50 g/L)
LDH	250	(100–250 U/L)	250	(100–250 U/L)
Alk Phos	102	(0–120 U/L)	102	(0–120 U/L)
AST	7	(0–55 U/L)	7	(0–55 U/L)
GGTP	40	(0–50 U/L)	40	(0–50 U/L)
Bilirubin	1.5	(0.0–1.5 mg/dL)	25.7	(0–25.7 µmol/L)
Bilirubin, direct	0.18	(0.02–0.18 mg/dL)	3.1	(0.34–3.08 µmol/L)

Table 1.3 Electrolytes

			SI units	
Na	135	(134–143 mEq/L)	135	(134–143 mmol/L)
K	4.4	(3.5–4.9 mEq/L)	4.4	(3.5–4.9 mmol/L)
Cl	97	(95–108 mEq/L)	97	(95–108 mmol/L)
CO_2	27	(21–32 mEq/L)	27	(21–32 mmol/L)

Table 1.4 Arterial blood gases

			SI units	
pH	7.51 H	(7.35–7.45)	7.51 H	(7.35–7.45)
PCO_2	29 L	(32–46 mmHg)	3.86 L	(4.26–6.13 kPa)
PO_2	87	(74–108 mmHg)	11.6	(9.86–14.4 kPa)
HCO_3^-	24	(21–29 mEq/L)	24	(21–29 mmol/L)

Table 1.5 Special hematology

			SI units	
Retic	1.7	(0.1–2.0%)	1.7	(0.1–2.0%)
Iron	24 L	(42–135 µg/dL)	4.3 L	(7.5–24.2 µmol/L)
TIBC	90 L	(280–400 µg/dL)	16.1 L	(50.1–71.6 µmol/L)
Ferritin	845 H	(5–139 ng/mL)	845 H	(5–139 µg/L)

Table 1.6 Microbiology

Blood cultures:	Pending
Sputum culture:	Pending

Table 1.7 Urinalysis

Within normal limits

Table 1.8 Angiotensin-converting enzyme (ACE)

			SI units	
ACE	50	(8–52 U/L)	0.85	(0.136–0.88 µkat/L)

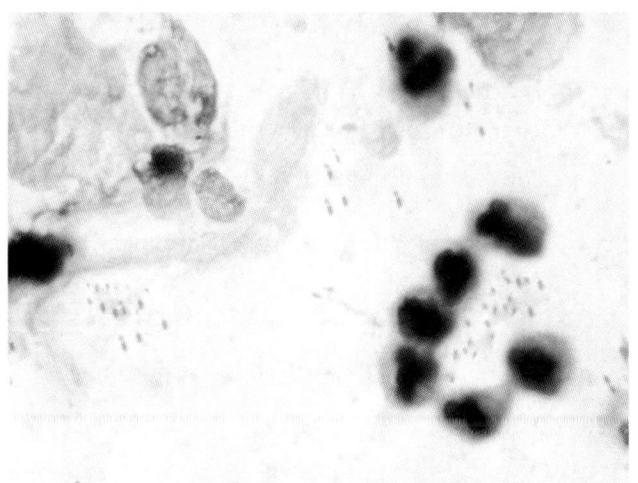

Figure 1.1 Sputum (patient). Gram stain.

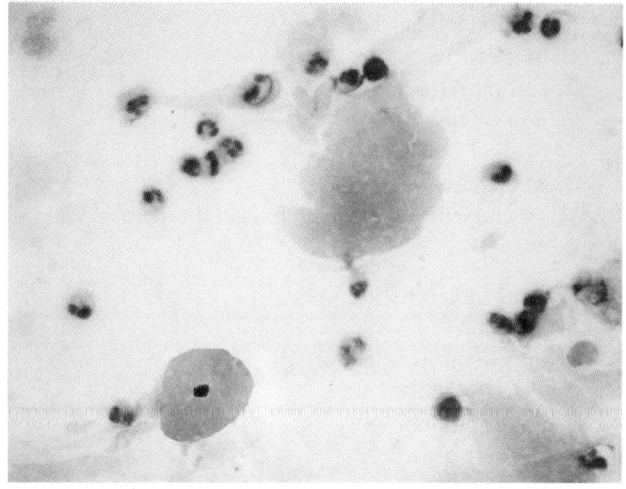

Figure 1.2 Sputum (normal). Gram Stain.

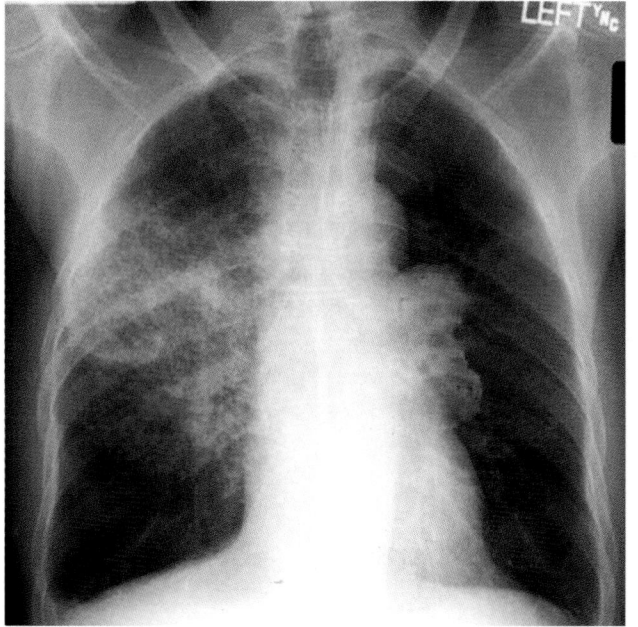

Figure 1.3 Chest X-ray, A-P view (patient).

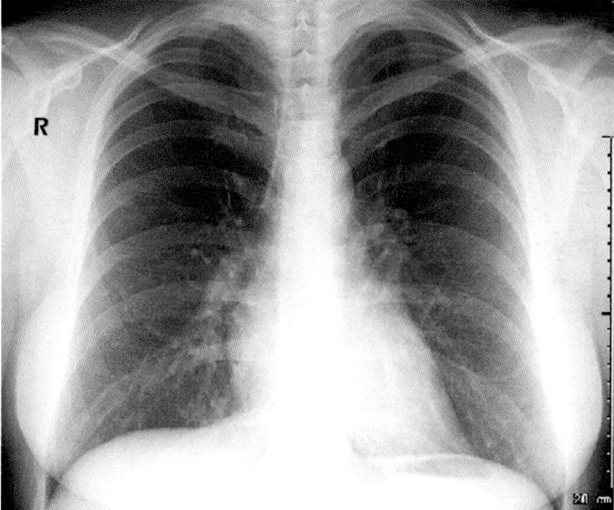

Figure 1.4 Chest X-ray, A-P view (normal).

Questions

Based on the above information you can best conclude the following:

BASIC

1. The most likely cause of this patient's anemia is:

    a. chronic gastrointestinal bleeding
    b. vitamin B_{12} deficiency
    c. iron deficiency
    d. chronic renal failure
    e. none of the above

ADVANCED

2. The increased serum ferritin level in this patient could be related to:

    a. acute inflammation
    b. infection
    c. the presence of a chronic disease
    d. all of the above
    e. none of the above

INTERMEDIATE

3. The hypoproteinemia and hypoalbuminemia seen in this patient may be etiologically associated with all of the following EXCEPT:

    a. malnutrition
    b. fever
    c. dehydration
    d. infection

INTERMEDIATE

4. Arterial blood gases in this patient are best interpreted as indicating:

    a. metabolic acidosis
    b. respiratory acidosis
    c. respiratory alkalosis
    d. metabolic alkalosis

INTERMEDIATE

5. The Gram stain of the patient's sputum (Fig. 1.1):

    a. shows acute inflammatory cells and no microorganisms
    b. shows chronic inflammatory cells and no microorganisms
    c. shows Gram-negative bacilli and acute inflammatory cells
    d. shows Gram-positive cocci and acute inflammatory cells
    e. shows none of the above

INTERMEDIATE

6. Which of the following findings is seen in this patient's chest X-ray (Fig. 1.3)?

    a. emphysema
    b. no abnormal findings
    c. pulmonary edema
    d. a left pleural effusion
    e. hilar lymphadenopathy

Clinical course

The sputum culture was positive for *Klebsiella pneumoniae* and the blood cultures were reported as "no growth." The patient was started on antibiotics and her condition improved. A repeated chest X-ray, however, showed persistent pulmonary changes. CT scan of the chest (Table 1.9) was performed. The patient underwent an additional work-up including mediastinoscopy with mediastinal biopsy (Figs 1.5–1.8). CT scans of abdomen and pelvis were performed and no other lesions were identified.

Table 1.9 CT scan of the chest

The patient's chest CT scan confirmed the radiographic findings seen on the chest X-ray (Fig. 1.3) and showed narrowing of the left main stem bronchus

---

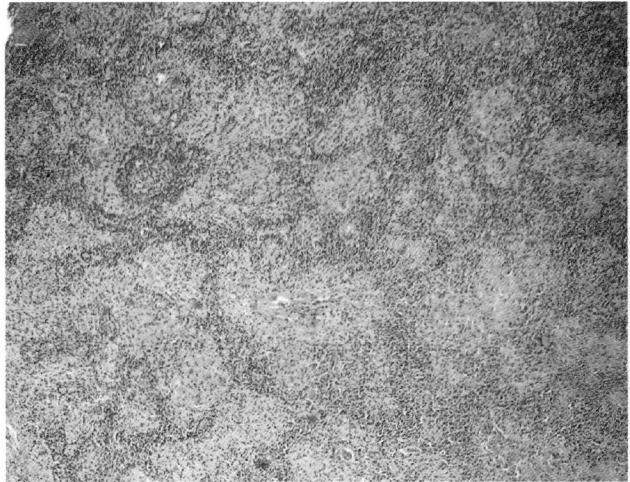

Figure 1.5 Biopsy of mediastinal mass (patient). Hematoxylin & eosin stain.

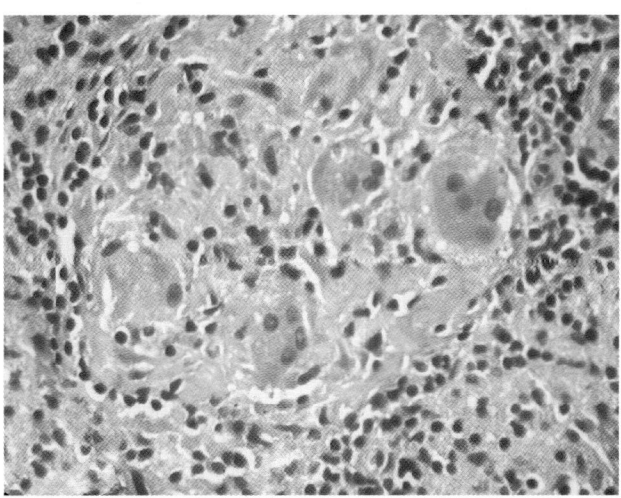

Figure 1.6 Biopsy of mediastinal mass (patient). Hematoxylin & eosin stain.

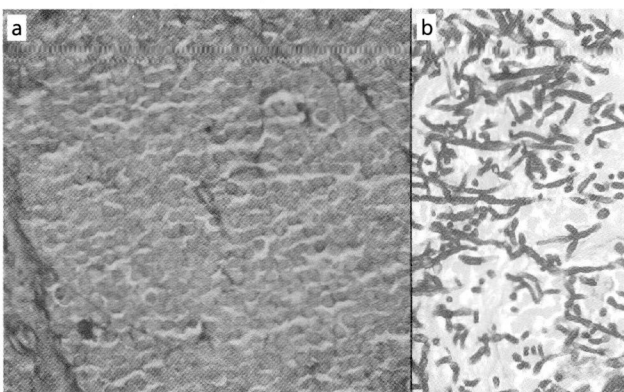

Figure 1.7 Biopsy of mediastinal mass (patient "a" and positive control "b"). Periodic acid-Schiff (PAS) stain (fungal stain).

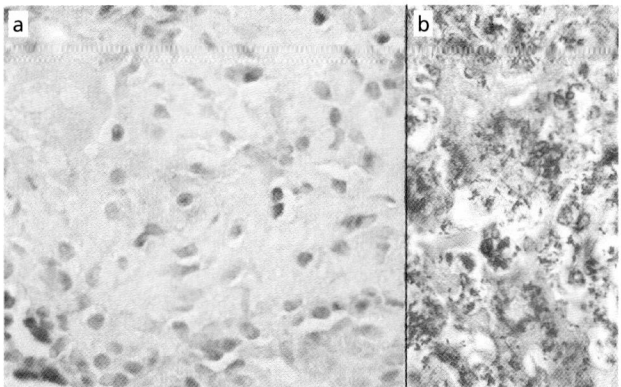

Figure 1.8 Biopsy of mediastinal mass (patient "a" and positive control "b"). Acid-fast bacilli (AFB, Ziehl-Neelsen) stain.

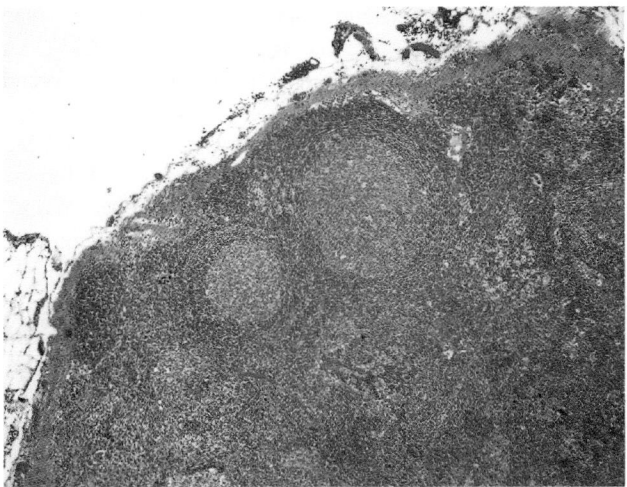

Figure 1.9 Biopsy of mediastinal lymph node (normal). Hematoxylin & eosin stain.

Questions

INTERMEDIATE

7. The mediastinal biopsy (Figs 1.5–1.8) shows:

   a. an abscess
   b. a granulomatous disease
   c. a metastatic squamous cell carcinoma
   d. a non-specific acute inflammatory process
   e. none of the above

INTERMEDIATE

8. The H & E, acid-fast bacilli and fungal stains of the mediastinal biopsy (Figs 1.5–1.8) revealed the presence of:

   a. a mycobacterial infection
   b. a fungal infection
   c. foreign bodies
   d. none of the above

INTERMEDIATE

9. A morphological finding similar to that seen in the patient's mediastinal biopsy (Figs 1.5–1.8) may be noted with:

   a. fungal infection
   b. mycobacterial infection
   c. berylliosis
   d. sarcoidosis
   e. all of the above

ADVANCED

10. The immunological abnormalities associated with the disease process depicted in Figs 1.5–1.8 in general include all of the following EXCEPT:

   a. an increased number of CD4+ lymphocytes in the bronchial lavage
   b. an elevated level of soluble IL-2 receptors in the serum
   c. a decreased level of soluble IL-2 receptors in the bronchial lavage
   d. the presence of activated alveolar macrophages in the bronchial lavage
   e. none of the above

INTERMEDIATE

11. All of the following statements regarding the disease process depicted in Figs 1.5–1.8 are true EXCEPT:

   a. it may present as a skin lesion
   b. it seldom affects the spleen
   c. it usually involves lymph nodes
   d. it may lead to pulmonary fibrosis
   e. it is of an unknown etiology

ANSWERS AND FURTHER INFORMATION

Figure descriptions

Figure 1.1 Sputum (patient). Gram stain.
Several neutrophils and numerous Gram-negative rods can be seen in this photomicrograph. The Gram-negative rods have a length of four to five times their width. This morphology is consistent with *Klebsiella pneumoniae*, and that identification was confirmed on culture.

Figure 1.2 Sputum (normal). Gram Stain.
Several neutrophils and a single epithelial cell in a mucoid background are seen in this image. The specimen also showed a mixed bacterial flora composed of Gram-positive and Gram-negative rods and cocci (not seen in this photomicrograph).

Figure 1.3 Chest X-ray, A-P view (patient).
Right upper lobe pneumonia and bilateral hilar adenopathy: Frontal radiograph of the chest demonstrating an infiltrate in the right upper lobe and bilateral hilar adenopathy.

Figure 1.4 Chest X-ray, A-P view (normal).
Normal chest X-ray: This is a normal chest X-ray in a middle-aged female showing clear lung fields.

Figure 1.5 Biopsy of mediastinal mass (patient). Hematoxylin & eosin stain.
Non-caseating granulomas, consistent with sarcoidosis: This photomicrograph shows an enlarged mediastinal lymph node, in which the lymph node architecture is effaced (compare with Fig. 1.9). The lymph node architecture is replaced by numerous non-caseating granulomas. Some granulomas exhibit a hyaline fibrous scar and no central necrosis. These morphological findings are suggestive but not diagnostic of sarcoidosis.

Figure 1.6 Biopsy of mediastinal mass (patient). Hematoxylin & eosin stain.
Non-caseating granuloma, consistent with sarcoidosis: A higher magnification of one of the granulomas shown in Fig. 1.5, shows a non-caseating granuloma composed of a cluster

of epithelioid cells with multiple Langhans giant cells. The granuloma is surrounded by an ill-defined rim of mononuclear cells, an infiltrate of lymphocytes, and plasma cells.

Figure 1.7 Biopsy of mediastinal mass (patient "a" and positive control "b"). Periodic Acid-Schiff (PAS) stain (fungal stain).
The image on the left (a) is a section from the patient's mediastinal mass. No evidence of fungal infection is noted in this section of the mediastinal lymph node stained for fungus by the Periodic acid-Schiff (PAS) stain. The image on the right (b) is a section from tissue with fungal infection (positive control).

Figure 1.8 Biopsy of mediastinal mass (patient "a" and positive control "b"). Acid-fast bacilli (AFB, Ziehl-Neelsen) stain.
The image on the left (a) is a section from the patient's mediastinal mass. No evidence of mycobacterial infection is noted in this section of the mediastinal lymph node stained for acid-fast microorganisms by an acid-fast bacilli (Ziehl-Neelsen) stain. The image on the right (b) is a section from tissue with mycobacterial infection (positive control).

Figure 1.9 Biopsy of mediastinal lymph node (normal). Hematoxylin & eosin stain.
This is a section from a normal lymph node. It shows part of the lymph node capsule, the subcapsular sinus, the peripheral cortex with its lymphoid follicles and a part of the medullary cords. Each follicle contains a pale-staining germinal center. The germinal center is surrounded by a mantle of small B lymphocytes. The parafollicular zones contain T lymphocytes. Medullary cords can be see in the lower right corner of this photomicrograph.

Answers

1. E. This patient has anemia with normal red blood cell indices. The iron studies in this patient revealed a lower than normal level of serum iron, decreased total iron-binding capacity (TIBC), and an increased level of serum ferritin. The percentage of reticulocytes is normal. These findings are not consistent with any of the options listed; chronic gastrointestinal bleeding would lead in time to iron deficiency, which would be manifested by microcytic anemia, low serum iron, and increased TIBC; vitamin B_{12} deficiency leads to macrocytic anemia and an increased serum iron level; the patient's findings are most consistent with anemia of chronic disease. There is no indication of renal failure (BUN and serum creatinine are normal).

2. D. Ferritin is a protein–iron complex that serves as the major body iron storage compound. Most of the ferritin is stored within parenchymal cells and mononuclear phago-

cytes, and only a small amount circulates in plasma. Under normal circumstances serum ferritin is a good indication of the adequacy of iron stores. Certain conditions, however, can elevate serum ferritin levels (ferritin is considered to be an acute-phase reactant). Such conditions include inflammation, infections, and a variety of chronic diseases. On the basis of the physical findings, laboratory values, chest X-ray, and the sputum analysis, one can conclude that our patient has an acute infectious, inflammatory lung condition. In addition, the recurrent pneumonia, weight loss, and hilar lymphadenopathy raise a suspicion of an underlying chronic pathological process; both processes could be contributing to the elevation of serum ferritin.

3. C. This patient has a decreased level of total serum protein and of serum albumin. The only condition that would not be manifested by such a decrease is dehydration, which on the contrary, would cause a relative increase in protein and albumin levels. Fever, inflammation, and infection lead to an increased catabolism and/or impaired synthesis of serum protein and albumin. Malnutrition leads to inadequate intake of protein.

4. C. Since the plasma pH is increased, we know that the patient has an alkalosis. This is not a metabolic alkalosis, driven by an increase in HCO_3^- with a reduction of non-volatile acids, since the HCO_3^- is reduced, as is the P_aCO_2. If we take the expected HCO_3^- as the average of the reference range values, or 25 mEq/L (25 mmol/L), we have a net reduction of only 1 mEq/L (1 mmol/L) in HCO_3^-, associated with a reduction of P_aCO_2 of 10 mmHg (1.37 kPa) below its expected value. This relatively slight reduction in the HCO_3^- level, which is within the reference range, suggests an acute rather than a chronic respiratory alkalosis without compensation by reduction of HCO_3^- regeneration in the kidneys.

5. C. The Gram stain of the patient's sputum shows Gram-negative bacilli and acute inflammatory cells (neutrophils). Chronic inflammatory cells (lymphocytes) and Gram-positive cocci are not seen in this sputum.

6. E. The patient's X-ray (Fig.1.3) shows a patchy infiltrate within the right upper lobe and a density with poorly defined margins in the hilar area. There is no evidence of emphysema, pulmonary edema, or a left pleural effusion.

7. B. The microscopic appearance of the tissue obtained by the mediastinal biopsy shows non-necrotizing granulomas, (see the descriptions of Figs 1.5–1.8). These represent a form of chronic inflammation, consisting of activated macrophages, transformed into epithelium-like cells, surrounded by a collar of mononuclear leukocytes (lymphocytes and some plasma cells). Abscess is a localized lesion that has a central area of tissue necrosis that is surrounded by neutrophils. Non-specific acute inflammation is characterized by the presence of a granulocytic (neutrophilic) infiltrate. No epithelial malignant cells suggestive of metastatic carcinoma are seen, and there is no suggestion of acute inflammatory cells or of abscess formation.

8. D. Figures 1.5 and 1.6 show non-caseating granulomas with no foreign bodies. Stains for acid-fast bacilli and fungus (Figs 1.8 and 1.7) are negative.

9. E. The lesion depicted in Figs 1.5–1.8 is a non-caseating granuloma. Mycobacterial infection, fungal infection, chronic low-dose exposure to beryllium compounds and sarcoidosis lead to granuloma formation. In the case of infection with *Mycobacterium tuberculosis*, the granuloma is called a tubercle and it is characterized by a central necrosis (caseous necrosis).

10. C. The patient has sarcoidosis. Sarcoidosis is associated with a variety of immunological abnormalities. These include the presence of activated alveolar macrophages, an increased number of CD4+ lymphocytes in the bronchial lavage, and an elevated level of soluble IL-2 receptors in the serum and in the bronchial lavage.

11. B. Sarcoidosis is a systemic disease of unknown etiology that produces non-caseating granulomas. Lymph nodes are involved in almost every case. Lung, spleen, liver, bone marrow, and skin involvement are also common. It may also affect other organs such as eye and salivary glands. In the lung, there is a strong tendency for granulomas to heal by fibrosis, causing pulmonary fibrosis.

Final diagnosis and synopsis of the case

- Sarcoidosis
- Acute bacterial pneumonia
- Anemia of chronic disease

A 64-year-old, previously healthy woman, presented with her third episode of pneumonia in the last 3 months and with a weight loss. In addition to her pneumonia she was found to be anemic, and she had hypoalbuminemia. The arterial blood gases pointed to acute respiratory alkalosis. The chest X-ray showed a right upper lobe infiltrate and an ill-defined hilar lymphadenopathy; her sputum culture was positive for

Klebsiella pneumoniae. The patient responded well to the antibiotic therapy. A CT scan of the chest confirmed the presence of the hilar lymphadenopathy and showed two nodules at the base of the left lung. Work-up for her hilar lymphadenopathy included mediastinoscopy and biopsy. The microscopic examination was consistent with sarcoidosis. The CBC (FBC) and blood iron studies suggested that the patient's anemia is most likely an anemia of chronic disease. The mildly elevated calcium was thought to be secondary to her sarcoidosis. The patient will be followed-up by her physician.

Lab tips

Blood cultures
The phlebotomy site must be cleansed with an alcohol pad and swabbed with iodine, to avoid contamination of the specimen by the skin flora. Blood for blood cultures is collected directly into blood culture bottles. Two sets of aerobic and anaerobic blood cultures should be collected from different sites and/or at different times. Blood for aerobic blood culture should be collected first.

Sputum
The patient must rinse his/her mouth with water to remove oral flora. Ask the patient to cough deeply, to produce a lower respiratory specimen which is required for adequate evaluation.

The sputum will be **examined macroscopically** for:
- color
- odor
- consistency

It will be **examined microscopically** for:
- cells
- microorganisms

Microscopic examination may be performed on an unstained wet mount or, as is more usual, a smear is prepared, dried, and stained by any of several **different stains**, i.e.
- Gram stain for bacteria
- acid-fast stain for mycobacteria
- Wright stain for blood cells
- Papanicolaou stain for malignant cells

The sputum will then be submitted for **culture**. An ideal sputum sample for culture should have less than 10 squamous cells/low-power field. Bronchial epithelial cells as well as alveolar macrophages may be present. An inadequate sputum sample has more than 25 squamous epithelial cells/low-power field.

A 5-year-old girl with a painful hip

CASE AND MCQS

Clinical history and presentation

A 5-year-old girl presented with a history of pain in her right hip for about 6 weeks. She had been seen by an orthopedist and diagnosed as having a viral synovitis. Her pain became progressively worse, and now she complains of groin pain and of tenderness to touch of the right hip. Her medical history is otherwise unremarkable, her immunizations are up-to-date, and neither she nor her parents recall any trauma to the area. Physical examination revealed a well-developed, thin, and pale child. She was afebrile. The pertinent findings included pain on internal and external rotation of the right hip and tenderness to palpation of the right hip. She was limping while walking, favoring the right leg. The rest of the physical examination was unremarkable.

Admission data

Table 2.1 Hematology

			SI Units	
WBC	4.1	(4.0–11.0 thou/µL)	4.1	(4.0–11.0 × 10⁹/L)
Neut	32 L	(37–75%)	32 L	(37–75%)
Lymph	61 H	(12–50%)	61 H	(12–50%)
Mono	6	(0–6%)	6	(0–6%)
RBC	3.21 L	(3.8–5.2 mill/µL)	3.21 L	(3.8–5.2 × 10¹²/L)
HGB	9.0 L	(12.0–16.0 g/dL)	90 L	(120–160 g/L)
HCT	28.1 L	(35.0–47.0%)	0.281 L	(0.35–0.47)
MCV	87.5	(80.0–100.0 fL)	87.5	(80.0–100.0 fL)
MCH	28.0	(27.0–34.0 pg)	28.0	(27.0–34.0 pg)
MCHC	32.0	(28.0–37.1 g/dL)	320	(280–370 g/L)
Plts	212	(150–400 thou/µL)	212	(150–400 × 10⁹/L)

Table 2.2 Chemistry

			SI Units	
Glucose	96	(65–110 mg/dL)	5.3	(3.6–6.11 mmol/L)
BUN	11	(7–22 mg/dL)	3.9	(2.50–7.8 mmol/L)
Creatinine	0.3 L	(0.5–1.2 mg/dL)	26.5 L	(44.2–106 µmol/L)
Uric acid	4.7	(2.0–6.5 mg/dL)	0.27	(0.12–0.39 mmol/L)
Calcium	11 H	(8.7–10.7 mg/dL)	2.75 H	(2.17–2.63 mmol/L)
Phosphorus	6.3 H	(2.4–4.3 mg/dL)	2.03 H	(0.78–1.39 mmol/L)
Protein	6.9	(6.1–8.0 g/dL)	69	(61–80 g/L)
Albumin	4.2	(3.5–4.8 g/dL)	42	(35–48 g/L)
Alk Phos	124	(100–300 U/L)	124	(100–300 U/L)
GGTP	14	(0–23 U/L)	14	(0–23 U/L)
ALT	29	(7–40 U/L)	29	(7–40 U/L)
LDH	504 H	(150–300 U/L)	504 H	(150–300 U/L)
AST	45	(12–45 U/L)	45	(12–45 U/L)
Bilirubin	0.9	(0.1–1.2 mg/dL)	15.4	(0.5–20.5 µmol/L)

Table 2.3 Erythrocyte sedimentation rate

ESR	80 H		(0–20 mm/hr)

Table 2.4 Coagulation

APTT	26.1	(24.6–34.8 s)
PT	10.6	(10.2–12.4 s)
INR	0.816	

Table 2.5 Urinalysis

Color	Yellow	(Yellow)
pH	7.5	(5.0–7.5)
Glucose	Neg	(Neg)
Bilirubin	Neg	(Neg)
Ketones	Neg	(Neg)
Sp. grav.	1.015	(1.010–1.035)
Blood	Neg	(Neg)
Protein	Neg	(Neg)
Nitrites	Neg	(Neg)
WBC	1–3/HPF	(0–5)

Table 2.6 X-rays of pelvis and of the right femur

A-P pelvis examination demonstrated diffuse demineralization of all of the visualized osseous structures. No focal lytic or sclerotic lesions are seen. The sacroiliac and hip joints appear normal. There are some questionable associated metaphyseal lucencies in the femoral necks. Views of the right femur show some mild generalized osteopenia. There is no widening of the growth plates to suggest rickets. A mild relative femoral metaphyseal lucency is present.

Questions

On the basis of the preceding information, you can best conclude the following:

1. Which of the following conditions is NOT likely to cause a painful hip in a child?

    a. Ewing's sarcoma
    b. juvenile rheumatoid arthritis
    c. Lyme disease
    d. psoriatic arthritis
    e. trauma

2. The patient's CBC (FBC) is abnormal. Which of the following tests would LEAST likely contribute to your diagnosis of the RBC abnormalities?

    a. vitamin B_{12} serum level
    b. peripheral blood smear evaluation
    c. reticulocyte count
    d. serum haptoglobin
    e. direct antiglobulin test (Coombs' test)

3. The abnormalities seen in the WBC count of this patient:

    a. are typical of a leukemoid reaction
    b. are typical of those associated with tissue destruction
    c. are consistent with allergic reactions
    d. are commonly associated with viral infections
    e. are characteristic of most acute bacterial infections

ADVANCED

4. The chemistry profile shows increased values for serum LDH, calcium, and phosphorus, and a decreased value for serum creatinine. Based on these findings, your most reasonable action at this time would be:

    a. to request the PTH (parathyroid hormone) serum level

    b. to inquire in the laboratory whether the "normal" ranges are adjusted for the age of the child
    c. to suspect a hemolytic specimen and request a new analysis on a fresh blood sample
    d. to collect a 24-hour urine specimen for calcium and phosphate measurement

INTERMEDIATE

5. A markedly elevated erythrocyte sedimentation rate in this patient may reflect any of the following EXCEPT:

    a. systemic infection
    b. collagen vascular disease
    c. a neoplastic process
    d. an acute allergic reaction

Clinical course

The child was seen by a hematologist after the following test results became available (Table 2.7). A bone marrow aspirate and biopsy were obtained (Figs 2.3, 2.5 and 2.6). The bone marrow aspirate was sent for immunophenotyping (Table 2.8) and chromosome analysis (not shown here). The patient's prognostic factors were evaluated, and treatment was initiated.

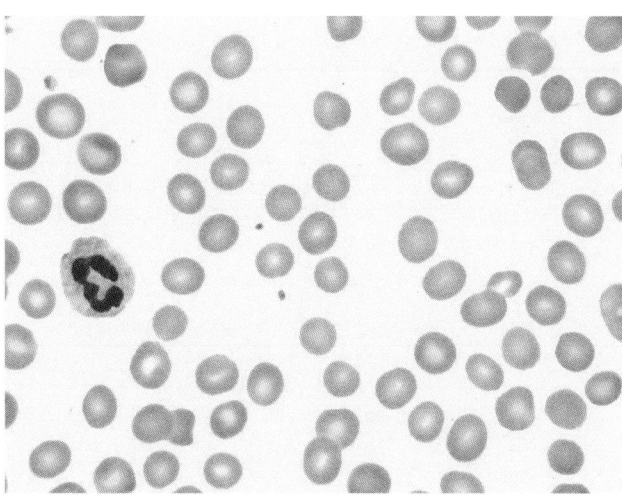

Figure 2.1 Peripheral blood smear (patient). Wright/Giemsa stain.

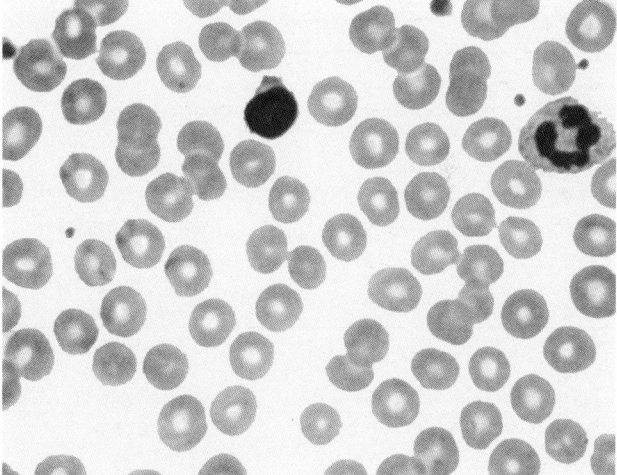

Figure 2.2 Peripheral blood smear (normal). Wright/Giemsa stain.

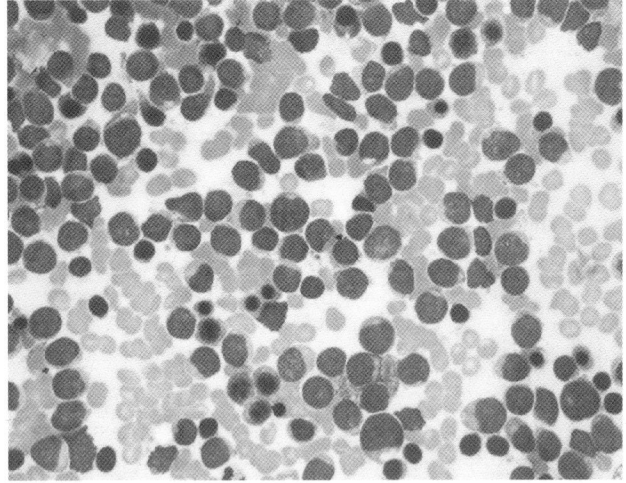

Figure 2.3 Bone marrow aspiration (patient). Wright/Giemsa stain.

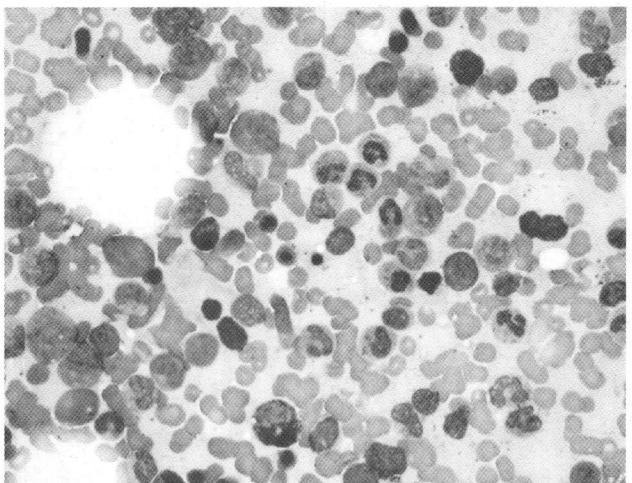

Figure 2.4 Bone marrow aspiration (normal). Wright/Giemsa stain.

Table 2.7 Additional tests

			SI Units	
Reticulocytes	2 H	(0.3–1.5%)	2 H	(0.3–1.5%)
Haptoglobin	220 H	(27–139 mg/dL)	2200 H	(270–1390 mg/L)
Anti IgG (Coombs' test)	Neg	(Neg)		
Anti C3 (Coombs' test)	Neg	(Neg)		
ANA	Neg	(Neg)		
Lyme disease serology	Neg	(Neg)		

Table 2.8 Immunophenotyping of bone marrow aspirate

Cluster designation	(Reactivity)	% of positive cells "lymphoid gate"
CD45	(Pan-leukocytic)	89.1
CD2	(Pan-T-cell)	3.1
CD3	(T-cell; receptor)	1.7
CD4	(T-cell; helper)	0.2
CD8	(T-cell; suppressor)	0.2
CD5	(T-cells/B CLL)	0.3
CD19	(Pan-B cell)	98.6
CD10	(Early B cell)	79.7
CD20	(B cell)	5.1
CD21	(B cell)	4.7
CD24	(B cell)	99.6
Kappa	(Mature B cell)	0.5
Lambda	(Mature B cell)	0.3
CD5/CD19	(B CLL)	0.1
HLA DR	(Diverse)	99.7
CD14	(Myelomonocytic)	5.4
CD13	(Myelomonocytic)	43.9
CD33	(Myelomonocytic)	73.4
CD34	(Progenitor cell)	99.2

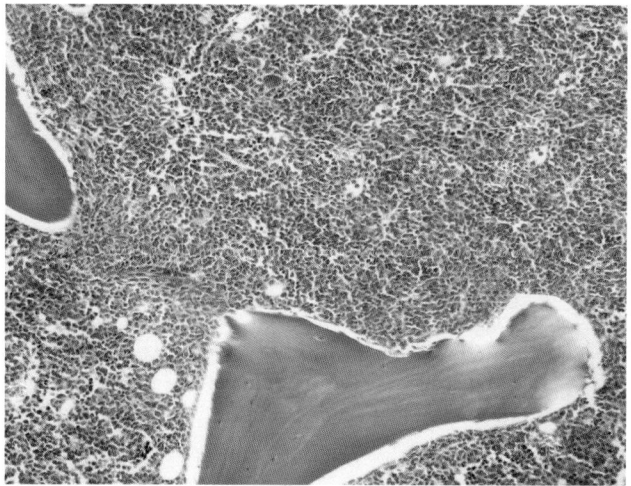

Figure 2.5 Bone marrow biopsy (patient). Hematoxylin & eosin stain.

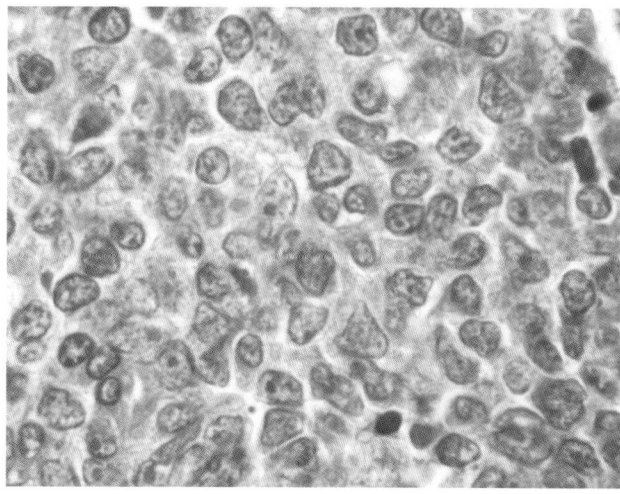

Figure 2.6 Bone marrow biopsy (patient). Hematoxylin & eosin stain.

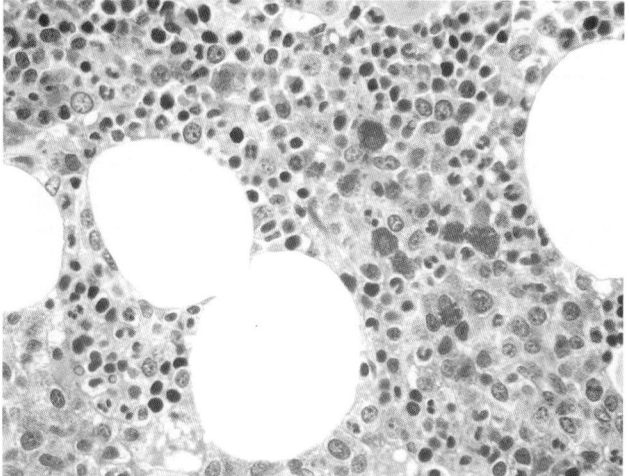

Figure 2.7 Bone marrow biopsy (normal). Hematoxylin & eosin stain.

Questions

INTERMEDIATE

6. Based on the laboratory test results in Tables 2.1 and 2.7 you conclude:

   a. the increased haptoglobin level reflects this patient's underlying problem

   b. the increased haptoglobin level is suggestive of hemolysis

   c. the negative Coombs' test indicates that this patient's anemia is not due to hemolysis

   d. all of the above statements are correct

INTERMEDIATE

7. Identify the INCORRECT statement:

   a. the diagnosis of the patient's main underlying problem is evident from the peripheral blood smear

   b. the diagnosis of the patient's main underlying problem is evident from the bone marrow biopsy appearance

   c. the diagnosis of the patient's main underlying problem is evident from the immunophenotypic analysis of the bone marrow aspirate

   d. anemia in this patient is due to impaired bone marrow function

8. Identify the correct proportions of hematopoietic cells in a normal ADULT bone marrow:

	Granulocytes & precursors	Lymphocytes & precursors	Erythroid precursors	Unidentified cells
a.	10%	40%	40%	10%
b.	80%	10%	10%	0–1%
c.	10%	10%	80%	0–1%
d.	30%	30%	30%	10%
e.	60%	10%	20%	10%

9. Normal bone marrow at the age of our patient:

a. is expected to be hematopoietically active throughout the skeleton

b. is not the sole source of hematopoiesis

c. has about the same ratio of fat cells/hematopoietic cells as in the healthy adult

d. all of the above statements are correct

10. The flow cytometric analysis of cells in the lymphocytic gate shows all of the following EXCEPT:

a. the absence of mature B cells

b. normal relative proportions of T and B cells

c. co-expression of lymphocytic and myelomonocytic markers

d. a pattern consistent with a lymphoproliferative disorder

11. Identify the INCORRECT statement about the underlying disease of this patient.

a. it affects children more commonly than adults

b. it is usually not associated with numerical or structural chromosomal changes

c. it is almost always associated with anemia

d. it is often manifested by bone or joint pain

e. the prognosis of this disease in general is better in children than in adults

12. Which of the following statements concerning this disease is correct?

a. peripheral blood must be involved by this process in order to confirm the diagnosis

b. in the bone marrow at least 25% of nucleated marrow cells must be blasts in order to establish the diagnosis

c. the morphologic type seen in this bone marrow is the most common type seen in both children and adults

d. the immunophenotype suggesting a mixed lineage variant of the disease is the most common phenotype in both children and adults

e. thrombocytopenia is not a feature of this disease

ANSWERS AND FURTHER INFORMATION

Figure descriptions

Figure 2.1 Peripheral blood smear (patient). Wright/Giemsa stain.
Red blood cells are apparently reduced in number, as compared with Fig. 2.2, and show mild aniso-poikilocytosis (different size and shape). The average size of the red blood cells appears normal as compared with the size of the neutrophil present. Platelets are present in this field. This blood smear and the CBC (FBC) data (Table 2.1) are consistent with a diagnosis of normocytic, normochromic anemia.

Figure 2.2 Peripheral blood smear (normal). Wright/Giemsa stain.
This is a photomicrograph of a normal blood smear for comparison. The red blood cells' size is approximately equal to that of the lymphocyte and to two-thirds of that of the neutrophil (present on the right side)

Figure 2.3 Bone marrow aspiration (patient). Wright/Giemsa stain.
Acute lymphoblastic leukemia: Hypercellular bone marrow showing a monotonous cell population. Except for a few normoblasts and one eosinophil, normal hematopoietic cells are absent. Most of the cells in this image are relatively small lymphoblasts with scant cytoplasm (L1 lymphoblasts). The rest of the lymphoblasts are larger with more cytoplasm and indented nuclei (L2 lymphoblasts).

Figure 2.4 Bone marrow aspiration (normal). Wright/Giemsa stain.
Normal bone marrow aspiration: A heterogeneous cell population showing myelocytes at different maturation stages and normoblastic erythropoiesis. Megakaryocytes (not seen in this image) were adequate in number.

Figure 2.5 Bone marrow biopsy (patient). Hematoxylin & eosin stain.

This is a hypercellular bone marrow, even for a 5-year-old girl. The marrow space is almost completely replaced by a monotonous cell population. Although, at this magnification, the cellular and nuclear details are not clear, this morphological finding is consistent with a diagnosis of an acute leukemia.

Figure 2.6 Bone marrow biopsy (patient). Hematoxylin & eosin stain.

At a higher magnification the leukemic infiltrate appears to be composed predominantly of small lymphoblasts with scant cytoplasm, occasional indentation of the nuclear membrane, and small inconspicuous nucleoli.

Figure 2.7 Bone marrow biopsy (normal). Hematoxylin & eosin stain.

This is a normal bone marrow from a 5-year-old child. It is approximately 80–90% cellular (hematopoietic cellularity), as it should be at this age. The erythroid maturation is normoblastic. There is an orderly myeloid maturation. Megakaryocytes, although not shown in this photomicrograph, are adequate in number

Answers

1. D. Psoriatic arthritis may involve the large joints such as hips or knees, but it is not a disease of childhood. It manifests between the ages of 35 and 45. Ewing's sarcoma, a primary malignant bone tumor, affects children, and the femur and bones of the pelvis are commonly involved. Juvenile rheumatoid arthritis is a connective tissue disease of children and may affect the hip joint. Lyme disease may occur at any age, and Lyme arthritis primarily affects large joints. Trauma may occur at any age.

2. A. This patient has an anemia with normal red blood cell indices. The major differential here should be hemolysis and bone marrow dysfunction. Vitamin B$_{12}$ deficiency would classically lead to a macrocytic anemia, which is not apparent in this patient. The blood smear examination is essential in all cases of anemia. The reticulocyte count is a very important indicator and helps to distinguish between hypoproliferative and hyperproliferative anemias (for example, distinguishing anemia due to bone marrow replacement from anemia due to hemolysis). Serum haptoglobin is a useful indicator of hemolysis, since haptoglobin binds free hemoglobin released from intravascular cell destruction and the hemoglobin–haptoglobin complex is removed from circulation by the liver. Therefore, serum haptoglobin levels are low in hemolysis. The direct antiglobulin test (Coombs' test) aids in the diagnosis of hemolytic anemias, which may result from an autoimmune

reaction or from a reaction to certain drugs. It detects the presence of immunoglobulins or serum complement components on patients' red blood cells.

3. D. This patient has a relative lymphocytosis associated with a normal WBC count. The most common etiology of such a finding is a viral infection. A leukemoid reaction is defined as a non-leukemic WBC count larger than 50 000 cells per μL (50×10^9/L), which is not true of our patient. Tissue destruction (hemorrhage, infarction, abscess, etc.) is often accompanied by neutrophilic leukocytosis, not apparent in this patient. Allergic reactions are most typically associated with eosinophilia, which is not seen in this case. Acute bacterial infections most typically cause leukocytosis with neutrophilia and the presence of band neutrophils, not seen in this case.

4. B. The normal values for serum calcium and phosphorus are higher in children than in the adult population due to rapid bone growth. The normal serum levels of LDH are one to two times higher in children than those of adults. The normal serum creatinine level for a child of our patient's age is less than 0.8 mg/dL (70.7 μmol/L). The chemistry profile of this patient is normal, with the possible exception of increased LDH. None of the other options (PTH serum level, hemolytic specimen, or 24-hour urine collection for calcium and phosphorus excretion) would explain all findings detected as being "outside" of the normal range.

5. D. The erythrocyte sedimentation rate (ESR) measures the time required for erythrocytes to settle to the bottom of a vertical tube. It is a non-specific test, affected by factors involving both the red blood cells and plasma. Plasma proteins, especially fibrinogen, which is an acute phase reactant, cause changes in the ESR. A marked elevation of the ESR occurs in infectious diseases, neoplasia, and non-infectious inflammatory conditions such as collagen vascular diseases. An acute allergic reaction does not increase the ESR.

6. A. There is no indication that this patient's anemia is due to hemolysis. The serum haptoglobin level would be low or absent in the presence of increased free hemoglobin due to hemolysis. Our patient's haptoglobin level is increased; this is best explained by the fact that haptoglobin (an α$_2$ globulin) is one of the "acute phase reactant" proteins that are increased by infection, tissue injury or by malignant processes. A negative direct Coombs' test indicates that the patient's red blood cells are not coated with antibodies or serum complement components. It is useful in identification of anemias due to immune hemolysis, but a negative test does not exclude hemolysis due to other causes.

7. A. The peripheral blood smear does not show any significant abnormalities on which the diagnosis of this patient's disease could be based. The bone marrow biopsy shows the marrow replaced by a leukemic cell population (see the description of Fig. 2.5). The immunophenotyping also provides the definitive answer, characterizing virtually all bone marrow cells as highly immature cells of B lineage comprising some myelo-monocytic antigens. It is of interest that some myeloid-associated surface antigens are co-expressed on these leukemic cells. The anemia is due to abnormally functioning bone marrow, which is infiltrated by leukemic cells. The reticulocyte count is not significantly increased, which further supports the etiology of this anemia.

8. E. Normal adult bone marrow contains about 60% of granulocytes and their precursors, 20% of erythroid precursors, 10% of lymphocytes, monocytes, and their precursors, and about 10% of unidentified cells. The normal myeloid/erythroid ratio is about 3:1.

9. A. By the time of birth the bone marrow becomes virtually the sole source of all forms of blood cells and a major source of lymphocyte precursors. Until the age of puberty all marrow throughout the skeleton is hematopoietically active. The hematopoietic cellularity of pediatric marrow differs from that of an adult person. During the first decade of life about 80% of the marrow cells are hematopoietic cells and 20% are fat cells; in a 30-year-old adult this changes to about 50% of hematopoietic cells and 50% of fat cells, and in the 70-year-old the hematopoietic cellularity is lower than 50%.

10. B. The flow cytometric analysis of a normal bone marrow would show that the majority of cells in the "lymphocytic" gate are T lymphocytes, while the B lymphocyte proportion is usually below 20% of the total lymphocytic population. Among B lymphocytes a majority of cells should be mature (express surface immunoglobulin kappa and lambda light chains in a ratio of about 2–3:1 respectively). In this patient's bone marrow there are virtually no T cells present, and B cells lack surface immunoglobulin light chain expression. All cells of B lineage are immature, as indicated by the expression of the hematopoietic progenitor cell antigen CD34 and of the CALLA (CD10) antigen. A majority of cells of B lineage co-express a myelomonocytic marker CD33, and many of these

cells also co-express another myelomonocytic marker CD13. These are distinctly abnormal findings, consistent with the diagnosis of a lymphoproliferative disorder of immature cells of B lineage (pre-B-cells) such as acute lymphoblastic leukemia (ALL).

11. B. The patient has a variant of acute lymphoblastic leukemia (ALL), characterized by expression of both lymphoid- and myeloid-associated cell-surface markers on the same cells (mixed lineage or biphenotypic leukemia). The disease has its highest incidence under 10 years of age. The prognosis, in general, is better in children than in adults, and it is best in the age group between 2 and 10 years of age. Most patients (90%) show abnormalities in their leukemic cells of chromosomal numbers and chromosomal structure. Cytogenetic analysis and immunophenotyping are currently very powerful prognostic tools. Most symptoms and signs of ALL are due to failure of production of normal blood cells (anemia belongs to this category) or due to proliferation and accumulation of leukemic cells (bone and joint pain belongs to this category and results from both bone marrow expansion and infiltration of subperiosteum with leukemic cells).

12. B. The bone marrow in patients with acute lymphoblastic leukemia is usually hypercellular with 60–100% of blast cells. It is generally accepted that at least 25% of nucleated bone marrow cells must be blasts to establish the diagnosis of acute leukemia. Replacement of normal marrow elements by leukemic cells leads to two of the most common features of ALL, anemia and thrombocytopenia. Peripheral blood is usually involved, and lymphoblasts are evident in the peripheral blood smear. In some cases, however, lymphoblasts are not apparent, and such cases are known as "aleukemic" leukemia. Our patient belongs in this category. A majority of blasts in our patient's bone marrow (over 90%) display L1 morphology, which is rather typical of childhood ALL. Only 7% of blasts are of L2 morphology, which is predominantly seen in adult ALL. An immunophenotype suggesting a mixed lineage is relatively uncommon both in adults and in children (less than 20% of acute lymphoblastic leukemias). The prognostic significance of this phenotype is at present unclear.

Final diagnosis and synopsis of the case

- Acute lymphoblastic leukemia of mixed lineage
- Anemia
- Bone pain due to infiltration by leukemic cells

A 5-year-old girl presented with persistent hip pain that progressively worsened over a period of 6 weeks. The initial impression was that she had a viral synovitis. The work-up, however, revealed a demineralization of pelvic bones and metaphyseal femoral lucencies on X-ray, an increased erythrocyte sedimentation rate, relative lymphocytosis, normocytic normochromic anemia, and no abnormal white blood cells in the peripheral blood smear. Her reticulocyte count was not increased, and the work-up for hemolytic anemia was negative. The bone marrow biopsy and aspirate showed that the marrow was replaced by a leukemic cell population, which constituted 98% of nucleated marrow elements. Most of the leukemic blasts were of L1 morphology. Immunophenotyping of blasts identified them as biphenotypic pre-B-cells co-expressing some myelomonocytic antigens. The anemia in this patient reflected inadequate erythropoiesis due to replacement of normal bone marrow by a leukemic infiltrate. It is of interest that the peripheral blood smear did not show any lymphoblasts; such rare cases are called "aleukemic leukemia." The hip pain was caused by leukemic infiltration and expansion of the marrow space by leukemic cells.

A 64-year-old woman with shortness of breath and ill-fitting shoes

CASE AND MCQS

Clinical history and presentation

A 64-year-old woman was brought to the emergency room because of increasing shortness of breath and weakness. Her current problems started a few days ago when she noticed difficulty in fitting on her shoes and shortness of breath on minimal exertion. She has a history of ischemic heart disease for which she has been medically treated, and of multiple episodes of transient ischemic attacks. She denied smoking and drinking alcohol. Her family history is positive for carcinoma of the lung (mother) and carcinoma of the colon (father). Physical examination revealed a lethargic and pale woman, with a blood pressure of 165/90 mmHg, a pulse of 98/min and regular, and a respiratory rate of 22/min. Her temperature was 99.8°F (37.7°C.) The jugular veins were distended; femoral and radial pulses were full and equal bilaterally; the heart apical impulse was displaced laterally. There were diffuse crackling rales at the lung bases. The abdomen was distended and there was shifting dullness to percussion. The liver was palpable about 5 cm below the right costal margin. Examination of the lower extremities showed pitting edema of both legs. The rest of the physical examination was unremarkable except for a guaiac-positive stool on rectal exam.

Admission data

Table 3.1 Hematology

			SI Units	
WBC	6.3	(3.3–11.0 thou/μL)	6.3	(3.3–11.0 × 10⁹/L)
Neut	53	(44–88%)	53	(44–88%)
Lymph	42	(12–43%)	42	(12–43%)
Mono	3	(2–11%)	3	(2–11%)
Eos	1	(0–5%)	1	(0–5%)
Baso	1	(0–2%)	1	(0–2%)
RBC	3.8 L	(3.9–5.0 mill/μL)	3.8 L	(3.9–5.0 × 10¹²/L)
HGB	8.5 L	(11.6–15.6 g/dL)	85 L	(116–156 g/L)
HCT	28.2 L	(37.0–47.0%)	0.282 L	(0.37–0.47)
MCV	72.3 L	(79.0–99.0 fL)	72.3 L	(79.0–99.0 fL)
MCH	22.3 L	(26.0–32.6 pg)	22.3 L	(26.0–32.6 pg)
MCHC	30.1 L	(31.0–36.0 g/dL)	301 L	(310–360 g/L)
Plts	85 L	(130–400 thou/μL)	85 L	(130–400 × 10⁹/L)
Retic	0.8	(0.1–2.0%)	0.8	(0.1–2.0%)

Table 3.2 Chemistry

			SI Units	
Glucose	87	(65–110 mg/dL)	4.8	(3.6–6.11 mmol/L)
Creatinine	2.0 H	(0.7–1.4 mg/dL)	176 H	(61.9–123.7 µmol/L)
BUN	68 H	(7–24 mg/dL)	24.3 H	(2.50–8.57 mmol/L)
Uric acid	8.3	(3.0–8.5 mg/dL)	0.49	(0.18–0.51 mmol/L)
Cholesterol	175	(150–200 mg/dL)	4.52	(3.88–5.17 mmol/L)
Calcium	8.6	(8.5–10.5 mg/dL)	2.15	(2.13–2.65 mmol/L)
Protein	6.2	(6–8 g/dL)	62	(60–80 g/L)
Albumin	3.3 L	(3.7–5.0 g/dL)	33 L	(37–50 g/L)
LDH	220	(100–250 U/L)	220	(100–250 U/L)
Alk Phos	54	(0–120 U/L)	54	(0–120 U/L)
AST	24	(0–55 U/L)	24	(0–55 U/L)
GGTP	12	(0–50 U/L)	12	(0–50 U/L)
Bilirubin	1.0	(0.0–1.5 mg/dL)	17.1	(0–25.7 µmol/L)
Bilirubin-direct	0.10	(0.02–0.18 mg/dL)	1.7	(0.34–3.08 µmol/L)
B-type natriuretic peptide (BNP)	950 H	(<100 pg/mL)	950 H	(<100 ng/L)

Table 3.3 Electrolytes

			SI Units	
Na	135	(134–143 mEq/L)	135	(134–143 mmol/L)
K	4.4	(3.5–4.9 mEq/L)	4.4	(3.5–4.9 mmol/L)
Cl	97	(95–108 mEq/L)	97	(95–108 mmol/L)
CO_2	27	(21–32 mEq/L)	27	(21–32 mmol/L)

Table 3.4 Arterial blood gases

			SI Units	
pH	7.26 L	(7.35–7.45)	7.26 L	(7.35–7.45)
PCO_2	53 H	(32–46 mmHg)	7.06 H	(4.26–6.13 kPa)
PO_2	52 L	(74–108 mmHg)	6.93 L	(9.86–14.4 kPa)
HCO_3^-	22	(21–29 mEq/L)	22	(21–29 mmol/L)
O_2 saturation	81 L	(92–100%)	81 L	(92–100%)

Table 3.5 Urinalysis

pH	5	(5.0–7.5)
Protein	Neg	(Neg)
Glucose	Neg	(Neg)
Ketone	Neg	(Neg)
Color	Yellow	(Yellow)
Clarity	Clear	(Clear)
Sp. grav.	1.015	(1.010–1.035)
WBC	5	(0–5/HPF)
RBC	2	(0–2/HPF)
Casts	Neg	(Neg)
Bacteria	Neg	(Neg)

Table 3.6 Cardiac enzymes

			SI Units	
CK	106	(0–130 U/L)	106	(0–130 U/L)
CK-MB	4	(0–4%)	0.04	(0–0.04)
Troponin I	0.02	(0–0.5 ng/mL)*	0.02	(0–0.5 µg/L)*
LDH	220	(100–225 U/L)	220	(100–225 U/L)
LDH_1	22	(17–27%)	0.22	(0.17–0.27)
LDH_2	37	(28–38%)	0.37	(0.28–0.38)
LDH_3	20	(18–28%)	0.20	(0.18–0.28)
LDH_4	11	(5–15%)	0.11	(0.05–0.15)
LDH_5	9	(5–15%)	0.09	(0.05–0.15)

*Troponin I: < 0.05 = normal, 0.05–0.5 = possible myocardial injury, ≥ 0.5 = acute MI.

Table 3.7 Electrocardiogram

Sinus tachycardia and non-specific ST-T changes

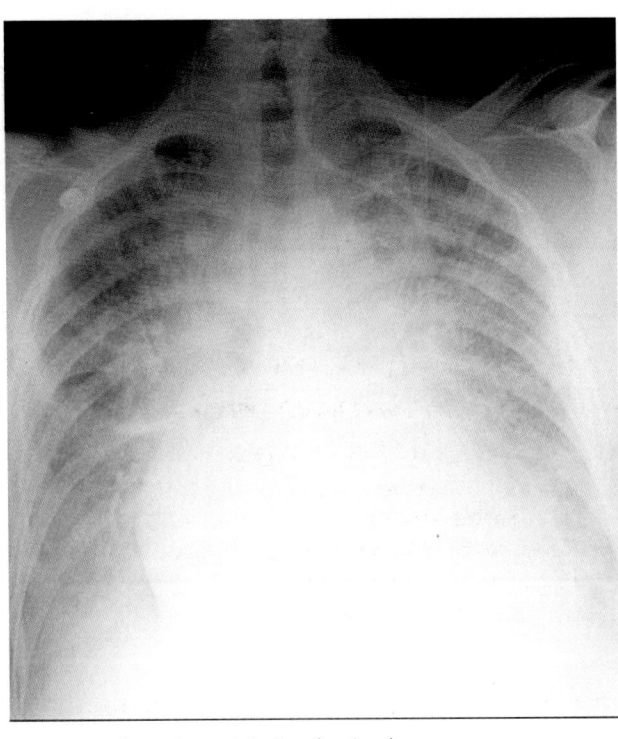

Figure 3.1 Chest X-ray, A-P view (patient).

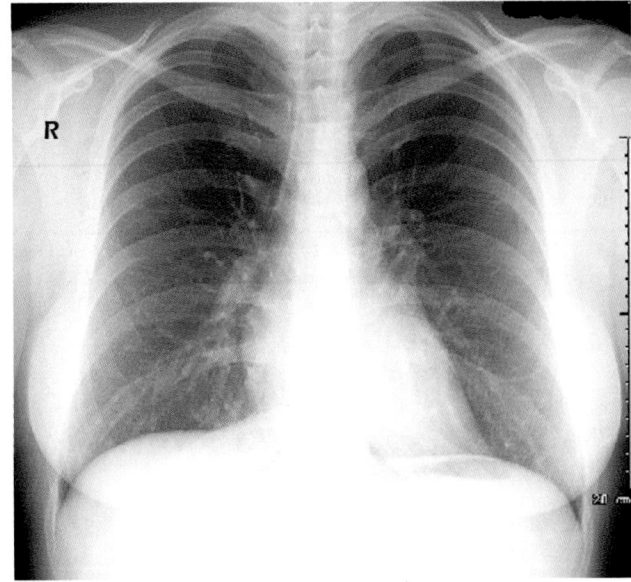

Figure 3.2 Chest X-ray, A-P view (normal).

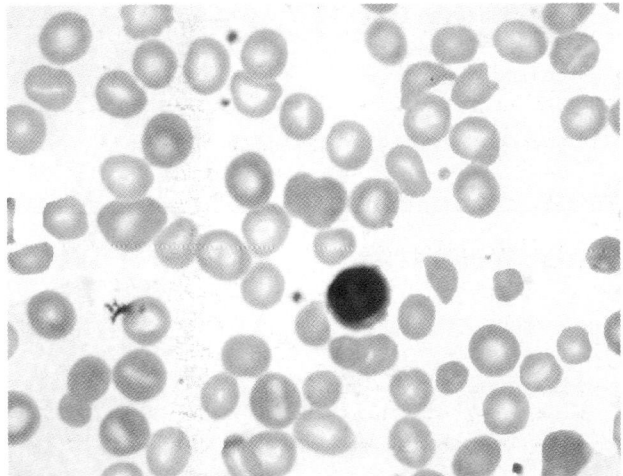

Figure 3.3 Peripheral blood smear (patient). Wright/Giemsa stain.

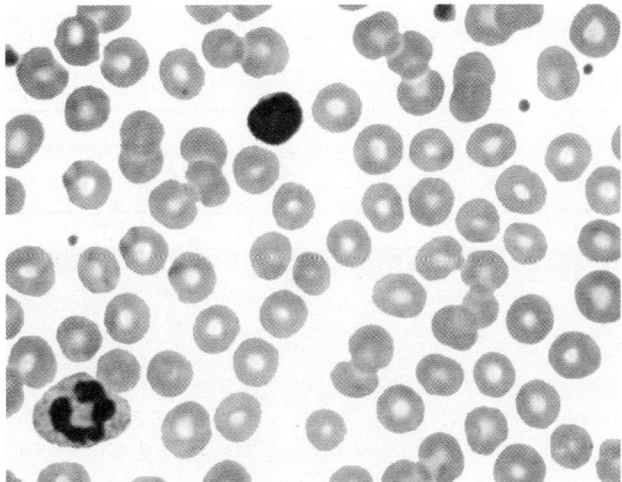

Figure 3.4 Normal peripheral blood smear. Wright/Giemsa stain.

Questions

Based on the above information you can best conclude the following:

1. Arterial blood gases in this patient are best interpreted as:

   a. metabolic acidosis
   b. respiratory acidosis
   c. respiratory alkalosis
   d. metabolic alkalosis

2. This patient's abnormal BUN and creatinine levels are most likely due to:

   a. decreased renal blood flow
   b. laboratory error
   c. hepato-renal syndrome
   d. none of the above

3. The pathogenesis of this patient's pulmonary findings (Fig. 3.1), lower limb edema, and ascites is associated with all of the following EXCEPT:

   a. decreased cardiac output
   b. increased central venous pressure
   c. increased venous hydrostatic pressure
   d. decreased production of antidiuretic hormone (ADH)

4. The patient's peripheral blood smear (Fig. 3.3) and CBC (FBC) are suggestive of:

   a. leukemoid reaction
   b. megaloblastic anemia
   c. iron reutilization defect
   d. chronic blood loss
   e. none of the above

Clinical course

The patient was admitted to the intensive care unit. After treatment, the patient's dyspnea and edema improved and this was reflected in an improvement of her blood gases (not shown). A colonoscopy was performed and the findings are depicted in Figs 3.5–3.8 (Fig. 3.9 is for comparison). The results were discussed with the patient and she was referred to a specialist for further management.

Table 3.8 Carcinoembryonic antigen (CEA)

			SI Units	
CEA	6.2 H	Non-smoker: 0–3.0 ng/mL Smoker:0–5.0 ng/mL	6.2 H	Non-smoker: 0–3.0 µg/L Smoker:0–5.0 µg/L

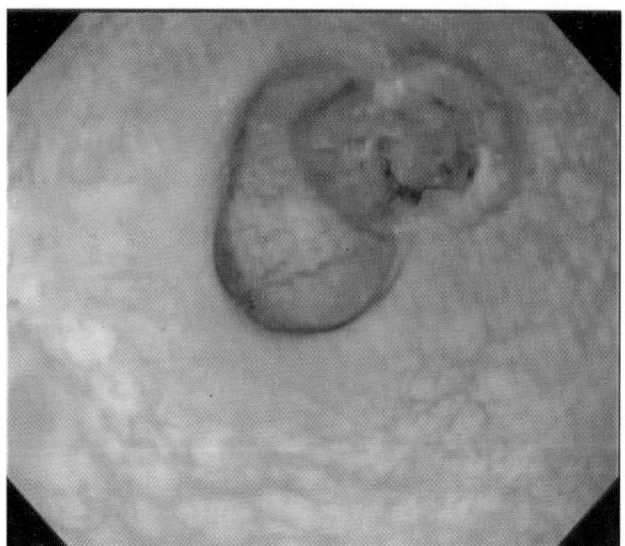

Figure 3.5 Colonoscopy (patient).

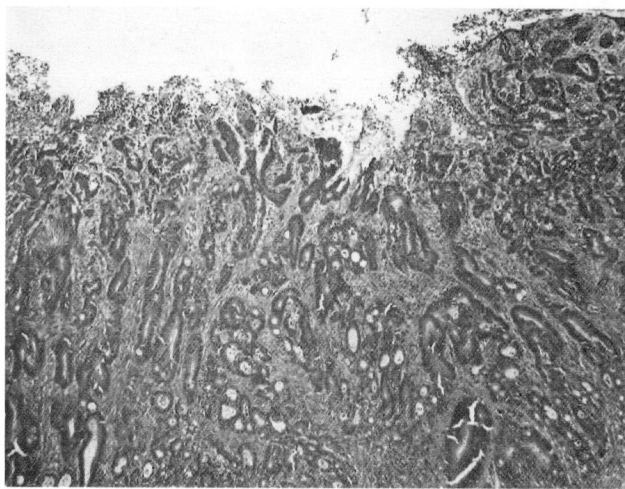

Figure 3.6 Colon biopsy (patient). Hematoxylin & eosin stain.

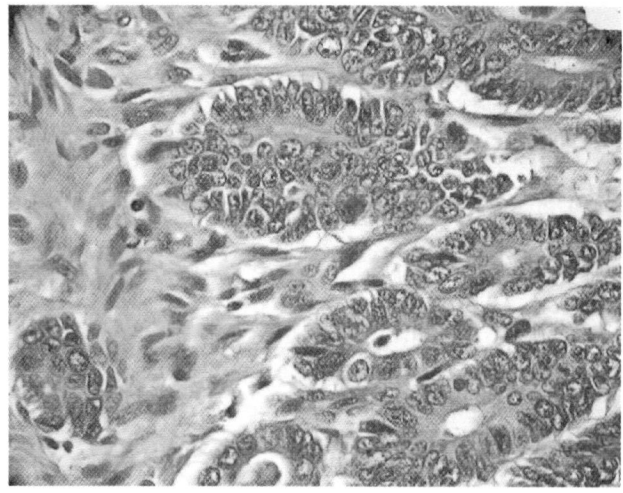

Figure 3.7 Colon biopsy (patient). Hematoxylin & eosin stain.

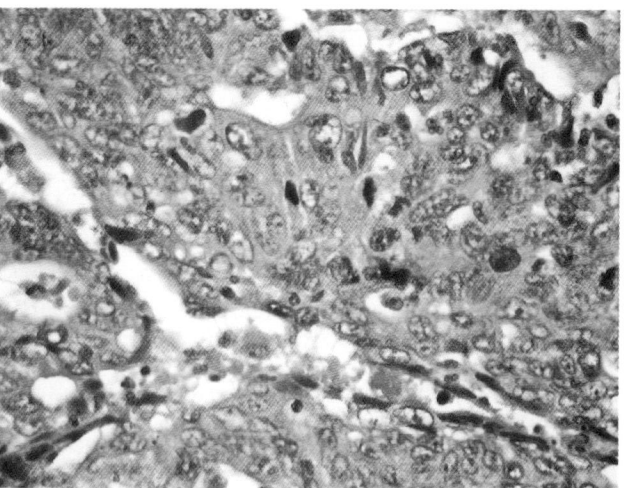

Figure 3.8 Colon biopsy (patient). Hematoxylin & eosin stain.

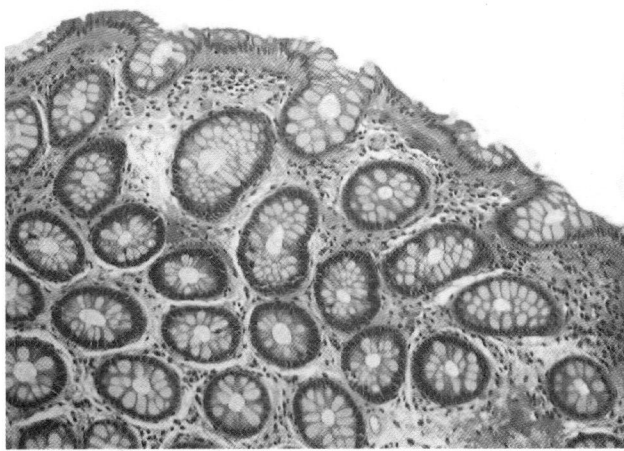

Figure 3.9 Colon biopsy (normal). Hematoxylin & eosin stain.

Questions

5. The indication(s) for colonoscopy and colon biopsy in this patient is/are:

    a. a positive fecal occult blood (guaiac) test
    b. a microcytic hypochromic anemia
    c. her age
    d. her family history
    e. all of the above

6. The colonic biopsy (Figs 3.6–3.8) shows which of the following intestinal problems?

    a. diverticulitis
    b. a benign colonic polyp
    c. a foreign body granuloma
    d. an invasive neoplasm
    e. a benign ulcer

7. In general, risk factors for this patient's colonic problem include all of the following EXCEPT:

    a. family history
    b. high fiber diet
    c. inflammatory bowel disease
    d. polyposis syndromes
    e. physical inactivity

8. Which of the following statements regarding such a colonic lesion is INCORRECT?

    a. its peak incidence is between 60 and 70 years of age
    b. it usually starts as an *in situ* lesion
    c. dietary habits constitute a predisposing factor
    d. it usually presents at multiple sites

9. Carcinoembryonic antigen level (CEA, shown in Table 3.8):

    a. is useful to monitor recurrence of colorectal carcinoma
    b. is increased in some benign conditions such as inflammatory bowel disease
    c. is increased in pancreatic, gastric, and lung carcinoma
    d. all of the above statements are correct

ANSWERS AND FURTHER INFORMATION

Figure descriptions

Figure 3.1 Chest X-ray, A-P view (patient).
Congestive heart failure: This frontal radiograph of the chest shows the presence of diffuse bilateral infiltrates, pulmonary vascular congestion, and cardiomegaly. Increased density at both lung bases is also seen and is consistent with pleural effusions. These findings are characteristic of congestive heart failure.

Figure 3.2 Chest X-ray, A-P view (normal).
A normal frontal radiograph of the chest in a female patient.

Figure 3.3 Peripheral blood smear (patient). Wright/Giemsa stain.
Microcytic hypochromic anemia: The patient's peripheral blood smear shows mild to moderate aniso-poikilocytosis (red blood cells of different size and shape). The red blood cells are microcytic (small in size) as compared with the normal lymphocyte present in the lower half of this photomicrograph. The red blood cells are also hypochromic with a prominent central pallor. This pattern is consistent with a diagnosis of microcytic hypochromic anemia.

Figure 3.4 Normal peripheral blood smear. Wright/Giemsa stain.
The red blood cells are similar in size and shape, and hemoglobinization appears normal. A normal lymphocyte and neutrophil are present, and the platelets are adequate in number and uniform in size.

Figure 3.5 Colonoscopy (patient).
Colonic adenocarcinoma: This endoscopic picture demonstrates a polypoid ulcerated mass in the ascending colon, measuring 3.5 cm.

Figure 3.6 Colon biopsy (patient). Hematoxylin & eosin stain.
Colonic adenocarcinoma: This low-power photomicrograph of the colonic biopsy shows an ulcerated, well to moderately differentiated adenocarcinoma of the colon. The tumor is composed of glands of different size and shape exhibiting a cribriform pattern and back-to-back arrangement. The tumor involves the colonic mucosa and submucosa, and the superficial portion of the muscularis propria (not shown).

Figure 3.7 Colon biopsy (patient). Hematoxylin & eosin stain.
Colonic adenocarcinoma: A higher magnification of the colonic adenocarcinoma showing glands lined by cells exhibiting large hyperchromatic nuclei, an increased nuclear/cytoplasmic ratio, and nuclear pleomorphism. Note the back-to-back arrangement of the malignant glands and desmoplastic stroma.

Figure 3.8 Colon biopsy (patient). Hematoxylin & eosin stain.
Colonic adenocarcinoma: This photomicrograph shows malignant glands lined by multiple layers of cells exhibiting hyperchromatic vesicular nuclei. There are numerous mitotic figures noted in this field.

Figure 3.9 Colon biopsy (normal). Hematoxylin & eosin stain.
Normal colon biopsy with a normal crypt architecture, showing colonic glands lined by a single layer of mucus-producing columnar epithelium.

Answers

1. B. This patient's arterial blood gases show reduced pH, pointing to acidosis. The presence of a low pH, elevated arterial PCO_2 and normal HCO_3^- are diagnostic of uncompensated respiratory acidosis resulting from inadequate alveolar ventilation and retention of CO_2. Metabolic acidosis, on the other hand, would show a reduced pH, normal arterial PCO_2, and reduced HCO_3^-.

2. A. The presence of elevated BUN and creatinine with a high BUN/creatinine ratio points to prerenal azotemia (i.e. impaired renal function, due to decreased renal blood flow, in the absence of organic renal disease). The most common causes of prerenal azotemia are heart failure and volume depletion. In both conditions there is sodium and water retention in order to compensate for the decreased effective blood volume. Hepato-renal syndrome is defined as a prerenal azotemia in patients with severe liver disease. Since this patient's liver function tests are within normal limits, a hepato-renal syndrome can be ruled out as the cause of this patient's abnormal renal function.

3. D. This patient presented with signs and symptoms of both left- and right-sided congestive heart failure (CHF). CHF results in the reduction of cardiac output, effective arterial blood volume, renal blood flow, and venous return. Decreased renal blood flow stimulates the production of renin, which leads to secondary hyperaldosteronism and sodium and water retention. In addition, the reduced effective blood volume stimulates the production of antidiuretic hormone (ADH). The fluid retention resulting from these events does not improve renal perfusion, simply because the failing heart is incapable of increasing its output. Moreover, fluid retention leads to worsening of the edema. In congestive heart failure venous hydrostatic pressure is increased due to fluid retention and reduction of venous return.

4. D. This patient's CBC (FBC) and peripheral blood smear show a microcytic hypochromic anemia, most likely due to chronic blood loss. Her CBC (FBC) and peripheral blood smear do not show any features suggestive of a leukemoid reaction, or of a megaloblastic anemia. A leukemoid reaction is a reactive leukocytosis with accelerated release of immature leukocytes from the bone marrow. Megaloblastic anemia is a macrocytic anemia with asynchronism between the cytoplasmic and nuclear maturation (i.e. there is inadequate DNA synthesis with normal RNA and protein synthesis). Peripheral blood smear examination in megaloblastic anemia would reveal large RBCs (macrocytes), and enlarged hypersegmented neutrophils. Iron reutilization defect (anemia of chronic disease) would show a normocytic normochromic anemia.

5. E. The patient, admitted for the worsening of her congestive heart failure, was found to have a microcytic hypochromic anemia, and a positive guaiac test. She has a positive family history of colon cancer. The patient is 64 years old. The peak incidence of colorectal carcinoma is at 60 to 79 years of age. All the above facts are indications for colonoscopy.

6 D. Figures 3.6–3.8 depict an invasive adenocarcinoma (see figure description). There are no benign polyps, granulomas or diverticula present. Diverticulitis refers to inflammatory changes due to obstruction or perforation of diverticula. None of these are seen in this photomicrograph.

7. B. Risk factors for a colonic problem such as that of this patient (colorectal carcinoma) include: inflammatory bowel disease, polyposis syndrome, family history, and diet, such as a low content of vegetable fiber, high intake of red meat, a high caloric intake relative to requirement and physical inactivity. A high fiber diet, on the contrary, is recommended as a preventive measure.

8. D. Colonic carcinoma affects predominantly older people, with a peak incidence at 60–79 years of age. It starts as an *in situ* lesion but develops different growth patterns in the proximal and the distal colon. The microscopic characteristics of those patterns are, however, similar. Cecum and ascending colon are the most frequent sites of colorectal carcinoma (38%), followed by sigmoid (35%) and descending colon (18%). Only about 1% of tumors are present at multiple sites. Dietary habits constitute a predisposing factor for the development of colorectal carcinoma.

9. D. CEA was the first tumor marker to be used clinically. It is a complex glycoprotein, which is associated with the plasma membrane of tumor cells. An abnormal CEA blood level is not diagnostic for colon cancer or for any malignancy. CEA levels are elevated in a variety of cancers including colonic, pancreatic, gastric, lung, and breast carcinoma. It is also elevated in benign conditions such as hepatic cirrhosis, pancreatitis, and inflammatory bowel disease. CEA level may also be elevated in smokers and in the healthy population. Due to its low positive predictive value, CEA is not recommended as a screening test. On the other hand, CEA is used to monitor recurrence of colorectal cancer and it serves as a prognostic indicator for patients with colorectal carcinoma.

Final diagnosis and synopsis of the case

- Congestive heart failure (CHF)
- Microcytic hypochromic anemia
- Colonic adenocarcinoma

A 64-year-old woman presented with an acute exacerbation of her congestive heart failure (dyspnea, distended jugular veins, ascites, edema, and hepatomegaly). Her chest X-ray revealed pulmonary edema, which was also reflected in her arterial blood gases. The work-up for acute myocardial infarc-tion was negative. The patient's cardiac condition improved considerably with supportive treatment of her heart failure. The rest of her laboratory work-up showed prerenal azotemia, most likely due to her congestive heart failure (reduced cardiac output and renal perfusion), microcytic hypochromic anemia, and a positive fecal occult blood (guaiac) test. Colonoscopy was performed and a colonic adenocarcinoma was diagnosed. The patient was referred to a specialist for further management.

B-type natriuretic peptide (BNP)

B-type natriuretic peptide is a 32-amino acid peptide secreted by the left ventricle in response to increased wall tension. This peptide promotes natriuresis, diuresis, and vasodilatation. The concentration of BNP serves as an indicator of high left ventricular end-diastolic pressure, a chief sign of congestive heart failure.

A low level of BNP will rule out congestive heart failure as an etiology of dyspnea. BNP level correlates with clinical severity of congestive heart failure, and serves as a prognostic indicator of CHF. Because of the short half-life of BNP (18–22 min), it will help to monitor a patient's response to therapy. BNP levels can be also elevated in primary pulmonary hypertension, renal failure, ascitic cirrhosis, and primary hyperaldosteronism.

Fecal occult blood test (guaiac test)

The guaiac test is a non-invasive, low-cost laboratory test that detects the presence of occult blood in stool. The test will be positive in conditions that lead to gastrointestinal bleeding. The guaiac test is one of several chemical indicators that will detect the peroxidase and the pseudoperoxidase activity of erythrocytes. A positive guaiac test indicates the presence of 5–10 mL of blood loss/day (normal gastrointestinal blood loss is approximately 2 mL/day).

False positive results can occur from ingested meats, certain vegetables and fruits, and a number of medications. False negative results have been noted with antioxidant ingestion (vitamin C, etc.).

This test is an important screening procedure for the early detection of colorectal carcinoma.

Test procedure:

1. Patient should have a high fiber diet with no meat, fish, turnips, horseradish, bananas, black grapes, pears, or plums for 2 to 3 days preceding and during the test (these foods have peroxidase activity).

2. Drugs that increase GI bleeding should be withheld (i.e. aspirin, iron compounds, steroids, indomethacin, etc.).

3. Three stool specimens are collected. A small amount of stool is placed on the test paper and mixed with water and reagents. The appearance of dark-blue color within 5 min represents a positive test for occult blood.

A 50-year-old psychologist who feels dizzy

CASE AND MCQS

Clinical history and presentation

The patient is a 50-year-old man who presented with complaints of dizziness and extreme weakness. He underwent a partial gastrectomy for peptic ulcer disease about 10 years ago; he also has a history of labyrinthitis and of alcohol abuse. His family history is non-contributory. His blood pressure is 134/82 mmHg; he is afebrile, and the pulse is 86/min and regular. Lungs are clear to auscultation. The abdomen is soft, showing a surgical scar. No organomegaly is noted, and there is no tenderness to palpation. Bowel sounds are normal. The rectal examination shows an enlarged prostate and a guaiac-positive stool. The neurological examination is unremarkable.

Admission data

Table 4.1 Hematology

			SI Units	
WBC	5.93	(3.3–11.0 thou/µL)	5.93	(3.3–11.0 × 10⁹/L)
Neut	61	(44–88%)	61	(44–88%)
Lymph	30	(12–43%)	30	(12–43%)
Mono	4	(2–11%)	4	(2–11%)
Eos	4	(0–5%)	4	(0–5%)
Baso	1	(0–2%)	1	(0–2%)
RBC	3.81 L	(3.9–5.0 mill/µL)	3.81 L	(3.9–5.0 × 10¹²/L)
HGB	7.9 L	(11.6–15.6 g/dL)	79 L	(116–156 g/L)
HCT	25.2 L	(37.0–47.0%)	0.252 L	(0.37–0.47)
MCV	66 L	(79.0–99.0 fL)	66 L	(79.0–99.0 fL)
MCH	20.7 L	(26.0–32.6 pg)	20.7 L	(26.0–32.6 pg)
MCHC	31.4	(31.0–36.0 g/dL)	314	(310–360 g/L)
Plts	306	(130–400 thou/µL)	306	(130–400 × 10⁹/L)
RDW	18.5 H	(11.5–14.5%)	18.5 H	(11.5–14.5%)

Table 4.2 Chemistry

			SI Units	
Glucose	93	(65–110 mg/dL)	5.16	(3.6–6.11 mmol/L)
BUN	7	(7–24 mg/dL)	2.5	(2.50–8.57 mmol/L)
Creatinine	0.8	(0.7–1.4 mg/dL)	70.7	(61.9–123.7 µmol/L)
Uric acid	3.0	(3.0–8.5 mg/dL)	0.178	(0.18–0.51 mmol/L)
Calcium	8.5	(8.5–10.5 mg/dL)	2.13	(2.13–2.63 mmol/L)
Protein	7.0	(6–8 g/dL)	70	(60–80 g/L)
Albumin	4.0	(3.7–5.0 g/dL)	40	(37–50 g/L)
Cholesterol	181	(150–200 mg/dL)	4.68	(3.88–5.17 mmol/L)
Alk Phos	123 H	(0–120 U/L)	123 H	(0–120 U/L)
GGTP	136 H	(0–50 U/L)	136 H	(0–50 U/L)
LDH	165	(100–250 U/L)	165	(100–250 U/L)
AST	19	(0–55 U/L)	19	(0–55 U/L)
Bilirubin	0.1	(0.0–1.5 mg/dL)	1.71	(0–25.7 µmol/L)
Bilirubin-direct	0.04	(0.02–0.18 mg/dL)	0.7	(0.34–3.08 µmol/L)

Table 4.3 Electrolytes

			SI Units	
Na	140	(134–143 mEq/L)	140	(134–143 mmol/L)
K	4.2	(3.5–4.9 mEq/L)	4.2	(3.5–4.9 mmol/L)
Cl	106	(95–108 mEq/L)	106	(95–108 mmol/L)
CO_2	28	(21–32 mEq/L)	28	(21–32 mmol/L)

Table 4.4 Special hematology

			SI Units	
Retic	4 H	(0.1–2.0%)	4 H	(0.1–2.0%)
Iron	6 L	(42–135 µg/dL)	1.07 L	(7.5–24.2 µmol/L)
TIBC	411 H	(280–400 µg/dL)	73.6 H	(50.1–71.6 µmol/L)
Transferrin sat.	2 L	(15–50%)	2 L	(15–50%)
Ferritin	6 L	(7–350 ng/mL)	6 L	(7–350 µg/L)

Table 4.5 Urinalysis

Sp. grav.	1.010	(1.010–1.035)
pH	7.5	(5.0–7.5)
Protein	Neg	(Neg)
Glucose	Neg	(Neg)
Bile	Neg	(Neg)
Ketone	Neg	(Neg)
Blood	Neg	(Neg)
Color	Yellow	(Pale yellow)
Clarity	Clear	(Clear)
WBC	0	(0–5/HPF)
RBC	0	(0–2/HPF)
Bacteria	0	(0)
Urobilinogen	Neg	(Neg)

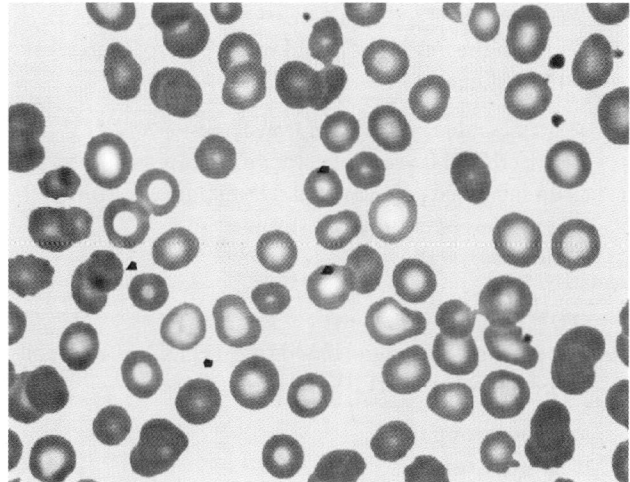

Figure 4.1 Peripheral blood smear (patient). Wright/Giemsa stain.

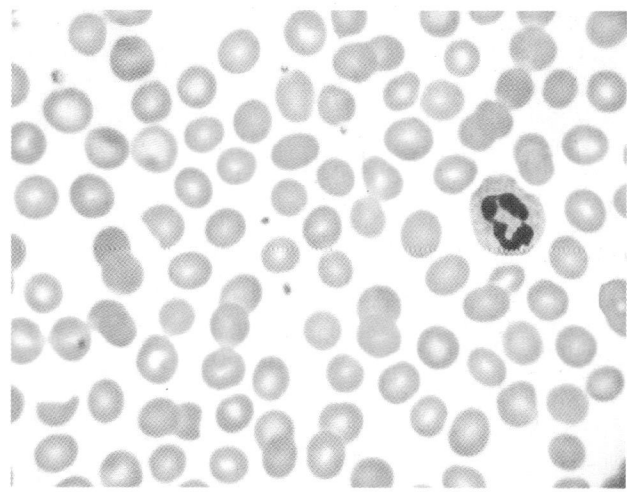

Figure 4.2 Peripheral blood smear (normal). Wright/Giemsa stain.

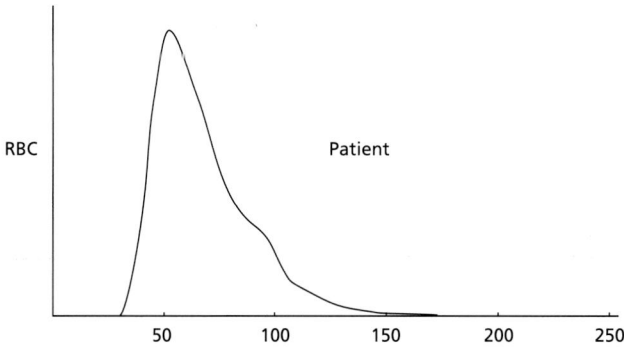

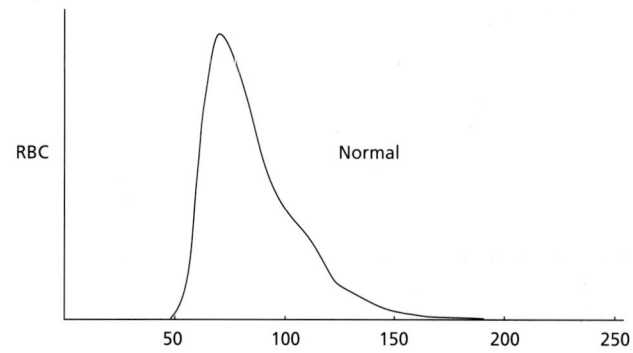

Figure 4.3 Red blood cell volume distribution histograms.

Questions

Based on the above information, you can best conclude the following:

1. The patient has a history of partial gastrectomy. The long-term complications of this procedure include all of the following EXCEPT:

   a. reduction in gastric acidity
   b. loss of gastric reservoir function
   c. the development of a gastrinoma
   d. rapid intestinal transit
   e. impaired absorption of iron

2. The LEAST likely contributory factor to this patient's abnormal hematological findings is:

   a. decreased production of erythropoietin
   b. blood loss through the gastrointestinal tract
   c. malabsorption of iron due to partial gastrectomy
   d. decreased production of gastric hydrochloric acid

3. The increase in serum gamma glutamyl transferase (GGTP) in this patient is most likely related to:

   a. his gastrointestinal bleeding
   b. a history of alcohol abuse
   c. hemolysis of red blood cells
   d. iron deficiency
   e. decreased liver synthesis of transferrin

4. This patient has a low red cell mean corpuscular volume (MCV) and a high red cell distribution width (RDW). Which of the following options concerning one or both of these parameters is correct?

    a. a high RDW is always associated with a low MCV
    b. a normal RDW is a typical finding in patients with anemia of vitamin B_{12} deficiency
    c. patients with hereditary spherocytosis have an exceptionally high RDW
    d. all of the above statements are correct
    e. none of the above statements is correct

5. Which of the following would you expect to be present in this patient?

    a. an increased synthesis of transferrin
    b. a decreased free erythrocyte protoporphyrin level
    c. an increased parenchymal cell storage of ferritin
    d. a prolonged erythrocyte survival
    e. none of the above

6. The patient's peripheral blood smear (Fig. 4.1) shows all of the following EXCEPT:

    a. hypochromia
    b. anisocytosis
    c. microcytosis
    d. poikilocytosis
    e. basophilic stippling

Clinical course

The patient was transfused with packed red blood cells. His hemoglobin and hematocrit were closely monitored. An upper endoscopy with gastric biopsy and colonoscopy were performed. The patient was started on iron supplement treatment and will also undergo a course of treatment for his gastric condition.

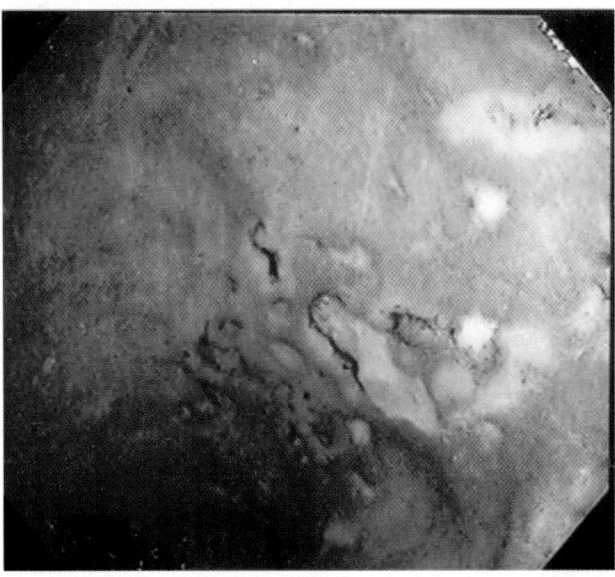

Figure 4.4 Gastric endoscopy (patient).

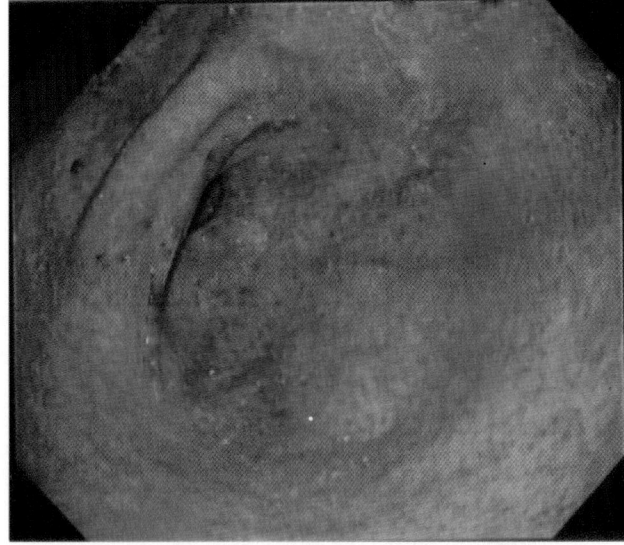

Figure 4.5 Gastric endoscopy (normal).

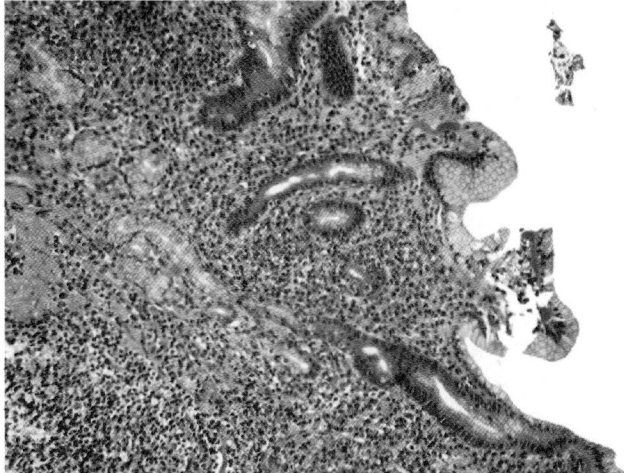

Figure 4.6 Endoscopic gastric biopsy (patient). Hematoxylin & eosin stain.

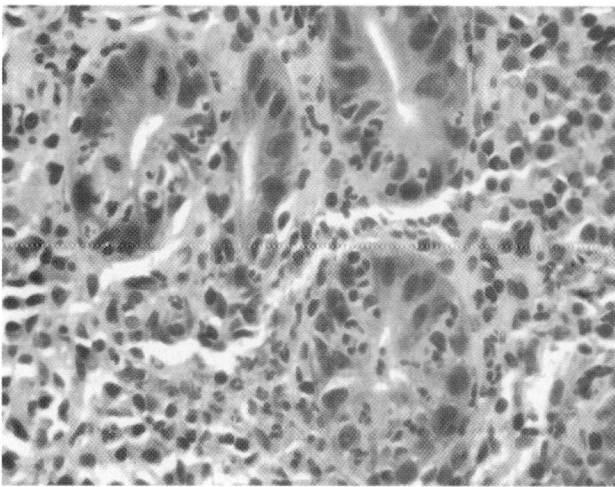

Figure 4.7 Endoscopic gastric biopsy (patient). Hematoxylin & eosin stain.

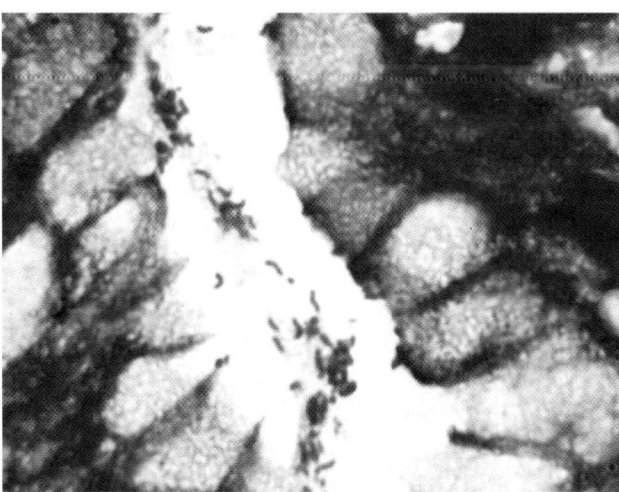

Figure 4.8 Endoscopic gastric biopsy (patient). Giemsa stain.

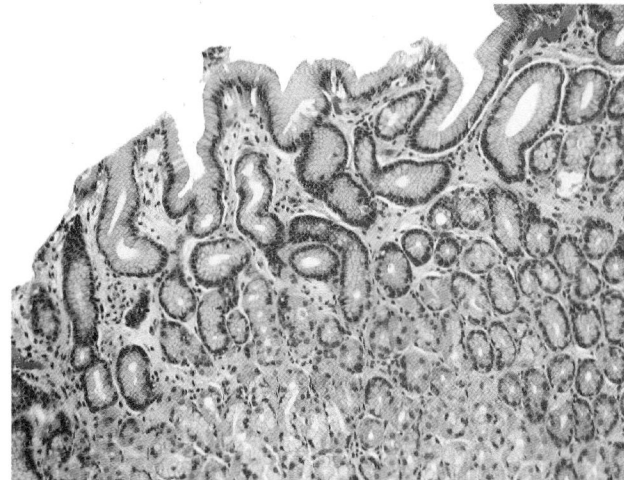

Figure 4.9 Endoscopic gastric biopsy (normal). Hematoxylin & eosin stain.

Questions

7. The microscopic appearance of the patient's gastric biopsy (Figs 4.6–4.8) shows all of the following EXCEPT:

   a. signs of acute inflammation
   b. signs of chronic inflammation
   c. the presence of a microbial agent
   d. changes characteristic of gastric carcinoma

8. The etiological agent of this patient's gastric condition (shown in Fig. 4.8):

   a. is usually present in the superficial mucous layer on the luminal mucosa
   b. grows faster in areas of the stomach with intestinal metaplasia
   c. is mainly present in the area of the gastro-esophageal junction
   d. increases the risk of developing squamous cell carcinoma of the esophagus
   e. does none of the above

9. Which abnormality would appear first in the development of this patient's condition?

   a. decreased blood hemoglobin
   b. decreased bone marrow iron stores
   c. increased red blood cell distribution width (RDW)
   d. decreased MCV (mean corpuscular volume)
   e. decreased transferrin saturation

10. In general, which of the following combinations of findings favors the diagnosis of anemia of chronic disease over anemia of iron deficiency?

	Serum iron	Serum ferritin	Storage iron	TIBC
a.	D	D	D	I
b.	D	I	D	I
c.	D	I	I	D
d.	N	D	N	I
e.	N	N	I	I

D, decreased; I, increased; N, normal

11. Identify the INCORRECT statement about this patient's problems:

   a. the "dizziness" and weakness are symptoms of anemia
   b. the patient should receive a course of antibiotic treatment
   c. the patient most likely has more than one contributing factor to his iron deficiency
   d. the patient's long-term prognosis is guarded because of the malignant character of his gastric lesion
   e. impaired iron absorption is likely to be an ongoing problem

---

ANSWERS AND FURTHER INFORMATION

Figure descriptions

Figure 4.1 Peripheral blood smear (patient). Wright/Giemsa stain.
Microcytic hypochromic anemia: The patient's peripheral blood smear shows aniso-poikilocytosis (red blood cells of different size and shape). The red blood cells are microcytic (small in size), hypochromic, and with prominent central pallor. Platelets are adequate in number and uniform in size.

Figure 4.2 Peripheral blood smear (normal). Wright/Giemsa stain.
The red blood cells are similar in size and shape, and hemoglobinization appears normal with normal central pallor. A normal neutrophil is present and the platelets are adequate in number and uniform in size.

Figure 4.3 Red blood cell volume distribution histograms.
The left image shows the distribution histogram of the patient's red blood cell volume. In this patient's red blood cell volume histogram, the MCV (mean corpuscular volume) lies closer to 50 fL than to the 100 fL mark (actual MCV = 66 fL). The red cell distribution width (RDW) is an index of the variation in red blood cell volume. RDW = (standard deviation of red cell volume ÷ mean cell volume) × 100. The right image shows the distribution histogram of another patient with a normal red blood cell mean corpuscular volume (MCV) for comparison.

Figure 4.4 Gastric endoscopy (patient).
Gastritis: A photograph from the gastric endoscopy, showing moderate to severe gastritis with multiple small ulcers.

Figure 4.5 Gastric endoscopy (normal).
This is an endoscopic photograph of normal gastric mucosa for comparison.

Figure 4.6 Endoscopic gastric biopsy (patient). Hematoxylin & eosin stain.
Chronic active gastritis with focal mucosal ulceration: Gastric biopsy with a marked acute and chronic inflammatory cell infiltrate, consisting of neutrophils, plasma cells, and lymphocytes, involving the lamina propria. A small ulcer is noted on the surface epithelium. Note neutrophilic infiltrate of the gastric glands underneath the ulcer. There is mild focal mucosal congestion.

Figure 4.7 Endoscopic gastric biopsy (patient). Hematoxylin & eosin stain.
Chronic active gastritis: A higher magnification of the gastric biopsy showing a dense neutrophilic and lympho-plasmacytic infiltrate of the lamina propria. A marked neutrophilic

infiltrate of the gastric glands is evident in this photomicrograph.

Figure 4.8 Endoscopic gastric biopsy (patient). Giemsa stain.
Helicobacter pylori gastritis: Gastric biopsy stained with Giemsa stain showing numerous dark-blue, curvilinear "S-shaped" microorganisms, consistent with *Helicobacter pylori*. *Helicobacter pylori* is usually found in the mucus along the luminal surface of the gastric epithelium. This microorganism usually does not invade tissue.

Figure 4.9 Endoscopic gastric biopsy (normal). Hematoxylin & eosin stain.
Normal gastric mucosa: This image shows a normal gastric mucosa. There is no significant inflammatory cell infiltrate in the lamina propria. Gastric glands are intact. The surface epithelial cells are mucus-secreting cells.

Answers

1.C. Gastrinoma is a tumor of islet cells of pancreas, which produces gastrin and causes gastric hypersecretion leading to ulcerations. There is no known association between post-gastrectomy status and the development of this tumor. All other options (reduction in gastric acidity, loss of gastric reservoir function, rapid intestinal transit) are known complications of post-gastrectomy status and contribute or lead to the impaired absorption of iron.

2. A. The patient has a hypochromic microcytic anemia, which is due to iron deficiency as suggested by special hematology iron studies. Decreased production of erythropoietin by the kidney (which is the major source of erythropoietin) is not likely to be a cause or a factor contributing to his iron deficiency anemia. There are no signs or symptoms of renal failure, or of other conditions (protein malnutrition, etc.), associated with a decrease in erythropoietin production. The severe anemia of this patient should, on the contrary, stimulate erythropoietin production. The patient has a guaiac-positive stool, which most likely reflects gastrointestinal bleeding, contributing to iron loss and anemia. Malabsorption of iron and a decreased production of gastric hydrochloric acid are long-standing complications of partial gastrectomy and contribute to the development of iron deficiency.

3. B. An increase in serum gamma glutamyl transferase (GGTP) in this patient most likely reflects his abuse of alcohol, which is a potent inducer of GGTP synthesis. Gastrointestinal bleeding, hemolysis of red blood cells, and iron deficiency per se have no direct effect on the level of serum GGTP.

4 E. Red blood cell distribution width (RDW) provides a measurement of the distribution of erythrocyte volume and is automatically provided by modern cell counters. The difference in size between the normal and abnormal RBC is presented as a broadening of the normal histogram peak (a high RDW) or as more than one histogram peak. A high RDW is a measure of anisocytosis and can be associated with a low, normal, or high MCV. Patients with vitamin B_{12} deficiency develop megaloblastic anemia, with a considerable anisocytosis and poikilocytosis, leading to an abnormal, high RDW. In hereditary spherocytosis the erythrocytes are small and round, and the RDW is normal. Therefore, none of the options is correct.

5. A. This patient has a severe iron deficiency anemia. Transferrin, a glycoprotein synthesized in the liver, transports circulating iron to the cells. The synthesis of transferrin increases in iron deficiency anemia. Protoporphyrin IX (a heme precursor) forms a complex with iron, which is the last step in heme synthesis. If iron is not present, the protoporphyrin complexes with zinc instead. The zinc can be removed and "free" protoporphyrin is then measured. In iron deficiency anemia the level of "free" protoporphyrin is high due to deficiency of iron. Ferritin, a storage form of iron, is decreased in iron deficiency anemia, both in parenchymal cells and in the circulation. Erythrocyte survival in iron deficiency is normal or slightly reduced, but it is not prolonged.

6. E. The patient's blood smear shows changes consistent with microcytic hypochromic anemia (hypochromia, anisocytosis, microcytosis, and poikilocytosis). "Basophilic stippling" describes dark-blue structures derived from aggregated ribosomes or mitochondria and is typically seen in conditions such as lead poisoning or thalassemia.

7. D. The histology of the gastric biopsies does not indicate the presence of gastric carcinoma. Two of the images of the patient's gastric biopsy (Figs 4.6 and 4.7) show evidence of acute and chronic gastritis. Another (Fig. 4.8) shows the presence of a microbial agent, *Helicobacter pylori*, on the mucosal surface.

8. A. *Helicobacter pylori* (*H. pylori*) is a curvilinear (S-shaped) Gram-negative rod that is usually present in the superficial mucous layer of the stomach along the luminal surface of the gastric epithelium. It is a major cause of chronic gastritis affecting the antrum and the body. *H. pylori* is associated with gastric adenocarcinoma and a rare type of lymphocytic tumor of the stomach called MALT lymphoma. *H. pylori* is absent from areas of the stomach with intestinal metaplasia and it plays no role in the pathogenesis of squamous cell carcinoma.

9. B. The depletion of body iron goes through several stages before it causes anemia. At first, there is a decrease in bone marrow iron stores without any signs of iron deficiency. This is followed by a reduction in serum ferritin; the next stage is characterized by absent bone marrow iron, decreased hemoglobin, and decreased mean corpuscular volume (MCV). At this stage the transferrin saturation is decreased and anisocytosis appears (increased red blood cell distribution width – RDW). Untreated, this stage progresses to severe iron deficiency anemia.

10. C. Anemia of chronic disease is characterized by low serum iron, increased storage iron, a high serum ferritin level reflecting the increase in the storage iron, and by a reduced total iron binding capacity. This type of anemia is thought to develop due to a defect in the reutilization of iron, or by the effect of inflammatory cytokines (IL-1 and INF-γ) in inhibiting erythrocyte precursor proliferation, or the synthesis and release of erythropoietin by the kidney. The typical laboratory setting of iron deficiency anemia is depicted in option "A." It is characterized by ubiquitous iron deficiency and by an increased synthesis of transferrin reflected by increased TIBC and reduced transferrin saturation.

11 D. This patient has an iron deficiency anemia, which has several contributing factors, including an impaired absorption of iron due to previous partial gastrectomy and chronic gastrointestinal bleeding due to gastritis with mucosal erosions. Since the gastric biopsy showed the presence of *Helicobacter pylori*, the patient should be treated with antibiotics. This gastric lesion is not malignant and is curable. His anemia, however, will have to be monitored, since the absorption of iron will continue to be impaired.

Final diagnosis and synopsis of the case

- Gastritis; *Helicobacter pylori* infection
- Chronic blood loss
- Iron deficiency anemia

A middle-aged man with a long-standing history of labyrinthitis and peptic ulcer disease, status post partial gastrectomy 10 years ago, presented with complaints of dizziness and weakness. A CBC (FBC) showed him to be severely anemic. The work-up of his anemia revealed a severe and most likely long-standing iron deficiency. His stool was positive for occult blood. His esophago-gastroduodenoscopy revealed gastritis with signs of acute and chronic inflammation and erosion. There was also microscopic evidence of *Helicobacter pylori* infection. The colonoscopy did not show any abnormalities. The patient received a blood transfusion, and he will be treated with antibiotics for the *Helicobacter* infection and will receive iron supplements.

Lab tips

Typical iron studies patterns in anemia (Table 4.6)

Table 4.6

	MCV	Serum iron	TIBC	BM iron storage	Serum ferritin	Storage iron
Iron deficiency anemia	Low	D	I	D	D	D
Anemia of chronic disease	N	D	D	I	I	I
β-Thalassemia minor*	Very low	N	N	N	N	N

BM, bone marrow; D, decreased; I, increased; N, normal.
* There may be an increased level of Hb A_2.

Gastric biopsy

Gastric biopsies are obtained by endoscopy, after an 8-hour fast. During this procedure the patient is under mild sedation. The specimen is transported to the laboratory in formalin, grossly examined, processed, and embedded in paraffin, to produce histological sections. Following staining (initially by hematoxylin and eosin stain), it is examined by a pathologist.

A 74-year-old man with discomfort on eating

CASE AND MCQS

Clinical history and presentation

A 74-year-old man was seen by his family physician complaining of inability to chew on the right side of his mouth because of pain. He had poorly fitting dentures and a whitish area was noted on the right side of the mandibular gum area. He has a history of smoking two packs of cigarettes a day for 60 years and admits to heavy drinking. Physical examination revealed a well-developed male who was alert and co-operative, and in no acute distress. There was some tenderness in the right submandibular area, and there was a large firm nodule in the right side of the neck.

The oral cavity showed a whitish area on the buccal aspect of the mandibular gingiva on the right side, resistant to scraping off. The pulse rate was 76/min and regular, and the blood pressure was 150/90 mmHg. The abdomen showed an old appendectomy scar, no tenderness or organomegaly. Because of the findings in the gingiva, the patient was referred to a specialist for a biopsy of the right oral cavity and right neck mass. The results are shown in Figs 5.1–5.4. (Figure 5.5 shows a normal lymph node for comparison.)

Admission data

Table 5.1 Hematology

			SI Units	
WBC	10.1	(3.3–11.0 thou/µL)	10.1	(3.3–11.0 × 10⁹/L)
Neut	70	(44–88%)	70	(44–88%)
Band	0	(0–10%)	0	(0–10%)
Lymph	24	(12–43%)	24	(12–43%)
Mono	5	(2–11%)	5	(2–11%)
Eos	1	(0–5%)	1	(0–5%)
Baso	0	(0–2%)	0	(0–2%)
RBC	4.0	(3.9–5.0 mill/µL)	4.0	(3.9–5.0 × 10¹²/L)
HGB	12.1	(11.6–15.6 g/dL)	121	(116–156 g/L)
HCT	38.1	(37.0–47.0%)	0.381	(0.37–0.47)
MCV	95.2	(79.0–99.0 fL)	95.2	(79.0–99.0 fL)
MCH	30.3	(27.0–34.6 pg)	30.3	(27.0–34.6 pg)
MCHC	31.8	(31.0–37.1 g/dL)	318	(310–371 g/L)
Plts	285	(130–400 thou/µL)	285	(130–400 × 10⁹/L)

Table 5.2 Coagulation		
PT	12.9	(11–14 s)
APTT	28.0	(22–32 s)
INR	0.99	

Table 5.3 CT scan of neck with contrast

A 4 × 6 cm irregular mass is present in the right submandibular region. It extends laterally to the deep soft tissues, eroding the hyoid bone and displacing the airway to the left.

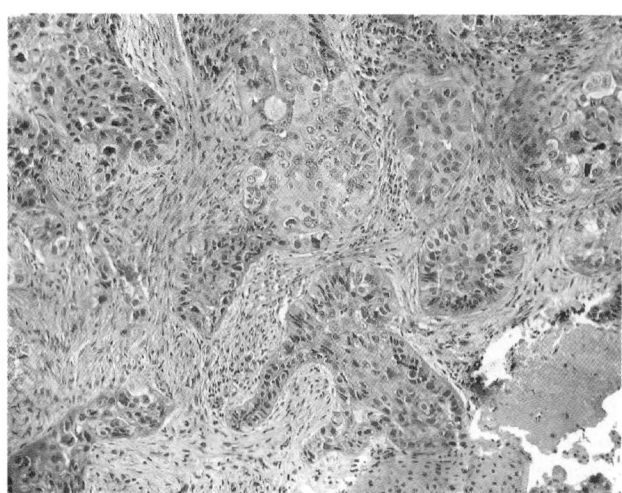

Figure 5.1 Biopsy of right oral cavity (patient). Hematoxylin & eosin stain.

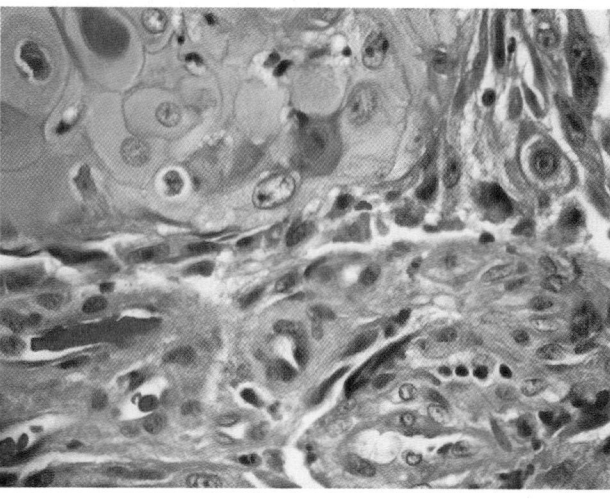

Figure 5.2 Biopsy of right oral cavity (patient). Hematoxylin & eosin stain.

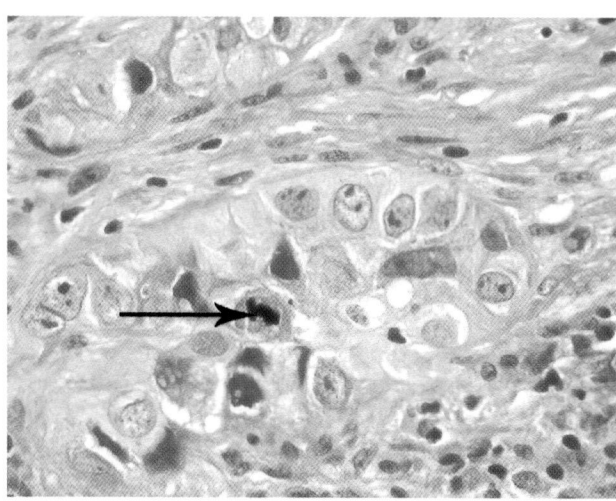

Figure 5.3 Biopsy of right oral cavity (patient). Hematoxylin & eosin stain.

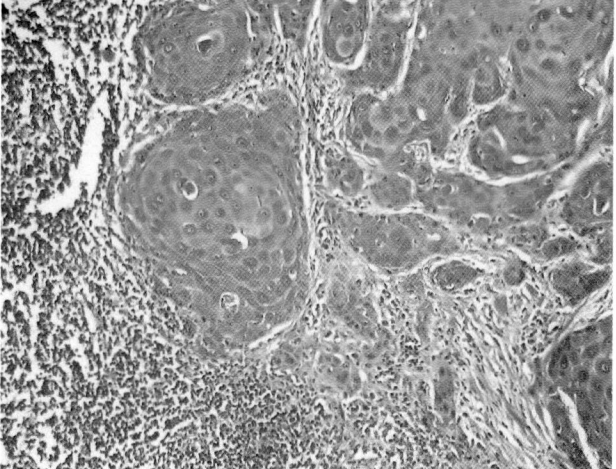

Figure 5.4 Biopsy of right neck mass (patient). Hematoxylin & eosin stain.

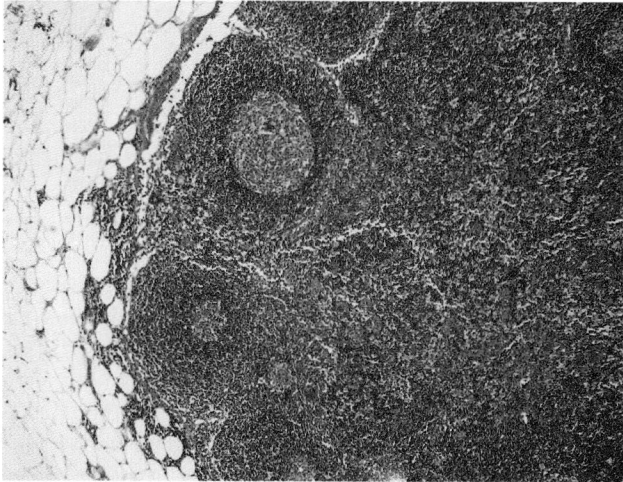

Figure 5.5 Lymph node (normal). Hematoxylin & eosin stain.

Questions

Based on the above information you can best conclude the following:

BASIC

1. Which of the following oral lesions typically appears as a white plaque?

   a. pyogenic granuloma
   b. aphthous ulcer "canker sore"
   c. leukoplakia
   d. all of the above
   e. none of the above

INTERMEDIATE

2. The lesion depicted in Figs 5.1–5.3 is consistent with:

   a. candidiasis
   b. pyogenic granuloma
   c. a papilloma
   d. a squamous cell carcinoma
   e. a chronic inflammatory process

INTERMEDIATE

3. Which of the following factors have been clearly implicated in the pathogenesis of such a lesion as that depicted in Figs 5.1–5.3?

   a. a high fiber diet
   b. tobacco and alcohol use
   c. vitamin C deficiency
   d. caffeine
   e. none of the above

BASIC

4. Which of the following lesions of the oral cavity are considered to be premalignant?

   a. leukoplakia
   b. aphthous ulcer "canker sore"
   c. pyogenic granuloma
   d. fibroma
   e. all of the above

INTERMEDIATE

5. The appearance of the biopsy of the right neck mass (Fig. 5.4) is consistent with:

   a. a metastatic carcinoma
   b. an acute non-specific lymphadenitis
   c. a keratinous cyst
   d. an abscess
   e. none of the above

INTERMEDIATE

6. The most common site for the development of lesions such as those depicted in Figs 5.2 and 5.3 is:

   a. the floor of the mouth
   b. tonsils
   c. uvula
   d. hard palate

ANSWERS AND FURTHER INFORMATION

Figure descriptions

Figure 5.1 Biopsy of right oral cavity (patient). Hematoxylin & eosin stain.
Moderately differentiated infiltrating squamous cell carcinoma: This photomicrograph shows many infiltrating solid nests of neoplastic cells in a desmoplastic stroma (a stromal response to tumor invasion that results in extensive fibrosis with scarring). Nuclear pleomorphism is apparent at this low magnification.

Figure 5.2 Biopsy of right oral cavity (patient). Hematoxylin & eosin stain.
Moderately differentiated infiltrating squamous cell carcinoma: This image clearly demonstrates the squamous nature of this tumor. The neoplastic cells are large with hyperchromatic nuclei and prominent nucleoli. Single cell keratinization is noted in this image.

Figure 5.3 Biopsy of right oral cavity (patient). Hematoxylin & eosin stain.
Moderately differentiated infiltrating squamous cell carcinoma: This image also shows the squamous nature of the infiltrating neoplastic cells. A mitotic figure (arrow) is seen in this field.

Figure 5.4 Biopsy of right neck mass (patient). Hematoxylin & eosin stain.
Cervical lymph node with metastatic squamous cell carcinoma: This photomicrograph shows a portion of a cervical lymph node almost completely replaced by metastatic squamous cell carcinoma.

Figure 5.5 Lymph node (normal). Hematoxylin & eosin stain.
Normal lymph node: This is a section of a normal reactive lymph node for comparison.

Answers

1. C. Leukoplakia produces a white plaque on the oral mucosa that cannot be scraped off. It can be a solitary lesion or it can produce multiple white patches. Microscopically it represents a wide spectrum of epithelial changes ranging from hyperkeratosis to dysplasia and squamous cell carcinoma *in situ*. Pyogenic granuloma is a highly vascular lesion. Aphthous ulcer is a painful hyperemic ulceration with an erythematous rim around its border.

2. D. The lesion represents a squamous cell carcinoma (see the descriptions for Figs 5.1–5.3) with clearly evident keratinization and stromal invasion. Its evident cytological malignancy excludes the diagnosis of papilloma. There is no evidence of candidiasis, chronic inflammation or of pyogenic granuloma, which is a form of capillary hemangioma.

3. B. The pathogenesis of oral squamous cell carcinoma is linked to tobacco smoking (especially chewing tobacco) and alcohol drinking. Heavy drinking and smoking use greatly (×6–15) increase the risk of oral carcinoma as compared to the control population. A high fiber diet, caffeine, and vitamin C deficiency are not known to play any role in the pathogenesis of oral squamous cell carcinoma.

4. A. Leukoplakia is considered to be a precancerous lesion, especially when it occurs on a high-risk site (floor of the mouth or the ventral surface of the tongue). Persistent lesions should be biopsied. Aphthous ulcer, fibroma, and pyogenic granuloma are benign lesions.

5. A. Figure 5.4 shows a portion of a cervical lymph node with metastatic squamous cell carcinoma. Squamous cell carcinoma of the oral cavity tends to infiltrate locally before it metastasizes to the lymph nodes, lung, liver, and bone. Once detected it must be treated. The success of treatment depends on many factors, the most important of which is early detection. Primary lesions less than 4 mm deep have a low propensity to metastasize. Most patients with lesions less than 2 cm in diameter can be cured. Squamous cell carcinoma of the oral cavity affects mostly people over 50 years of age. Acute non-specific lymphadenitis refers to acutely inflamed nodes, most commonly due to direct drainage of infected areas. Such nodes are tender to touch. Histologically, there is prominence of lymphoid follicles with large germinal centers. An abscess is characterized by a localized production of pus, consisting of neutrophils, necrotic tissue, and edema. Keratinous cysts are formed by down-growth and cystic expansion of the epidermis or of the epithelium forming the hair follicle. They are filled with keratin and lipid-containing macrophages and produce firm and movable nodules. None of the characteristics of acute lymphadenitis, abscesses, or keratinous cysts are present in the biopsy material shown in Fig. 5.4.

6. A. The most common site for the development of cancer in the mouth is the floor of the mouth, followed by the ventral surface of the tongue and the hard palate.

Final diagnosis and synopsis of the case

- Oral squamous cell carcinoma involving the mandible

A 74-year-old man was seen by his family physician for evaluation of a painful mass of the right lower gingival region. On biopsy a diagnosis of squamous cell carcinoma with cervical lymph node metastasis was made. A CT scan showed involvement of submandibular lymph nodes and mandibular bone. He was treated by resection of the lesion, with ipsilateral *en bloc* neck dissection, with reconstruction and repair using a metallic splint and skin flap. He tolerated these procedures quite well, and was discharged for follow-up.

A 49-year-old teacher with dysuria and fever

CASE AND MCQS

Clinical history and presentation

A 49-year-old female was admitted to the hospital with a chief complaint of left-sided abdominal pain, nausea, fever, and chills of two days' duration. Over the past year she had had episodes of painful and frequent urination. She has a history of non-insulin-dependent diabetes mellitus. Physical examination revealed an alert and oriented female. Her blood pressure was 135/90 mmHg, pulse was 100/min and regular, temperature was 102.8°F (39.3°C), and respiratory rate 26/min. Abdominal examination showed a marked tenderness in the left costovertebral area on deep palpation. The rest of the physical examination was unremarkable. Blood and urine were collected for cultures (Fig. 6.1) and a CT scan of the kidney was performed (Fig. 6.2).

Admission data

Table 6.1 Hematology

			SI Units	
WBC	17.5 H	(3.3–11.0 thou/µL)	17.5 H	(3.3–11.0 × 10⁹/L)
Neut	66	(44–88%)	66	(44–88%)
Band	18 H	(0–10%)	18 H	(0–10%)
Lymph	9 L	(12–43%)	9 L	(12–43%)
Mono	1 L	(2–11%)	1 L	(2–11%)
Eos	0	(0–5%)	0	(0–5%)
Baso	0	(0–2%)	0	(0–2%)
Myelocytes	4 H	(0)	4 H	(0)
Metamyelocytes	2 H	(0)	2 H	(0)
RBC	3.7 L	(3.9–5.0 mill/µL)	3.7 L	(3.9–5.0 × 10¹²/L)
HGB	8.6 L	(11.6–15.6 g/dL)	86 L	(116–156 g/L)
HCT	28.1 L	(37.0–47.0%)	0.281 L	(0.37–0.47)
MCV	76.2 L	(79.0–99.0 fL)	76.2 L	(79.0–99.0 fL)
MCH	23.2 L	(26.0–32.6 pg)	23.2 L	(26.0–32.6 pg)
MCHC	31.0	(31.0–36.0 g/dL)	310	(310–360 g/L)
Plts	335	(130–400 thou/µL)	335	(130–400 × 10⁹/L)

Table 6.2 Chemistry

			SI Units	
Glucose	95	(65–110 mg/dL)	6.27	(3.6–6.11 mmol/L)
BUN	19	(7–24 mg/dL)	6.78	(2.50–8.57 mmol/L)
Creatinine	1.1	(0.7–1.4 mg/dL)	97.2	(61.9–123.7 μmol/L)
Uric acid	4.2	(3.0–8.5 mg/dL)	0.25	(0.18–0.51 mmol/L)
Cholesterol	164	(150–200 mg/dL)	4.2	(3.88–5.17 mmol/L)
Calcium	9.2	(8.5–10.5 mg/dL)	2.3	(2.13–2.63 mmol/L)
Protein	7.1	(6–8 g/dL)	71	(60–80 g/L)
Albumin	4.5	(3.7–5.0 g/dL)	45	(37–50 g/L)
LDH	135	(100–250 U/L)	135	(100–250 U/L)
Alk Phos	86	(0–120 U/L)	86	(0–120 U/L)
AST	32	(0–55 U/L)	32	(0–55 U/L)
GGTP	23	(0–50 U/L)	23	(0–50 U/L)
Bilirubin	1.4	(0.0–1.5 mg/dL)	23.9	(0–25.7 μmol/L)

Table 6.3 Electrolytes

			SI Units	
Na	140	(134–143 mEq/L)	140	(134–143 mmol/L)
K	4.3	(3.5–4.9 mEq/L)	4.3	(3.5–4.9 mmol/L)
Cl	98	(95–108 mEq/L)	98	(95–108 mmol/L)
CO_2	26	(21–32 mEq/L)	26	(21–32 mmol/L)

Table 6.4 Urinalysis

Sp. grav.	1.020	(1.010–1.035)
pH	6	(5.0–7.5)
Protein	1+ H	(Neg)
Glucose	Neg	(Neg)
Ketone	Neg	(Neg)
Blood	1+ H	(Neg)
Color	Pale yellow	(Pale yellow)
Clarity	Clear	(Clear)
WBC	15 H	(0–5/HPF)
RBC	10 H	(0–3/HPF)
Casts	Leukocyte casts	(0)
Urobilinogen	Neg	(Neg)
Cells	Few squamous cells	(0)
Bacteria	3+ H	(neg)

Table 6.5 Microbiology

Blood culture	Pending
Urine culture	Pending

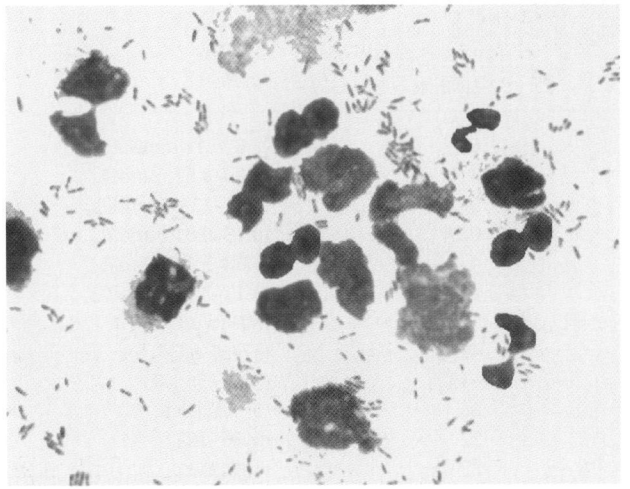

Figure 6.1 Urine sediment smear (patient). Giemsa stain.

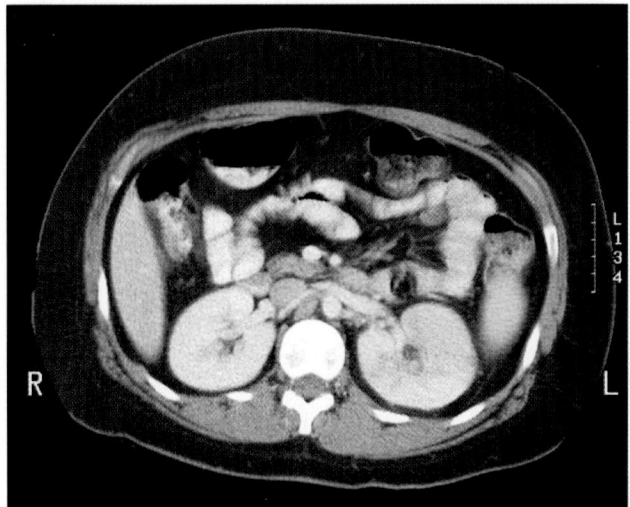

Figure 6.2 CT scan of the kidneys with contrast (patient).

Questions

Based on the above information you can best conclude the following:

BASIC

1. The WBC count reveals:

   a. absolute leukocytosis
   b. absolute granulocytosis
   c. relative lymphopenia
   d. all of the above
   e. none of the above

INTERMEDIATE

2. Which of the following causes could contribute to the proteinuria in this patient?

   a. infection of the renal pelvis or ureter
   b. contamination of urine with vaginal secretions
   c. fever
   d. all of the above
   e. none of the above

INTERMEDIATE

3. Which of the following statements about proteinuria in general is INCORRECT?

   a. the presence of protein in the urine is virtually diagnostic of a primary kidney disease
   b. proteinuria can be due to pre-renal causes
   c. the presence of WBCs in the urine can contribute to a positive protein reaction
   d. hyaline casts are composed of protein

INTERMEDIATE

4. Which of the following statements about hematuria is CORRECT?

   a. it is diagnostic of an inflammatory process involving the urinary bladder
   b. it is diagnostic of a neoplastic process involving the kidney
   c. it is diagnostic of an immunological process affecting the glomerulus
   d. it is diagnostic of an ischemic process affecting renal tubules
   e. it is not diagnostic of any of the above

INTERMEDIATE

5. Which of the following locations is the site of formation of leukocyte casts?

   a. urethra
   b. renal pelvis
   c. bladder lumen
   d. ureter
   e. renal tubular lumina

INTERMEDIATE

6. The appearance of the urine sediment (Fig. 6.1) is most consistent with:

   a. transitional cell carcinoma
   b. glomerulonephritis
   c. renal cell carcinoma
   d. urinary tract infection
   e. none of the above

7. The best evidence of kidney involvement in this patient's acute problem is:

a. pyuria
b. pyuria and hematuria

c. proteinuria
d. finding of leukocyte casts in the urine
e. positive microbial culture of urine

Clinical course

Her blood culture was negative, but her urine culture was positive for *E. coli* (>10^5 colonies/mL of urine). The patient was started on appropriate therapy and responded well. If a biopsy of the affected kidney had been performed, it would have looked like that shown in Figs 6.3–6.5. (Figure 6.6 is shown for comparison.)

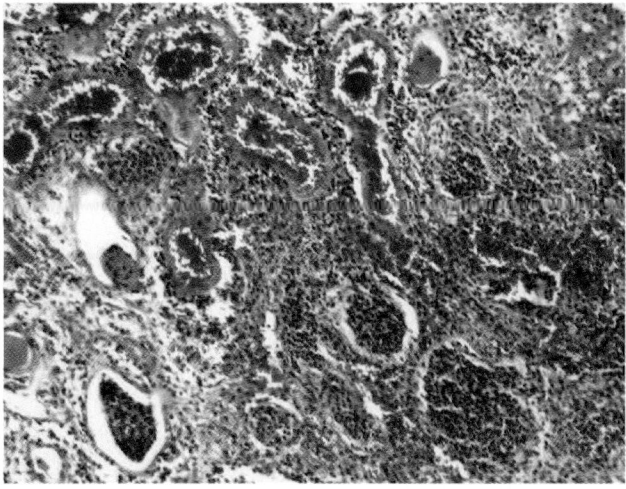

Figure 6.3 Portion of left kidney (from another patient). Hematoxylin & eosin stain.

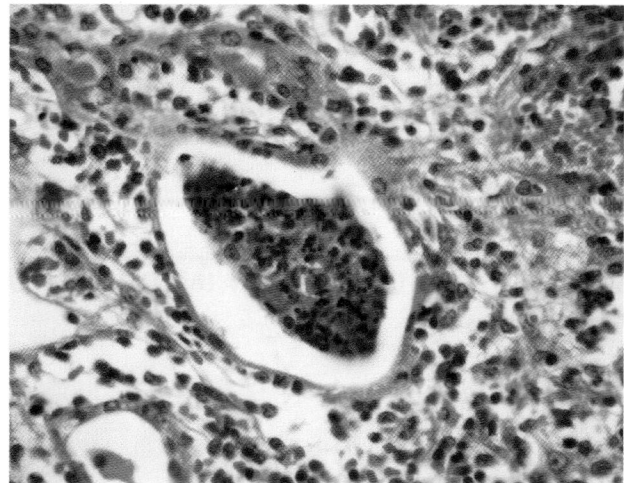

Figure 6.4 Portion of left kidney (from another patient). Hematoxylin & eosin stain.

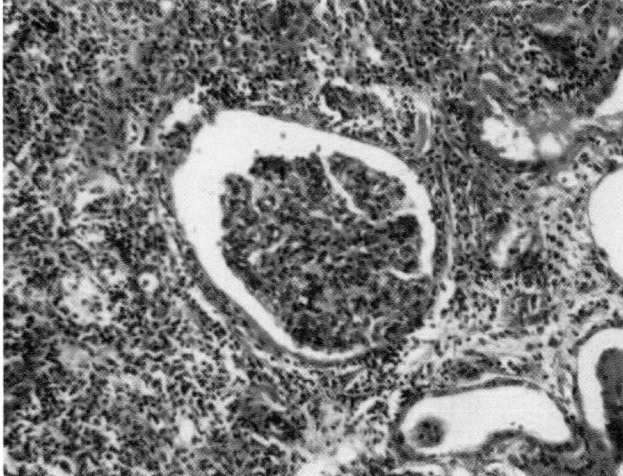

Figure 6.5 Portion of left kidney (from another patient). Hematoxylin & eosin stain.

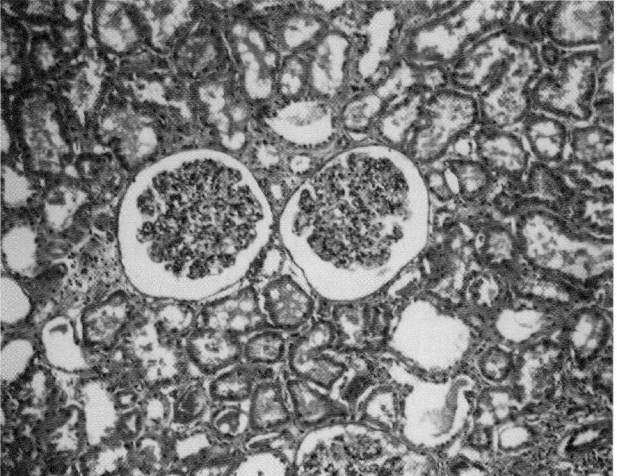

Figure 6.6 Portion of an unaffected area of the left kidney away from the lesion (from another patient). Hematoxylin & eosin stain.

Questions

8. The disorder depicted in Figs 6.3–6.5 most likely represents:

   a. an inflammatory process
   b. a neoplastic process
   c. an autoimmune disease
   d. a congenital malformation
   e. none of the above

9. In general, the most common cause of this patient's disorder is:

   a. ascending bacterial infection
   b. fungal infection of the vagina
   c. previous streptococcal infection of the throat
   d. immune complex deposition
   e. none of the above

10. The management of this patient should include:

   a. antineoplastic chemotherapy
   b. radiation therapy
   c. combined chemotherapy and radiation therapy
   d. steroid therapy
   e. antibiotics

11. Predisposing factors for such an acute renal problem include:

   a. a congenital or an acquired urinary obstruction
   b. diabetes mellitus
   c. immunosuppression
   d. instrumentation of the urinary tract
   e. all of the above

ANSWERS AND FURTHER INFORMATION

Figure descriptions

Figure 6.1 Urine sediment smear (patient). Giemsa stain.
Numerous neutrophils and large bacilli are seen in this image.

Figure 6.2 CT scan of the kidney with contrast (patient).
Acute pyelonephritis: This image from a contrast enhanced CT scan of the abdomen shows asymmetrically decreased enhancement of the left kidney. Also, mild perinephric stranding is seen, consistent with edema. This constellation of findings is compatible with the clinical picture of pyelonephritis.

Figure 6.3 Portion of left kidney (from another patient). Hematoxylin & eosin stain.
Acute pyelonephritis: At this magnification, one can recognize a marked tubular and interstitial inflammatory cell infiltrate, vascular congestion, and hemorrhage. In the lower portion of the image there are multiple dilated renal tubules filled with inflammatory cells.

Figure 6.4 Portion of left kidney (from another patient). Hematoxylin & eosin stain.
Acute pyelonephritis: This image shows tubular and interstitial neutrophilic (suppurative) infiltrate. Note the collection of neutrophils in the renal tubule in the center of this image. In acute pyelonephritis, inflammation may extend through the renal tubular lumina into the collecting tubules. Leuko-cytes inside the tubules are the source of urinary white blood cell casts.

Figure 6.5 Portion of left kidney (from another patient). Hematoxylin & eosin stain.
Acute pyelonephritis: This image shows an unaffected glomerulus situated in the middle of markedly inflamed renal parenchyma. Glomeruli, in general, appear to be resistant to bacterial infection; however, in large areas of necrosis glomerular destruction can be seen.

Figure 6.6 Portion of an unaffected area of the left kidney away from the lesion (from another patient). Hematoxylin & eosin stain.
This image represents a somewhat normal field for comparison. Two normal glomeruli are present in the middle of the image.

Answers

1. D. The patient has an absolute leukocytosis (WBC of 17.5 thou/μL, 17.5×10^9/L), a relative (and also absolute) lymphocytopenia (9% or 1.575 thou/μL, 1.575×10^9/L), and an absolute granulocytosis with left shift.

2. D. The patient has a 1+ proteinuria, which correlates with the excretion of about 100 mg of protein per deciliter of urine. There are many causes of proteinuria, some of which are directly associated with systemic or renal disease. Fever represents a relatively common cause of so-called pre-renal proteinuria; infection of the renal pelvis or ureter represents a cause of post-renal proteinuria, as does contamination with vaginal secretions. The patient has a fever, her urinalysis shows an increased number of WBCs, suggesting a urinary tract infection, and there are some squamous epithelial cells present in her urine, suggesting a contamination with vaginal secretions. Therefore all three factors (fever, infection of the renal pelvis or ureter, and contamination with vaginal secretion) could contribute to her proteinuria.

3. A. The presence of protein in the urine is not diagnostic of a primary kidney disease. Proteinuria can be of functional origin, not associated with systemic disease or kidney damage, or it can be of renal, pre-renal, or post-renal origin. The presence of WBCs and RBCs in the urine may cause a positive protein reaction. Protein is necessary for cast formation. Hyaline casts are composed of protein only; other casts, however, contain cellular component in addition to protein.

4. E. Hematuria refers to the presence of RBCs (>3 RBCs/HPF) in the urine. Several conditions may cause hematuria. Inflammation of the urinary tract, neoplasia, immunological processes affecting the glomeruli, and ischemic tubular damage may cause hematuria. But hematuria in itself is not diagnostic of any specific process. If persistent or intermittent, it should be further evaluated as to its cause.

5. E. Leukocyte casts are formed within the renal tubules. Protein is necessary for their formation. Stasis due to tubular obstruction and a highly concentrated urine are contributing factors for cast formation. Distal and collecting ducts are the main sites of cast formation.

6. D. Figure 6.1 shows neutrophils and bacilli (see the description of Fig. 6.1). No malignant cells or RBC casts are seen.

7. D. The best evidence of kidney involvement in this patient is the presence of leukocyte casts in her urine. These are formed in the renal tubules. All other findings could be associated with a non-renal etiology.

8. A. The lesions depicted in Figs 6.3–6.5 represent an inflammatory process (see the descriptions of Figs 6.3–6.5). There is no evidence of neoplastic, autoimmune, or congenital disorders.

9. A. The patient has acute pyelonephritis. The most common cause of such a disease is an ascending bacterial infection due to *E. coli*, followed by *Proteus* and *Klebsiella*. However, almost any bacterial or fungal agent can cause this disorder.

10. E. The treatment of choice for acute pyelonephritis is antibiotic therapy. There is no indication for antineoplastic chemotherapy, radiation therapy, combined chemotherapy and radiation therapy, or steroid therapy.

11 E. All mentioned factors (urinary tract obstruction, diabetes mellitus, immunosuppression, and instrumentation) are factors predisposing to urinary tract infection and acute pyelonephritis.

Final diagnosis and synopsis of the case

- Acute pyelonephritis

The patient presented with a classical clinical picture of acute pyelonephritis: fever, chills, left-sided abdominal and flank pain, dysuria, and frequent urination. Her urine cultures were positive for *E. coli*. Urinalysis revealed bacteria, pyuria, hematuria, and leukocyte casts. The patient's CBC (FBC) showed leukocytosis and granulocytosis with a left shift (increased number of myeloid precursors in the peripheral blood). During the last few years, she had several episodes of urinary tract infection. The patient has diabetes, which is a predisposing factor for the development of urinary tract infections. The patient responded well to antibiotic treatment.

Lab tips

Urinary casts
Site of formation:
- distal and collecting tubules

Factors contributing to cast formation:
- proteinuria
- concentrated urine
- urinary stasis

Significance varies according to:
- type of casts
- number of casts
- persistence of casts after treatment
- correlation of the presence of casts with clinical situation

Cast formation

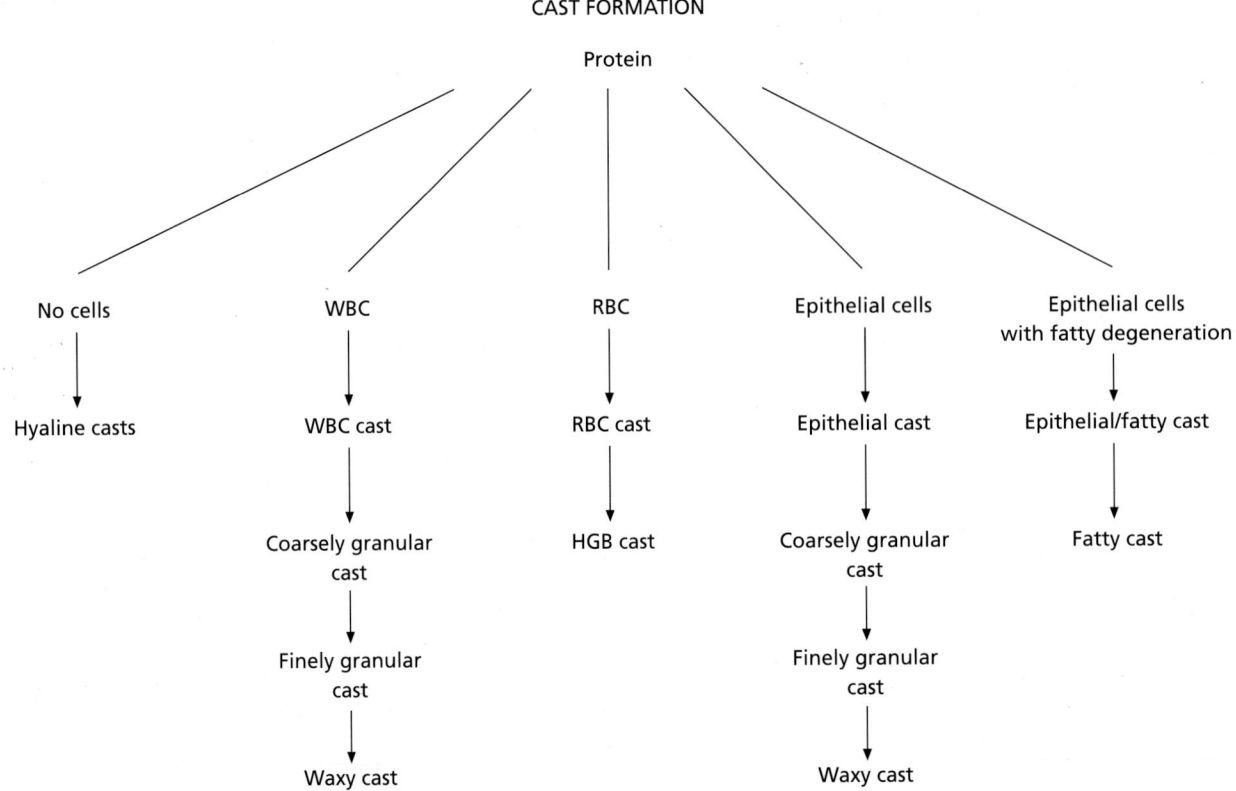

Figure 6.7 Modified from *Clinical Laboratory Medicine* by Richard Ravel, 6th edition, Mosby.

Clinical implications

WBC casts: Always significant; indicate infection or inflammation of renal parenchyma, most commonly pyelonephritis.

RBC casts: Always significant; indicate acute inflammation or vascular disorder in the glomerulus (acute glomerulonephritis, systemic lupus erythematosus, etc.).

Epithelial casts: When many are present, they indicate damage to the tubular epithelium (in nephritic syndrome, amyloidosis, etc.).

Fatty casts: Signify renal tubular damage with fatty degeneration of the tubular epithelial cells (in nephritic syndrome due to lipoid nephrosis, systemic lupus erythematosus, or in mercury poisoning).

Waxy casts: Are indicative of a serious renal problem involving prolonged stasis in renal tubules – they occur in chronic renal failure and indicate tubular inflammation and degeneration.

Hyaline casts: When alone, these casts have little clinical significance – usually they are a temporary finding.

A 70-year-old widow with severe pain in left shoulder

CASE AND MCQS

Clinical history and presentation

A 70-year-old widow presented with severe pain in her left shoulder of about 5 weeks' duration. This pain had become progressively worse and at present prevents the patient from engaging in her normal daily activities. The patient has a history of colon cancer for which she underwent surgery 9 years ago. She has been in good health since then, and she is not using any medications other than acetaminophen (paracetamol) for her shoulder pain. Physical examination revealed a frail woman making a visible effort to avoid movement of her left shoulder. Her vital signs were normal. Her chest was clear to auscultation and percussion, the abdomen was soft, with no organomegaly. Rectal examination was normal and stool was negative for occult blood. The left shoulder was tender to palpation and extremely painful on passive movement; there was no edema or redness. The rest of the physical examination was unremarkable. Admission data include an X-ray of the patient's left shoulder (Fig. 7.1).

Admission data

Table 7.1 Hematology

			SI Units	
WBC	2.9 L	(3.3–11.0 thou/μL)	2.9 L	(3.3–11.0 × 10⁹/L)
Neut	68	(44–88%)	68	(44–88%)
Lymph	23	(12–43%)	23	(12–43%)
Mono	4	(2–11%)	4	(2–11%)
Eos	1	(0–5%)	1	(0–5%)
Baso	0	(0–2%)	0	(0–2%)
Plasma cells	4 H	(0%)	4 H	(0%)
RBC	3.37 L	(3.9–5.0 mill/μL)	3.37 L	(3.9–5.0 × 10¹²/L)
HGB	10.4 L	(11.6–15.6 g/dL)	104 L	(116–156 g/L)
HCT	30.2 L	(37.0–47.0%)	30.2 L	(0.37–0.47)
MCV	89.4	(79.0–99.0 fL)	89.4	(79.0–99.0 fL)
MCH	30.09	(26.0–32.6 pg)	30.09	(26.0–32.6 pg)
MCHC	34.6	(31.0–36.0 g/dL)	346	(310–360 g/L)
Plts	120 L	(130–400 thou/μL)	120 L	(130–400 × 10⁹/L)

Table 7.2 Chemistry

			SI Units	
Glucose	109	(65–110 mg/dL)	5.99	(3.6–6.11 mmol/L)
Creatinine	3.7 H	(0.7–1.4 mg/dL)	327.1 H	(61.9–123.8 µmol/L)
BUN	44 H	(7–24 mg/dL)	15.74 H	(2.50–8.57 mmol/L)
Uric acid	8.4	(3.0–8.5 mg/dL)	0.49	(0.18–0.51 mmol/L)
Cholesterol	152	(150–200 mg/dL)	3.95	(3.88–5.17 mmol/L)
Calcium	12 H	(8.5–10.5 mg/dL)	3 H	(2.13–2.63 mmol/L)
Protein	8.3 H	(6–8 g/dL)	83 H	(60–80 g/L)
Albumin	3.7	(3.7–5.0 g/dL)	37	(37–50 g/L)
LDH	110	(100–250 U/L)	110	(100–250 U/L)
Alk Phos	115	(0–120 U/L)	115	(0–120 U/L)
AST	42	(0–55 U/L)	42	(0–55 U/L)
GGTP	35	(0–50 U/L)	35	(0–50 U/L)
Bilirubin	0.5	(0.0–1.5 mg/dL)	8.55	(0–25.7 µmol/L)
Bilirubin-direct	0.06	(0.02–0.18 mg/dL)	1.026	(0.34–3.08 µmol/L)

Table 7.3 Electrolytes

			SI Units	
Na	143	(134–143 mEq/L)	143	(134–143 mmol/L)
K	4.5	(3.5–4.9 mEq/L)	4.5	(3.5–4.9 mmol/L)
Cl	102	(95–108 mEq/L)	102	(95–108 mmol/L)
CO_2	32	(21–32 mEq/L)	32	(21–32 mmol/L)

Table 7.4 Urinalysis

pH	5	(5.0–7.5)
Protein	4+ H	(Neg)
Glucose	Neg	(Neg)
Ketone	Neg	(Neg)
Color	Yellow	(Yellow)
Clarity	Clear	(Clear)
Sp. grav.	1.013	(1.010–1.035)
WBC	4	(0–5/HPF)
RBC	2	(0–2/HPF)
Casts	Neg	(Neg)
Bacteria	Neg	(Neg)

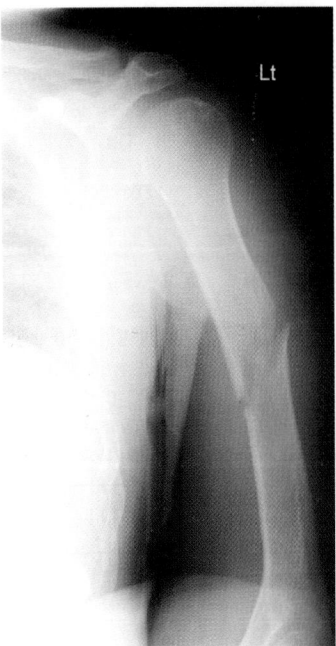

Figure 7.1 X-ray of left humerus (patient).

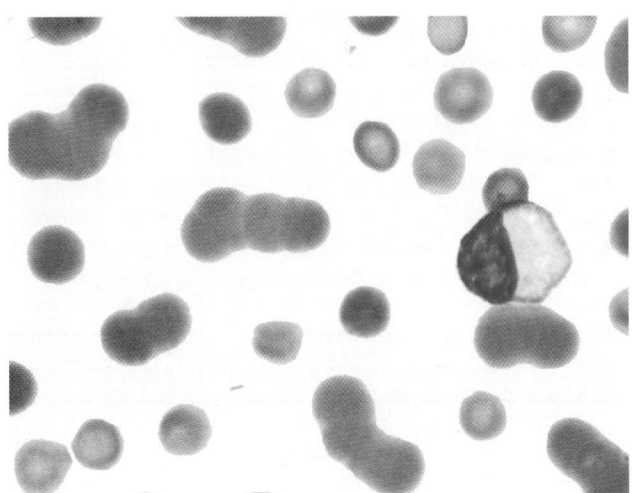

Figure 7.2 Peripheral blood smear (patient). Wright/Giemsa stain.

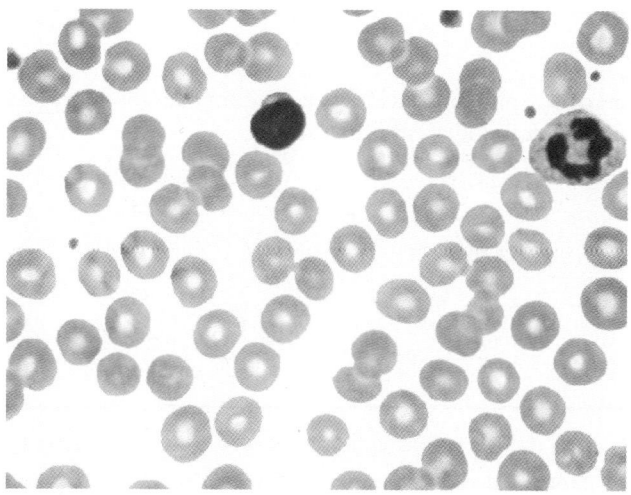

Figure 7.3 Peripheral blood smear (normal). Wright/Giemsa stain.

Questions

Based on the above information, you can best conclude the following:

INTERMEDIATE

1. The patient's anemia could be explained by:

   a. deficiency of erythropoietin
   b. neoplastic disease
   c. chronic renal disease
   d. a process involving bone marrow replacement
   e. any of the above

INTERMEDIATE

2. Pancytopenia, in general, can be a consequence of:

   a. bone marrow replacement
   b. drug therapy or chemical exposure
   c. viral infections
   d. ionizing radiation
   e. any of the above

INTERMEDIATE

3. Which of the following laboratory tests would provide the best information about the nature of the patient's hyperproteinemia?

   a. determination of 24-hour urine protein excretion
   b. serum electrophoresis
   c. liver function tests
   d. serum C-reactive protein level

INTERMEDIATE

4. The clinical effects of hypercalcemia, in general, do NOT include:

   a. fluid retention
   b. renal dysfunction
   c. changes on ECG
   d. peptic ulcer
   e. soft tissue calcification

INTERMEDIATE

5. The patient's peripheral blood smear (Fig. 7.2) shows:

   a. rouleaux formation
   b. a plasma cell
   c. aniso-poikilocytosis
   d. all of the above
   e. none of the above

INTERMEDIATE

6. The X-ray of the left humerus (Fig. 7.1) shows:

   a. a fracture
   b. an osteoid osteoma
   c. an aneurysmal bone cyst
   d. all of the above

Clinical course

The patient received special care for her painful shoulder and underwent an additional work-up. This included a bone marrow aspiration and biopsy and additional laboratory and radiological studies, shown below.

Table 7.5 Quantitative serum immunoglobulins

			SI Units	
IgA	60 L	(85–385 mg/dL)	600 L	(850–3850 mg/L)
IgG	2800 H	(564–1765 mg/dL)	28 000 H	(5640–17 650 mg/L)
IgM	50	(45–250 mg/dL)	500	(450–2500 mg/L)

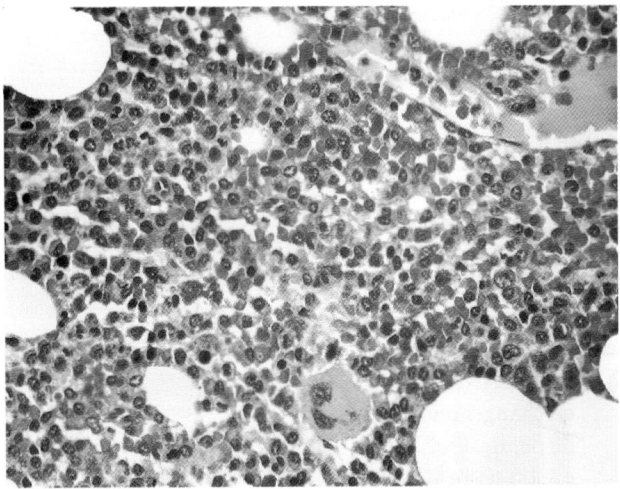

Figure 7.4 Bone marrow biopsy (patient). Hematoxylin & eosin stain.

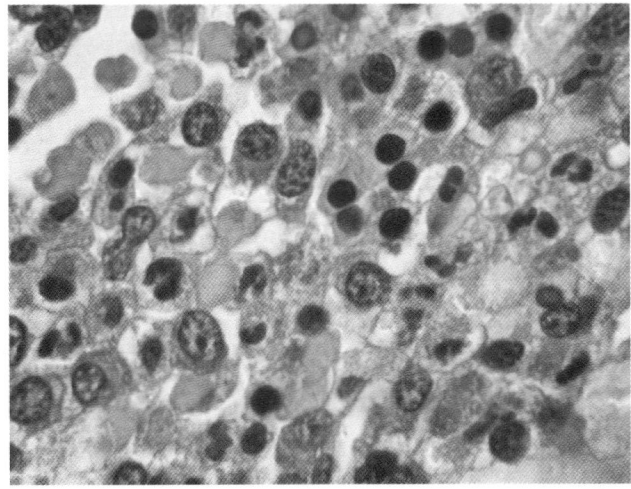

Figure 7.5 Bone marrow biopsy (patient). Hematoxylin & eosin stain.

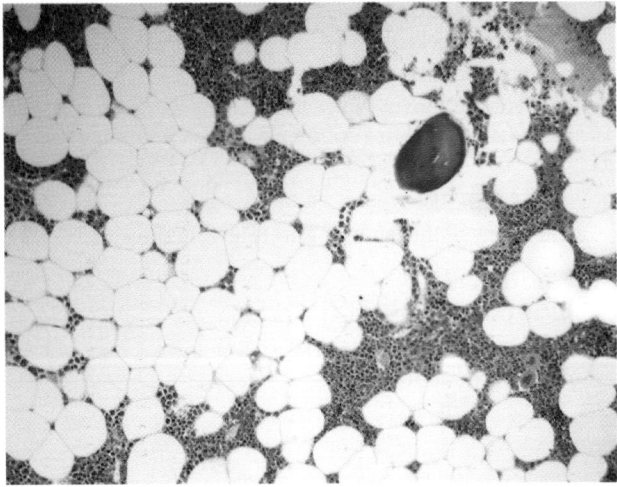

Figure 7.6 Bone marrow biopsy (normal). Hematoxylin & eosin stain.

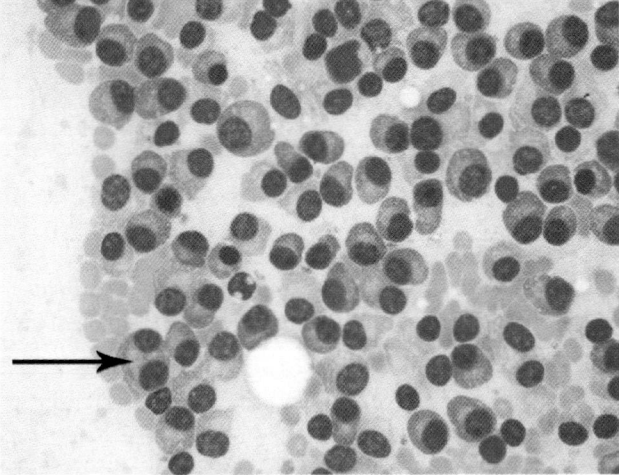

Figure 7.7 Bone marrow aspiration smear (patient). Wright/Giemsa stain.

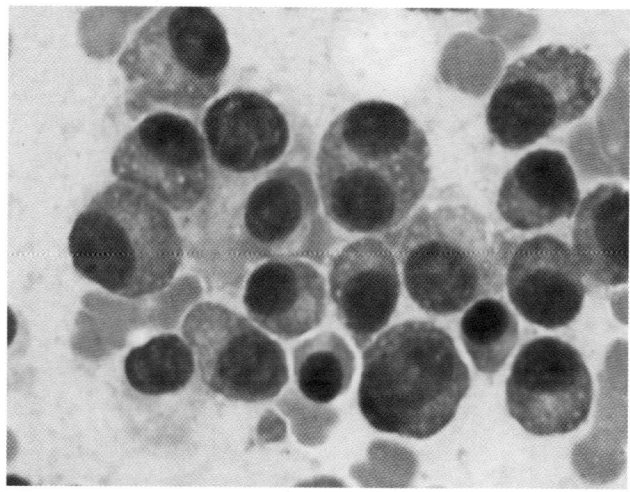

Figure 7.8 Bone marrow aspiration smear (patient). Wright/Giemsa stain.

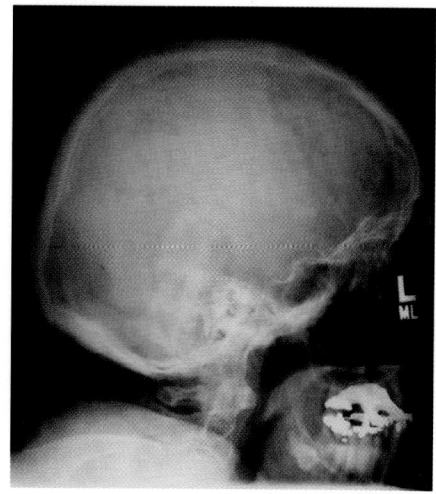

Figure 7.9 X-ray of skull lateral view (patient).

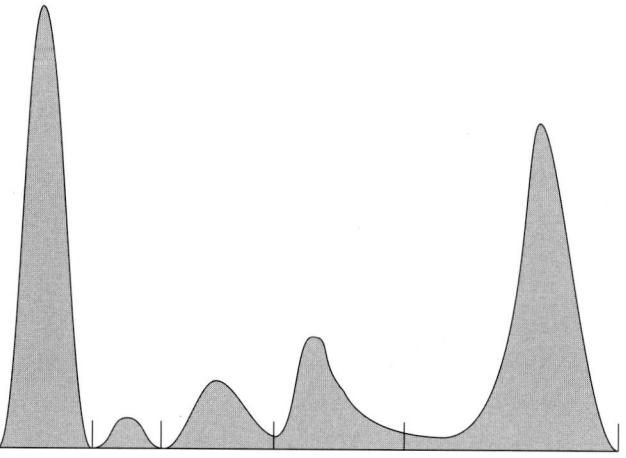

Figure 7.10 Serum protein electrophoresis (patient).

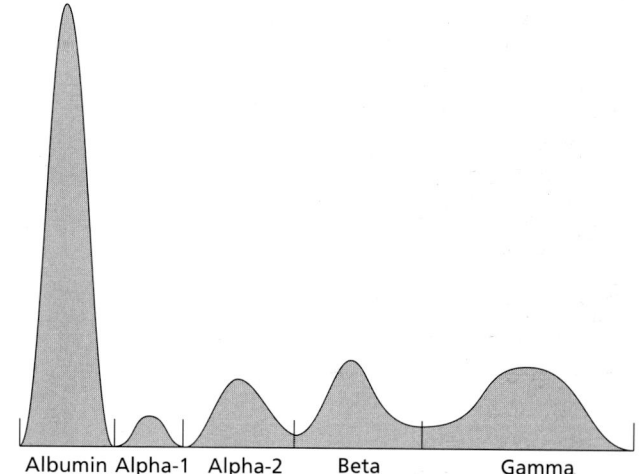

Albumin Alpha-1 Alpha-2 Beta Gamma

Figure 7.11 Serum protein electrophoresis (normal).

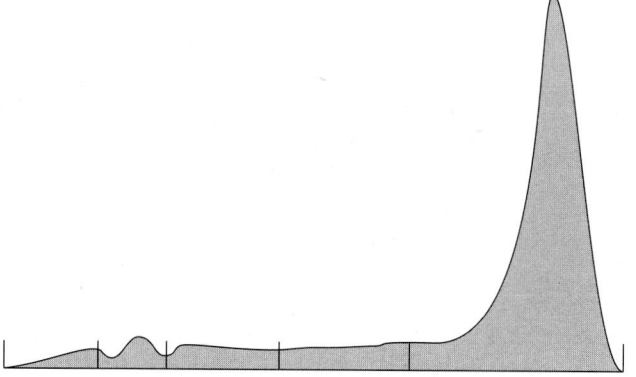

Figure 7.12 Urine protein electrophoresis (patient).

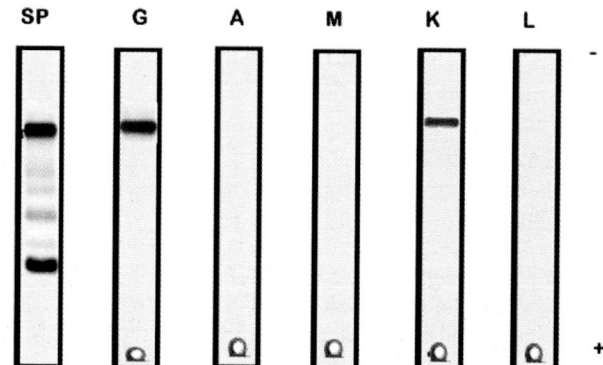

Figure 7.13 Immunofixation of serum protein (patient).

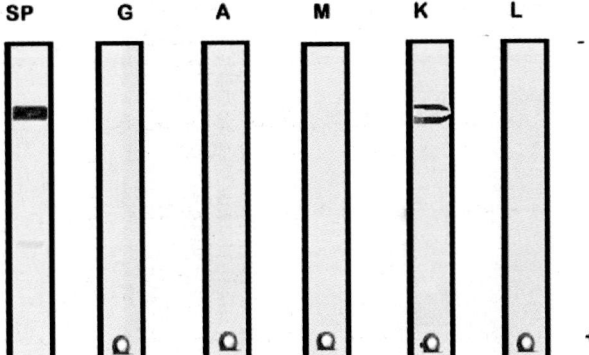

Figure 7.14 Immunofixation of urine protein (patient).

Questions

INTERMEDIATE

7. The patient's bone marrow biopsy and aspirate (Figs 7.4, 7.5, 7.7, and 7.8) show:

a. generally hypercellular bone marrow for a patient of this age

b. the presence of elements of the myeloid and erythroid series

c. an increased number of plasma cells

d. all of the above

ADVANCED

8. The best interpretation of serum protein electrophoresis (Fig. 7.10), quantitative serum immunoglobulins (Table 7.5), and of serum immunofixation (Fig. 7.13) is:

a. a pattern suggestive of an acute inflammatory process

b. a pattern characteristic of malabsorption

c. a pattern characteristic of a non-selective protein-losing syndrome

d. a pattern characteristic of nephrotic syndrome

e. none of the above

ADVANCED

9. The results of urine protein electrophoresis and immunofixation (Figs 7.12 and 7.14):

a. are characteristically found in a majority of patients with the same disease as that of our patient

b. are found only in conjunction with an increase in immunoglobulin levels in the serum

c. have no prognostic significance for the patient

d. all of the above statements are correct

e. none of the above statements is correct

INTERMEDIATE

10. The LEAST plausible statement concerning the patient's hyperuricemia is:

a. it may reflect fluid depletion

b. it may be a specific consequence of the patient's disease

c. it may contribute to the patient's nephropathy

d. it may be related to the effects of hypercalcemia

e. it is unrelated to the patient's underlying disease

ADVANCED

11. Which of the following factors could be related to the patient's hypercalcemia?

a. osteoclast stimulation by IL-1

b. secretion of IL-6 by bone marrow stromal cells

c. cytokines such as GM-CSF (granulocyte-macrophage colony-stimulating factor)

d. all of the above

e. none of the above

INTERMEDIATE

12. Which of the following renal tubular defects may be caused by the patient's disease?

a. obstruction of tubules by casts

b. accumulation of hyaline droplets in tubular cells

c. the accumulation of syncytial tubular cells and multinucleated giant cells

d. impairment of tubular transport of amino acids

e. all of the above

13. This patient's disease, in general, is characterized by all of the following features EXCEPT:

a. it is uncommon before the age of 40

b. it is increasing in incidence at an exponential rate after the age of 40

c. it is sometimes asymptomatic for a prolonged period

d. it is significantly more common in whites than in blacks

ANSWERS AND FURTHER INFORMATION

Figure descriptions

Figure 7.1 X-ray of left humerus (patient).
Pathological fracture: A mildly displaced transverse fracture through the mid-humeral shaft is seen extending through a portion of the humerus that shows relatively decreased density. This is consistent with a pathological fracture through a lytic lesion.

Figure 7.2 Peripheral blood smear (patient). Wright/Giemsa stain.
The patient's peripheral blood smear shows a mild normocytic normochromic anemia. The red blood cells exhibit aniso-poikilocytosis. There is multiple rouleaux formation (stacks or rolls of red blood cells) apparent in this image. In multiple myeloma rouleaux formation is due to the presence of high concentrations of abnormal globulins. A plasma cell with an eccentric oval nucleus is present. Also seen are a few platelets.

Figure 7.3 Peripheral blood smear (normal). Wright/Giemsa stain.
This is a photomicrograph of a normal blood smear for comparison. The red blood cells' size is approximately equal to that of the lymphocyte and to two-thirds of that of the neutrophil (present on the right side).

Figure 7.4 Bone marrow biopsy (patient). Hematoxylin & eosin stain.
Multiple myeloma: A hypercellular bone marrow (85% hematopoietic cellularity) for the patient's age. At this low magnification one can appreciate the increased mononuclear cell infiltrate and the reduced number of normal hematopoietic elements.

Figure 7.5 Bone marrow biopsy (patient). Hematoxylin & eosin stain.
Multiple myeloma: The morphological characteristics of the mononuclear cell infiltrate noted in Fig. 7.4 are apparent in this image with a higher magnification. It is predominantly composed of sheets of plasma cells. Atypical plasma cells, binucleated plasma cells, and plasmablasts are seen in this photomicrograph.

Figure 7.6 Bone marrow biopsy (normal). Hematoxylin & eosin stain.
This is a normocellular bone marrow from another patient in the same age group as our patient for comparison (30–35% hematopoietic cellularity). Trilineage hematopoiesis is evident in this image.

Figure 7.7 Bone marrow aspiration smear (patient). Wright/Giemsa stain.
Multiple myeloma: Virtually all the cells in this image are well-differentiated neoplastic plasma cells. They exhibit eccentric oval nuclei. Neoplastic plasma cells tend to stick together and form sheets. One binucleated plasma cell (arrow) is seen in this field.

Figure 7.8 Bone marrow aspiration smear (patient). Wright/Giemsa stain.
Multiple myeloma: Again all the cells in this field are plasma cells. They show cellular pleomorphism. Two binucleated plasma cells are seen in this field.

Figure 7.9 X-ray of skull lateral view (patient).
Multiple myeloma: The X-ray shows multiple ill-defined areas of decreased density, or "punched-out lesions." The lesions are seen in both the frontal and occipital regions on this lateral radiograph of the skull. These are compatible with lytic lesions in this patient with multiple myeloma.

Figure 7.10 Serum protein electrophoresis (patient).
Monoclonal gammopathy: A sharp peak in the gamma region is seen in this serum protein electrophoresis. This pattern is consistent with a diagnosis of monoclonal gammopathy.

Figure 7.11 Serum protein electrophoresis (normal).
This is a normal serum protein electrophoresis. The first sharp peak represents albumin. The other small peaks to the right of albumin represent alpha-1, alpha-2, beta, and gamma globulins respectively. No sharp peak is present in the gamma region.

Figure 7.12 Urine protein electrophoresis (patient).
A sharp peak in the gamma region corresponding to that seen in the serum electrophoresis is seen in this urine electrophoresis.

Figure 7.13 Immunofixation of serum protein (patient).
IgG kappa monoclonal gammopathy: In patients with an increased globulin fraction (total protein – albumin) serum protein electrophoresis is performed as an initial screening. Patients with an abnormal pattern should be further evaluated by serum immunofixation for identification of any monoclonal protein. The patient's serum is electrophoresed (SP), the heavy band at the top represents the monoclonal gamma globulin noted in the patient's serum protein electrophoresis (Fig. 7.10). This protein was identified as IgG kappa monoclonal globulin by the presence of a corresponding band in IgG and kappa channels.

Figure 7.14 Immunofixation of urine protein (patient).
In this urine immunofixation an irregular band in the kappa channel is present. This abnormal band indicates the presence of free kappa light chains in the urine (Bence-Jones protein).

Answers

1. E. The patient has a normocytic, normochromic anemia. Normocytic, normochromic anemias may be found with advanced neoplastic disease, chronic renal disease, or bone marrow replacement by neoplastic cells. All these conditions should be considered in this patient, because of her bone lesion, pancytopenia, hypercalcemia, abnormal BUN and creatinine levels, and proteinuria. Low levels of endogenous erythropoietin may occur in renal disease.

2. E. A common form of pancytopenia is due to bone marrow replacement by other cells, as in metastatic neoplasia. It can also be a consequence of exposure to ionizing radiation, or to chemicals such as benzene, to alkylating agents, or to chloramphenicol. Certain viral infections, such as hepatitis (especially hepatitis C), Epstein–Barr virus, and HIV-1, have also been implicated.

3. B. Serum protein electrophoresis is the best method to determine the non-albumin serum protein abnormalities. It allows one to identify areas where protein shifts occur. Other options do not provide such complex information. Determination of urinary protein excretion would provide information about the loss of protein in urine. Liver function tests would provide information about the variety of functions that the liver performs. Liver diseases affect serum protein levels but information about individual components of serum protein groups is provided by electrophoresis. The measurement of serum C-reactive protein level is used to detect and monitor acute inflammation and tissue destruction.

4. A. The clinical effects of hypercalcemia are related to its rate of progression, severity, and duration. The most frequent effects are gastrointestinal (nausea, vomiting, ulcer) and renal effects (decreased renal concentration, interstitial nephritis, renal failure). Changes on ECG (a shortened Q-T interval, ventricular arrhythmias) occur in the presence of moderate to severe hypercalcemia. Calcium deposits into soft tissues may occur. Patients with hypercalcemia tend to be dehydrated, due to polyuria, resulting from impaired renal concentration. Vomiting further aggravates this problem. Fluid retention, therefore, is not a consequence of hypercalcemia.

5. D. The peripheral blood smear shows all of the mentioned abnormal findings: rouleaux formation, plasma cell and aniso-poikilocytosis.

6. A. The X-ray shows a fracture in the middle of the humerus. An osteoid osteoma produces a characteristic X-ray appearance: a small radiolucent zone surrounded by a large sclerotic zone. On the X-ray, an aneurysmal bone cyst produces a well-circumscribed rarefied area surrounded by periosteal new bone formation.

7. D. All the features listed (a hypercellular bone marrow, the presence of elements of the myeloid and erythroid series, and an increased number of plasma cells) are present. The most striking feature is a diffuse infiltrate of plasma cells with the occasional formation of plasma cell nodules (see descriptions of Figs 7.4, 7.5, 7.7 and 7.8).

8. E. The serum protein electrophoresis (Fig. 7.10) shows the presence of monoclonal immunoglobulin in the gamma region. The quantitative immunoglobulin analysis (Table 7.5) shows a substantial increase in IgG, identified by immunofixation (Fig. 7.13) as IgG containing kappa light chains. All given options (A–D) in the question are incorrect. In an acute inflammatory process the gamma globulin region appears initially normal, the albumin band is normal or decreased, and α_1 and α_2 globulins show an increase. Malabsorption or malnutrition results in generalized hypoproteinemia. Non-selective protein-losing syndromes (such as seen, for example, in patients with severe burns) lead also to a decrease in all serum proteins. In the nephrotic syndrome, on the other hand, the loss of protein is selective. It shows a markedly decreased albumin, while the α_2 region is clearly increased due to the increase in the α_2 macroglobulin level; this protein is retained due to its large size, which prevents its loss in the urine through the damaged glomeruli.

9. A. The urinary protein electrophoresis (Fig. 7.12) shows the presence of a monoclonal component in the urine, identified by immunofixation (Fig.7.14) as a kappa light chain (Bence-Jones proteinuria), together with a small amount of other proteins. This is a common finding in patients with multiple myeloma (60–70% of patients have it); it may occur, however, without an increase in complete immunoglobulin molecules in the serum. The finding of Bence-Jones proteinuria has a negative prognostic significance, because the excreted light chains are often directly toxic to the tubular epithelial cells and contribute to the renal insufficiency.

10. E. The patient has multiple myeloma. It is unlikely that the patient's hyperuricemia is unrelated to her disease. The hypercalcemia of multiple myeloma may lead to dehydration, due to impaired renal concentration of urine. In the presence of a large tumor burden, tumor cell turnover and breakdown may lead to hyperuricemia, with precipitation of uric acid in the distal tubules and collecting ducts and consequent nephropathy.

11. D. All of the options (A–C) are correct. The patient has multiple myeloma. Myeloma cells produce IL-1β, which activates osteoclasts and depresses osteoblastic activity, leading to hypercalcemia. The growth of myeloma cells is stimulated by a variety of cytokines, such as IL-6 and granulocyte-macrophage colony-stimulating factor (GM-CSF).

12. E. The earliest specific tubular absorption defects have been ascribed to a nephrotoxic effect of some varieties of Bence-Jones proteins, which are reabsorbed by the proximal convoluted tubules. These defects consist of a variety of an adult Fanconi syndrome, a proximal tubular acidosis with loss of glucose, amino acids, and concentrating power. Less specific forms of nephrotoxicity are associated with tubular damage by lysosomal enzymes released as a consequence of protein reabsorption, and by the formation of casts formed by the combination of Bence-Jones proteins with urinary glycoprotein (Tamm–Horsfall protein) and by the development of epithelial syncytial cells and multinucleated giant cells (constituting the picture of the myeloma kidney).

13. D. Multiple myeloma is rare before the age of 40, and the incidence increases exponentially thereafter. In about 10% of patients with multiple myeloma the disease will have an indolent course, slowly progressing over many years. Blacks have twice the incidence of multiple myeloma as whites.

Final diagnosis and synopsis of the case

- Multiple myeloma
- Pathological bone fracture

A 70-year-old woman presented with a pathological fracture of the left humerus and with the typical findings of multiple myeloma: laboratory findings of anemia associated with leukopenia and thrombocytopenia, hypercalcemia, and abnormal renal function. Bone marrow biopsy showed a diffuse infiltrate of plasma cells with the formation of plasma cell nodules. Serum protein electrophoresis and immunofixation revealed a monoclonal gammopathy (IgG kappa), and there was Bence-Jones protein in the urine (kappa light chain). Impaired renal function is a frequent finding in patients with multiple myeloma; the pathogenesis includes multiple factors, of which Bence-Jones protein toxicity to renal tubular cells is the earliest and most specific. Her lytic bone lesion and pathological fracture resulted from the infiltration and destruction of the bone by neoplastic plasma cells. The hypercalcemia resulted from bone resorption. The patient received supportive treatment for her fracture, and her condition and a plan for chemotherapy were discussed with her.

Lab tips

The laboratory evaluation of hypergammaglobulinemia

The suspicion that a patient has elevated globulins arises when rouleaux are noted on the peripheral blood smear or when one finds an elevation in the total serum protein. This elevation is almost always due to globulins and in patients with hypoalbuminemia, elevated globulins may be present with the total serum protein lying within the normal range. A few of the laboratory procedures that are useful in confirming and identifying the nature of the elevated proteins are listed below.

Serum protein electrophoresis (SPE)
This test (see Fig. 7.10) is extremely useful to determine if the hypergammaglobulinemia is polyclonal or monoclonal in nature. A polyclonal increase in gamma-globulins is seen as a broad elevation in the gamma region, and if present usually no further testing is required. A sharp peak in the beta, pregamma, or gamma region suggests the presence of a monoclonal protein and further testing is usually necessary.

Quantitative immunoglobulin levels

Meaningful interpretation of the results obtained depends on one's awareness that the levels of the various classes of immunoglobulins will vary with age, sex, and race. Polyclonal elevations (all classes or selected classes) are seen in a number of infectious diseases and inflammatory states. When dealing with a monoclonal disorder, one usually finds elevation in one class and marked decreases in the other classes. This test is useful in identifying monoclonal proteins and in monitoring the course of disease and treatment.

Immunofixation (IEF)

When the results of quantitative immunoglobulin levels are not conclusive, the identification of a monoclonal component is done by immunofixation, which is a combination of electrophoresis and specific antibody binding. This test offers an ease of interpretation (bands are usually easily seen). It is also extremely sensitive in identifying monoclonal proteins (see Fig. 7.13). This technique can also be used for other body fluids, especially urine and cerebrospinal fluid.

A 61-year-old clerk with excruciating abdominal pain

CASE AND MCQS

Clinical history and presentation

A 61-year-old man was brought from his office to the emergency room because of acute abdominal pain of 6 hours' duration. The pain was increasing in intensity, was accompanied by an episode of vomiting and was localized to the right lower quadrant. The patient had no significant past medical history and did not take any medications. Physical examination revealed an alert man, in acute distress due to his abdominal pain. His blood pressure was 160/90 mmHg, pulse was 96/min and regular, temperature was 101.2°F (38.4°C), and respiratory rate 20/min. Pertinent physical findings included right-sided abdominal guarding. Bowel sounds were audible. Rectal examination was unremarkable and the stool was negative for occult blood. The rest of the physical examination was unremarkable. An abdominal X-ray was normal. The patient was admitted to the hospital.

Admission data

Table 8.1 Hematology

			SI Units	
WBC	10.1	(3.3–11.0 thou/μL)	10.1	(3.3–11.0 × 10⁹/L)
Neut	70	(44–88%)	70	(44–88%)
Band	22 H	(0–10%)	22 H	(0–10%)
Lymph	5 L	(12–43%)	5 L	(12–43%)
Mono	2	(2–11%)	2	(2–11%)
Eos	1	(0–5%)	1	(0–5%)
Baso	0	(0–2%)	0	(0–2%)
RBC	4.46	(3.9–5.0 mill/μL)	4.46	(3.9–5.0 × 10¹²/L)
HGB	14.1	(11.6–15.6 g/dL)	14.1	(116–156 g/L)
HCT	41.8	(37.0–47.0%)	0.418	(0.37–0.47)
MCV	93.7	(79.0–99.0 fL)	93.7	(79.0–99.0 fL)
MCH	31.7	(26.0–32.6 pg)	31.7	(26.0–32.6 pg)
MCHC	33.8	(31.0–36.0 g/dL)	338	(310–360 g/L)
Plts	242	(130–400 thou/μL)	242	(130–400 × 10⁹/L)

Table 8.2 Chemistry

			SI Units	
Glucose	106	(65–110 mg/dL)	6.88	(3.6–6.11 mmol/L)
Creatinine	1.2	(0.7–1.4 mg/dL)	106	(61.9–123.76 µmol/L)
BUN	15	(7–24 mg/dL)	5.36	(2.50–8.57 mmol/L)
Uric acid	6.3	(3.0–8.5 mg/dL)	0.37	(0.18–0.51 mmol/L)
Cholesterol	218 H	(150–200 mg/dL)	5.64 H	(3.88–5.17 mmol/L)
Calcium	8.5	(8.5–10.5 mg/dL)	2.13	(2.13–2.63 mmol/L)
Protein	6.2	(6–8 g/dL)	62	(60–80 g/L)
Albumin	4.2	(3.7–5.0 g/dL)	42	(37–50 g/L)
LDH	200	(100–250 U/L)	200	(100–250 U/L)
Alk Phos	75	(0–120 U/L)	75	(0–120 U/L)
AST	29	(0–55 U/L)	29	(0–55 U/L)
GGTP	44	(0–50 U/L)	44	(0–50 U/L)
Bilirubin	0.8	(0.0–1.5 mg/dL)	13.7	(0–25.7 µmol/L)
Bilirubin-direct	0.10	(0.02–0.18 mg/dL)	1.7	(0.34–3.08 µmol/L)
Amylase	25	(13–85 U/L)	0.42	(0.22–1.44 µkat/L)

Table 8.3 Electrolytes

			SI Units	
Na	135	(134–143 mEq/L)	135	(134–143 mmol/L)
K	4.0	(3.5–4.9 mEq/L)	4.0	(3.5–4.9 mmol/L)
Cl	95	(95–108 mEq/L)	95	(95–108 mmol/L)
CO_2	26	(21–32 mEq/L)	26	(21–32 mmol/L)

Table 8.4 Microbiology

Blood cultures	Pending

Table 8.5 Urinalysis

pH	6	(5.0–7.5)
Protein	Neg	(Neg)
Glucose	Neg	(Neg)
Ketone	Neg	(Neg)
Color	Yellow	(Yellow)
Clarity	Clear	(Clear)
Sp. grav.	1.017	(1.010–1.035)
WBC	0	(0–5/HPF)
RBC	0	(0–2/HPF)
Casts	Neg	(Neg)
Bacteria	Neg	(Neg)

Questions

Based on the above information you can best conclude the following:

INTERMEDIATE

1. Which of the following conditions occurs predominantly in adolescence?

   a. diverticulitis
   b. acute appendicitis
   c. acute cholecystitis
   d. gastroenteritis

INTERMEDIATE

2. This patient does not have an absolute leukocytosis. Such a finding virtually excludes which of the following problems?

   a. diverticulitis
   b. appendicitis
   c. acute cholecystitis
   d. gastroenteritis
   e. none of the above

3. The normal urinalysis at this stage of his problem is compatible with:

a. the diagnosis of acute appendicitis
b. the diagnosis of acute gastroenteritis
c. bacteremia
d. negative bacterial urine culture
e. all of the above

4. Which of the following diagnoses, based on the patient's clinical history and laboratory findings so far, would you most likely exclude?

a. urinary tract infection
b. diverticulitis
c. gastroenteritis
d. appendicitis

Clinical course

The pain remained localized to the right lower quadrant of the abdomen. The blood culture was positive for *Escherichia coli*, and the patient was started on antibiotic therapy. A repeated CBC (FBC) is shown in Table 8.6.

Table 8.6 Hematology

			SI Units	
WBC	19.9 H	(3.3–11.0 thou/μL)	19.9 H	(3.3–11.0 × 10⁹/L)
Neut	51	(44–88%)	51	(44–88%)
Band	40 H	(0–10%)	40 H	(0–10%)
Lymph	5 L	(12–43%)	5 L	(12–43%)
Mono	4	(2–11%)	4	(2–11%)
Eos	0	(0–5%)	0	(0–5%)
Baso	0	(0–2%)	0	(0–2%)
RBC	4.74	(3.9–5.0 mill/μL)	4.74	(3.9–5.0 × 10¹²/L)
HGB	13.9	(11.6–15.6 g/dL)	139	(116–156 g/L)
HCT	41.5	(37.0–47.0%)	0.415	(0.37–0.47)
MCV	87.5	(79.0–99.0 fL)	87.5	(79.0–99.0 fL)
MCH	29.3	(26.0–32.6 pg)	29.3	(26.0–32.6 pg)
MCHC	33.5	(31.0–36.0 g/dL)	335	(310–360 g/L)
Plts	211	(130–400 thou/μL)	211	(130–400 × 10⁹/L)

The patient underwent a surgical procedure. The pathological findings are depicted in Figs 8.1–8.4. The patient tolerated surgery well and was discharged several days later.

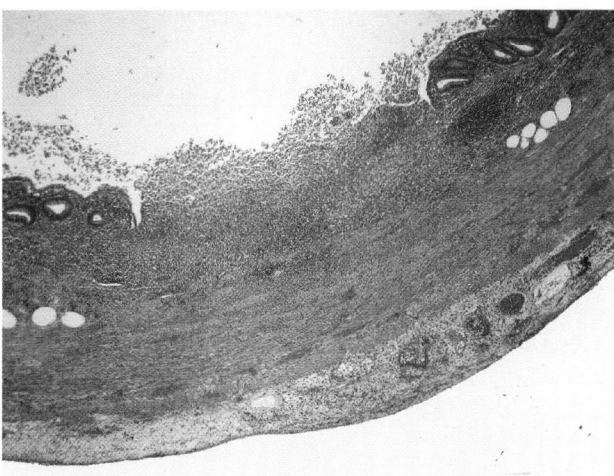

Figure 8.1 Appendix (patient). Hematoxylin & eosin stain.

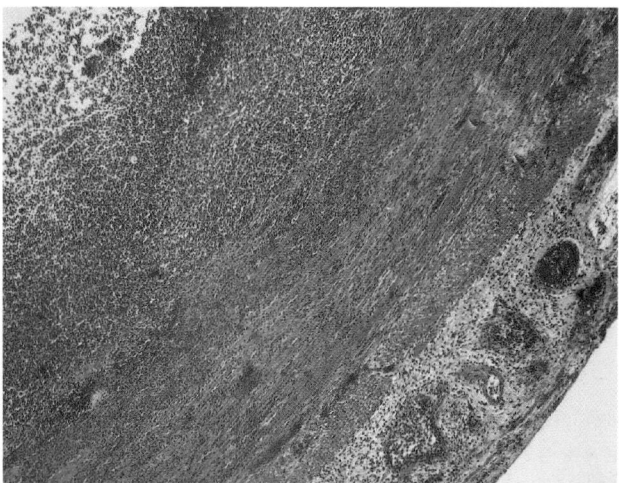

Figure 8.2 Appendix (patient). Hematoxylin & eosin stain.

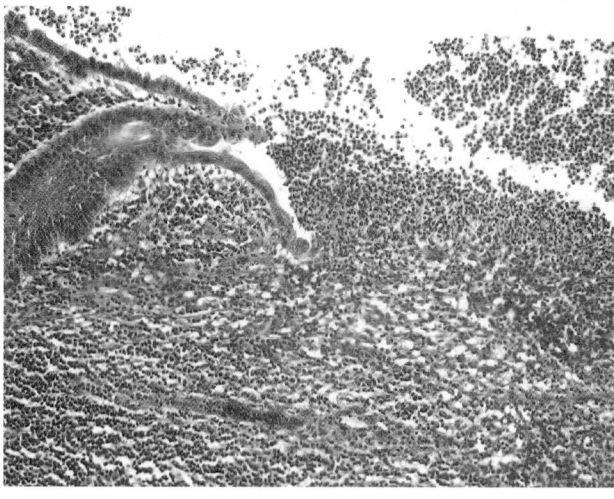

Figure 8.3 Mucosal surface of appendix (patient). Hematoxylin & eosin stain.

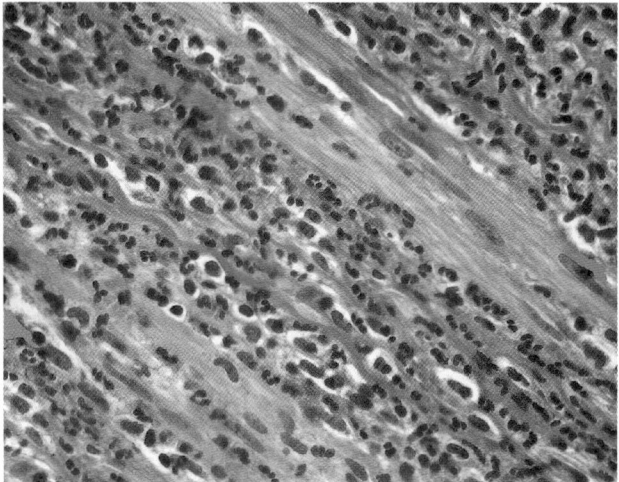

Figure 8.4 Muscularis externa of appendix (patient). Hematoxylin & eosin stain.

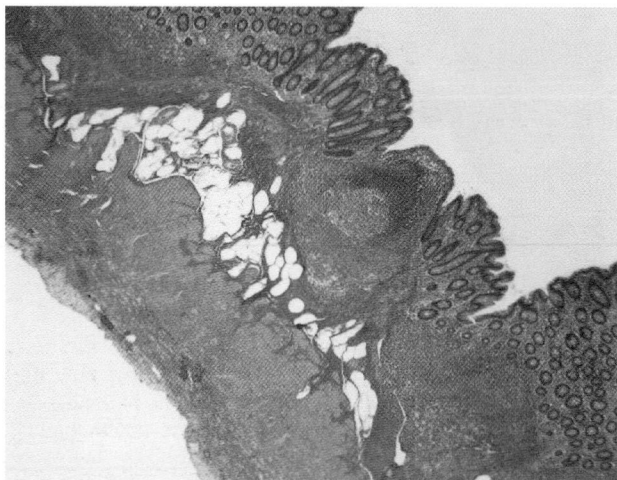

Figure 8.5 Appendix (normal). Hematoxylin & eosin stain.

Questions

5. The pathological process depicted in Figs 8.1–8.4 represents:

    a. a granulomatous inflammation
    b. a lymphoma
    c. an adenocarcinoma
    d. an acute suppurative inflammation
    e. a cystadenoma

6. Which of the following histologic findings in the affected organ is necessary for your diagnosis of this patient's problem?

    a. the presence of exudate in the lumen
    b. abundance of lymphoid tissue in the mucosa and submucosa
    c. neutrophilic infiltration of the muscularis
    d. transmural eosinophilic infiltrate
    e. none of the above

7. Which of the following factors, in general, is LEAST likely to contribute to the pathogenesis of such a problem as this patient has?

    a. distension of the affected organ by accumulation of mucus

    b. a localized delayed hypersensitivity reaction

    c. an increased number of lymphoid follicles within the mucosa and submucosa of the affected organ

    d. the presence of a fecalith within the lumen

    e. obstruction of the affected organ by tumor

ANSWERS AND FURTHER INFORMATION

Figure descriptions

Figure 8.1 Appendix (patient). Hematoxylin & eosin stain.
Acute transmural appendicitis: A section showing the full thickness of the vermiform appendix with mucosal ulceration and a transmural inflammatory cell infiltrate. The inflammatory cell infiltrate extends to involve the serosal surface. A few submucosal fat cells are evident.

Figure 8.2 Appendix (patient). Hematoxylin & eosin stain.
Acute transmural appendicitis: This is a higher magnification of the center of the previous image, again showing ulceration and a transmural acute inflammatory cell infiltrate. The inflammatory cell infiltrate extends to involve the serosal surface. Submucosal fat cells are not evident.

Figure 8.3 Mucosal surface of appendix (patient). Hematoxylin & eosin stain.
Acute transmural appendicitis: This image shows mucosal ulceration, and destruction of the appendiceal crypts by heavy acute suppurative inflammation.

Figure 8.4 Muscularis externa of appendix (patient). Hematoxylin & eosin stain.
Acute transmural appendicitis: Dense acute inflammatory cell infiltrate in the muscularis externa layer. The presence of acute inflammatory cells in the muscle layer of the appendix is the hallmark for the diagnosis of acute appendicitis.

Figure 8.5 Appendix (normal). Hematoxylin & eosin stain.
Normal appendix: This section shows a full thickness of the vermiform appendix with intact mucosa. A reactive germinal center and lymphoid aggregate are seen in this image. Note the normal thickness of the muscularis externa and the presence of submucosal fat. The serosal surface is also intact and shows no inflammation.

Answers

1. B. Acute appendicitis affects mainly adolescents and young adults, but it is not limited to those age categories. Gastroenteritis occurs in all age groups; the incidence of acute cholecystitis increases with age, as does the incidence of diverticulitis.

2. E. An absolute leukocytosis may be missing in early stages of all mentioned disorders: diverticulitis, appendicitis, acute cholecystitis, and gastroenteritis. The cell count should be repeated at a later stage.

3. E. The normal urinalysis is compatible with all of the mentioned problems: acute appendicitis, acute gastroenteritis, and bacteremia (it may arise from another focus of infection) and with a negative bacterial urinary culture.

4. A. The urinalysis on admission testing was normal. This makes the diagnosis of urinary tract infection unlikely. A normal urinalysis may be seen in all the other problems (diverticulitis, appendicitis, and gastroenteritis).

5. D. Figures 8.1–8.4 represent typical features of an acute suppurative inflammation of the appendix (see the descriptions for Figs 8.1–8.4). There are no findings pointing to the diagnosis of granulomatous inflammation or of a malignant or benign neoplasm.

6. C. A neutrophilic infiltration of the muscularis is the histologic criterion of acute appendicitis. Accumulation of exudate in the appendix could be a result of a drainage from an infection of the alimentary tract, not leading to a muscularis wall inflammation. The amount of lymphoid tissue is not diagnostic of an acute suppurative process.

7. B. Delayed hypersensitivity is not known to play a role in the pathogenesis of acute appendicitis. In the majority of cases, acute inflammation of the appendix is preceded by obstruction of the lumen by a fecalith or much less commonly by a tumor or by enlarged lymphoid follicles. An accumulation of mucus due to the obstruction leads to distension of the appendix, increased luminal pressure, ischemia (due to inadequate blood drainage and supply), and to bacterial proliferation. In a minority of cases, however, there is no evidence of luminal obstruction and the pathogenesis remains unknown.

Final diagnosis and synopsis of the case

- Acute appendicitis
- *Escherichia coli* bacteremia

This is a classical case of acute suppurative appendicitis and periappendicitis. The patient presented with a low-grade fever and acute abdominal pain of increasing intensity, which was later localized to the right lower quadrant. Initially the patient did not have a leukocytosis, but a few hours later he developed neutrophilia with a "shift to the left". An abdominal X-ray was normal. Blood culture was positive for *Escherichia coli*. The patient was started on antibiotics and an appendectomy was performed. There were no complications and the patient was discharged.

Lab tips

Leukocytosis
Leukocytosis is an increase in the total white blood cell count above the upper limit of the normal range for the person's age and sex.

Leukopenia
Leukopenia is a decrease in the total white blood cell count below the lower limit of the normal range for the person's age and sex.

Increases and decreases in the individual cell lines are indicated as:

Cell line	Increase	Decrease
1. Neutrophils	Neutrophilia	Neutropenia
2. Eosinophils	Eosinophilia	
3. Basophils	Basophilia	
4. Lymphocytes	Lymphocytosis	Lymphopenia
5. Monocytes	Monocytosis	Monocytopenia

Selected causes of non-neoplastic leukocytosis
Neutrophilia:
- Bacterial infection
- Physiologic stress (exercise, emotional stress, nausea & vomiting)
- Myocardial infarction
- Hemorrhage
- Hemolysis
- Tuberculosis
- Tumor necrosis
- Drugs (epinephrine, steroids, heparin, digitalis)
- Diabetic acidosis
- Gout

Lymphocytosis:
- Viral infection
- Infectious mononucleosis
- Tuberculosis

Eosinophilia:
- Allergic reactions
- Drugs (allopurinol, phenothiazine)
- Parasitic infestation
- Tuberculosis

A 75-year-old man who fell to the floor

CASE AND MCQS

Clinical history and presentation

A 75-year-old man presented with severe pain in his right arm. The patient stated that while preparing dinner he tripped over a footstool, lost his balance, fell, and landed on his right shoulder. The patient was in his usual state of health until approximately 2 years ago when a lung mass was found on routine X-ray and confirmed by a CT scan (Figs 9.1 and 9.3). Subsequently he underwent a right lobectomy and a mediastinal lymph node dissection (Figs 9.5, 9.6, and 9.8).

Physical examination on this admission revealed an alert and oriented man. Blood pressure was 116/70 mmHg, heart rate 90 beats/min and regular. Respiratory rate was 20/min. Auscultation of the chest revealed decreased breath sounds on the right side. He was unable to move his right arm, which was swollen and showed hematoma. No cyanosis or clubbing was noted.

Admission data

Table 9.1 Hematology

			SI Units	
WBC	7.8	(3.3–11.0 thou/μL)	7.8	(3.3–11.0 × 10⁹/L)
Neut	75	(44–88%)	75	(44–88%)
Band	5	(0–10%)	5	(0–10%)
Lymph	18	(12–43%)	18	(12–43%)
Mono	2	(2–11%)	2	(2–11%)
Eos	0	(0–5%)	0	(0–5%)
Baso	0	(0–2%)	0	(0–2%)
RBC	4.71	(3.9–5.0 mill/μL)	4.71	(3.9–5.0 × 10¹²/L)
HGB	13.2	(11.6–15.6 g/dL)	132	(116–156 g/L)
HCT	39.7	(37.0–47.0%)	0.397	(0.37–0.47)
MCV	84	(79.0–99.0 fL)	84	(79.0–99.0 fL)
MCH	28	(26.0–32.6 pg)	28	(26.0–32.6 pg)
MCHC	33.2	(31.0–36.0 g/dL)	332	(310–360 g/L)
Plts	159	(130–400 thou/μL)	159	(130–400 × 10⁹/L)

Table 9.2 Chemistry

				SI Units	
Glucose	150 H	(65–110 mg/dL)	8.33 H	(3.6–6.11 mmol/L)	
Creatinine	0.9	(0.7–1.4 mg/dL)	79.6	(61.9–123.7 µmol/L)	
BUN	26 H	(7–24 mg/dL)	9.28 H	(2.50–8.57 mmol/L)	
Uric acid	4.5	(3.0–8.5 mg/dL)	0.27	(0.18–0.51 mmol/L)	
Cholesterol	210 H	(150–200 mg/dL)	5.43 H	(3.88–5.17 mmol/L)	
Calcium	7.7 L	(8.5–10.5 mg/dL)	1.93 L	(2.13–2.63 mmol/L)	
Protein	6.0	(6–8 g/dL)	60	(60–80 g/L)	
Albumin	3.2 L	(3.7–5.0 g/dL)	32 L	(37–50 g/L)	
LDH	240	(100–250 U/L)	240	(100–250 U/L)	
Alk Phos	152 H	(0–120 U/L)	152 H	(0–120 U/L)	
AST	44	(0–55 U/L)	44	(0–55 U/L)	
GGTP	45	(0–50 U/L)	45	(0–50 U/L)	
Bilirubin	0.9	(0.0–1.5 mg/dL)	15.4	(0–25.7 µmol/L)	
Bilirubin-direct	0.08	(0.02–0.18 mg/dL)	1.37	(0.34–3.08 µmol/L)	

Table 9.3 Electrolytes

			SI Units	
Na	140	(134–143 mEq/L)	140	(134–143 mmol/L)
K	4.1	(3.5–4.9 mEq/L)	4.1	(3.5–4.9 mmol/L)
Cl	104	(95–108 mEq/L)	104	(95–108 mmol/L)
CO_2	26.5	(21–32 mEq/L)	26.5	(21–32 mmol/L)

Table 9.4 Urinalysis

pH	6	(5.0–7.5)
Protein	Neg	(Neg)
Glucose	Neg	(Neg)
Ketone	Neg	(Neg)
Color	Yellow	(Yellow)
Clarity	Clear	(Clear)
Sp. grav.	1.017	(1.010–1.035)
WBC	0	(0–5/HPF)
RBC	0	(0–2/HPF)
Casts	Neg	(Neg)
Bacteria	Neg	(Neg)

Table 9.5 Coagulation

PT	12.8	(11–14 s)
aPTT	27.1	(22–32 s)
INR	1.166	

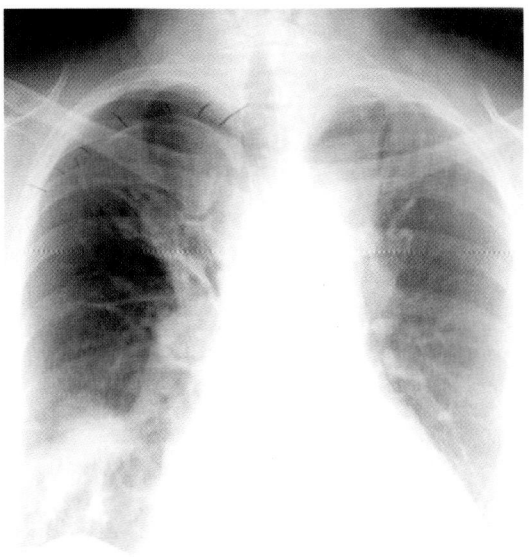

Figure 9.1 Chest X-ray, A-P view (patient, 2 years prior to the current admission).

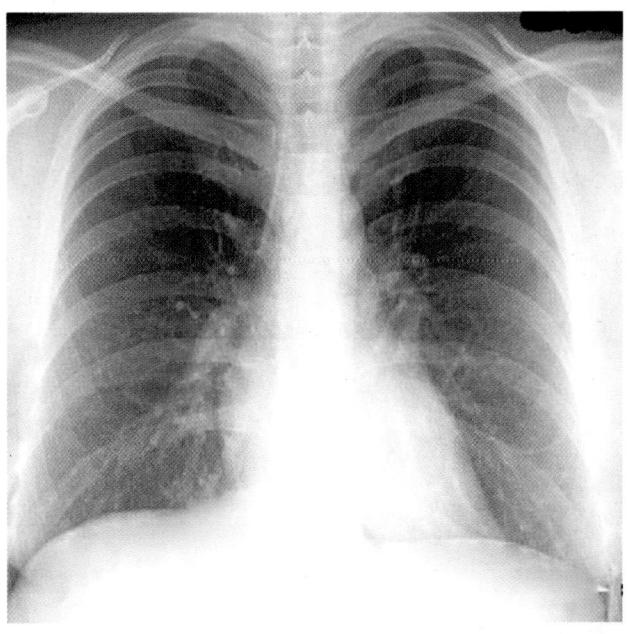

Figure 9.2 Chest X-ray, A-P view (normal).

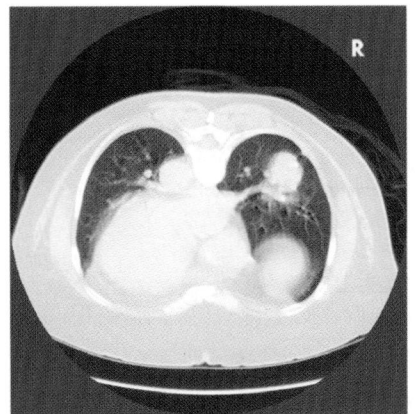

Figure 9.3 CT chest (patient, 2 years prior to the current admission).

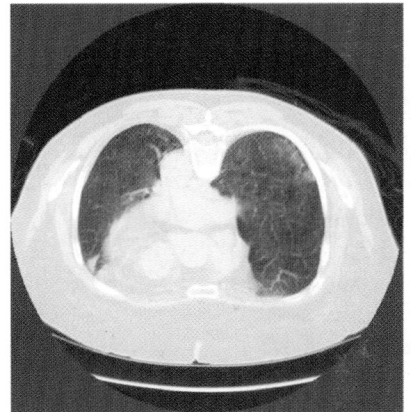

Figure 9.4 CT chest (normal).

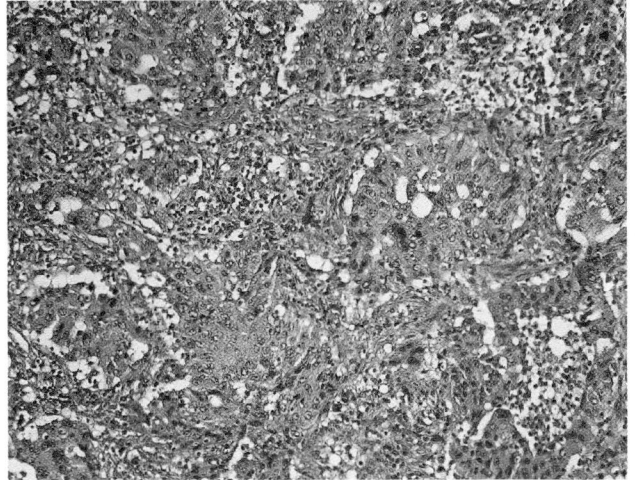

Figure 9.5 Lung biopsy (patient, 2 years prior to the current admission). Hematoxylin & eosin stain.

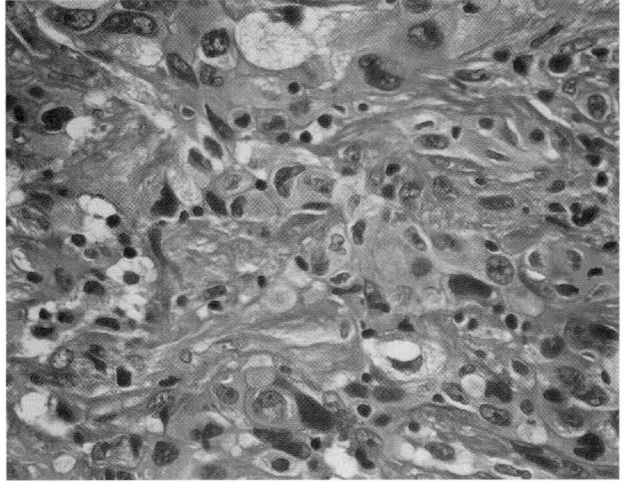

Figure 9.6 Lung biopsy (patient, 2 years prior to the current admission). Hematoxylin & eosin stain.

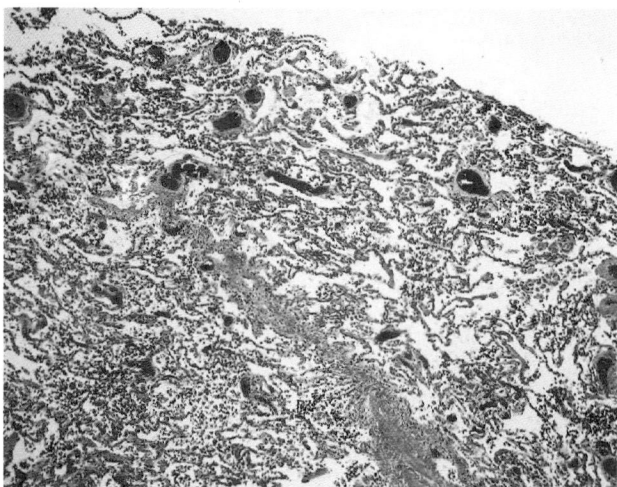

Figure 9.7 Lung biopsy (normal). Hematoxylin & eosin stain.

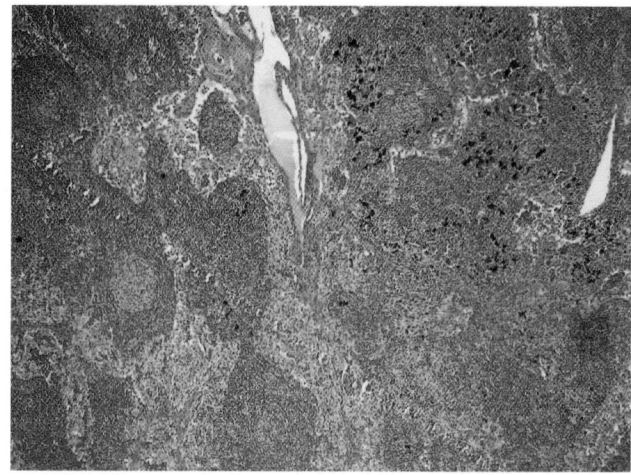

Figure 9.8 Mediastinal lymph node biopsy (patient). Hematoxylin & eosin stain.

Questions

Based on the above information, you can best conclude the following:

1. The patient's lung biopsy, 2 years prior to current admission (Figs 9.5 and 9.6), is consistent with:

   a. sarcoidosis
   b. tuberculosis
   c. a malignant neoplasm
   d. a lung abscess
   e. none of the above

2. In general, factors contributing to this patient's lung disease include all of the following, EXCEPT:

   a. cigarette smoking
   b. asbestos exposure
   c. pulmonary alveolar proteinosis
   d. radiation
   e. pulmonary scarring

3. Which of the following statements regarding the patient's elevated blood glucose is correct?

   a. such a finding is diagnostic of diabetes mellitus
   b. it could have been caused by malnutrition
   c. it could have been caused by acute stress
   d. none of the above statements is correct

4. Which of the following statements regarding this patient's hypocalcemia is true?

   a. it may be due to excess vitamin D
   b. it indicates a primary hyperparathyroidism
   c. it is due to renal failure
   d. none of the above

5. The patient's elevated level of serum alkaline phosphatase most likely suggests:

   a. bone metastasis
   b. biliary duct obstruction
   c. malnutrition
   d. none of the above

6. The patient's lung lesion depicted in Figs 9.5 and 9.6:

   a. arises from neuroendocrine cells of the lining bronchial epithelium
   b. frequently produces paraneoplastic syndromes due to ACTH production
   c. is most sensitive to chemotherapy
   d. none of the above

Clinical course

Upon admission, an X-ray of the right arm (Fig. 9.9) was performed. In addition, a CT scan of the abdomen and MRI examination of the brain were done. Subsequently the patient underwent intramedullary nailing of the humerus.

Bone from the preparatory reaming was submitted for examination (Fig. 9.10). The patient tolerated the procedure well and was discharged. An appointment was scheduled with his oncologist.

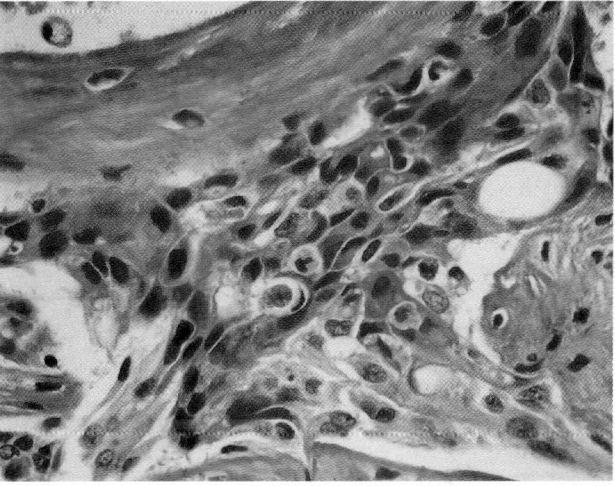

Figure 9.10 Bone biopsy from the reaming (patient). Hematoxylin & eosin stain.

Figure 9.9 X-ray of the right arm (patient).

Questions

INTERMEDIATE

7. The X-ray of the right arm (Fig. 9.9) and the bone biopsy from the reaming (Fig. 9.10) are consistent with:

a. multiple myeloma
b. traumatic fracture
c. osteosarcoma
d. pathological fracture

INTERMEDIATE

8. Lung lesions such as that of this patient:

a. represent the most common visceral malignancy in industrialized countries
b. show a decreasing incidence among women
c. tend to heal spontaneously by fibrosis
d. have a strong genetic predisposition

INTERMEDIATE

9. Choose the INCORRECT statement regarding lung lesions such as that of this patient:

a. they are strongly associated with cigarette smoking
b. they are the least common type of bronchogenic carcinoma
c. they may be associated with hypercalcemia
d. they frequently metastasize to the adrenal glands

INTERMEDIATE

10. Which of the following statements regarding this patient's problems is correct?

a. the cause of the patient's hyperglycemia should be evaluated
b. the elevated BUN level does not indicate renal parenchymal disease
c. the elevated serum alkaline phosphatase could be explained by the lesion noted in Fig. 9.10
d. all of the above statements are correct
e. none of the above statements is correct

ANSWERS AND FURTHER INFORMATION

Figure descriptions

Figure 9.1 Chest X-ray, A-P view (patient, 2 years prior to the current admission).
Lung mass, right lower lobe: This frontal radiograph of the chest demonstrates a rounded, speculated mass in the right lower lobe consistent with a neoplasm. Also, there is a moderate right-sided pneumothorax (black marks).

Figure 9.2 Chest X-ray, A-P view (normal).
This is a normal frontal radiograph of the chest in a male patient.

Figure 9.3 CT chest (patient, 2 years prior to the current admission).
Lung mass, right lower lobe: A CT scan of the lung bases in this patient shows a rounded nodular density in the right lower lobe measuring 5.2 cm. This mass is solid-appearing and is consistent with a neoplasm.

Figure 9.4 CT chest (normal).
A CT scan of the lung bases shows mild emphysematous changes but is otherwise free of solid parenchymal mass.

Figure 9.5 Lung biopsy (patient, 2 years prior to the current admission). Hematoxylin & eosin stain.
Non-small-cell bronchogenic carcinoma: Clusters of neoplastic cells infiltrating the lung parenchyma. An area with moderately differentiated adenocarcinoma and a solid tumor nest are seen in this image. The neoplastic cells show nuclear pleomorphism, hyperchromatic nuclei, and occasional nucleoli.

Figure 9.6 Lung biopsy (patient, 2 years prior to the current admission). Hematoxylin & eosin stain.
Non-small-cell bronchogenic carcinoma: This is a higher magnification of the tumor. The nuclear pleomorphism is clear in this image. This field of the tumor shows more poorly differentiated and anaplastic features than those seen in the previous image.

Figure 9.7 Lung biopsy (normal). Hematoxylin & eosin stain.
Normal lung biopsy: This is an image from the patient's lung away from the tumor. It shows congestion and a minimal inflammatory cell infiltrate.

Figure 9.8 Mediastinal lymph node biopsy (patient). Hematoxylin & eosin stain.
Mediastinal lymph node, negative for metastatic carcinoma: This image shows a reactive mediastinal lymph node with anthracotic pigment. No metastatic carcinoma is seen.

Figure 9.9 X-ray of the right arm (patient).
Pathological fracture: This X-ray shows a mildly displaced transverse fracture through the middle of the right humeral shaft. The fracture extends through a portion of the humerus that shows a relatively decreased density. This is consistent with a pathological fracture.

Figure 9.10 Bone biopsy from the reaming (patient). Hematoxylin & eosin stain.
Metastatic carcinoma: The bone marrow is infiltrated by poorly differentiated neoplastic cells.

Answers

1. C. The patient's lung biopsy (2 years prior to the current admission, Figs 9.5 and 9.6) shows an invasive non-small-cell carcinoma. No non-caseating granuloma suggesting sarcoidosis or caseating granulomas suggesting tuberculosis are seen in this lesion. Lung abscess would be characterized by the presence of tissue necrosis with the accumulation of neutrophils.

2. C. Factors contributing to the development of carcinoma of the lung include tobacco smoking, radiation, asbestos exposure, air pollution, genetic factors, and pulmonary scars. Pulmonary alveolar proteinosis is a disease of unknown etiology, characterized by the accumulation of dense granular material containing lipid and PAS-positive material in the intra-alveolar spaces. Pulmonary alveolar proteinosis is not a contributing factor for lung carcinoma.

3. C. The finding of abnormally elevated blood glucose level in itself is not diagnostic of diabetes mellitus. Malnutrition leads to hypoglycemia. Without any other information, acute stress would be the most likely cause for the patient's hyperglycemia.

4. D. Primary hyperparathyroidism and excess of dietary vitamin D lead to hypercalcemia. The patient does not have chronic renal failure, and his slightly elevated BUN is most likely due to a prerenal cause; his creatinine is normal. His hypocalcemia, however, could be explained by his hypoalbuminemia. Routine calcium assay measures the total calcium value; of that about 50% is bound to protein, mostly to albumin (the metabolically inactive fraction). The non-bound fraction (also known as "ionized" or "free" calcium) is the metabolically active fraction, not affected by the serum albumin level. Low serum albumin lowers the total serum calcium level by decreasing the metabolically inactive fraction. This

Table 10.2 Hematology

			SI Units	
WBC	14.2	(5.0–14.5 thou/µL)	14.2	(5.0–14.5 × 10^9/L)
Neut	60 H	(27–48%)	60 H	(27–48%)
Band	20 H	(0–7%)	20 H	(0–7%)
Lymph	15 L	(27–48%)	15 L	(27–48%)
Mono	4	(0–6%)	4	(0–6%)
Eos	0	(0–5%)	0	(0–5%)
Baso	0	(0–2%)	0	(0–2%)
Metamyelocytes	1 H	(0%)	1 H	(0%)
RBC	3.1 L	(3.8–5.2 mill/µL)	3.1 L	(3.8–5.2 × 10^{12}/L)
HGB	8.8 L	(11.0–14.0 g/dL)	88 L	(110–140 g/L)
HCT	27 L	(32.0–42.0%)	0.27 L	(0.32–0.42)
MCV	87	(75.0–87.0 fL)	87	(75.0–87.0 fL)
MCH	28.4	(25.0–31.0 pg)	28.4	(25.0–31.0 pg)
MCHC	32.6	(32.0–37.0 g/dL)	326	(320–370 g/L)
Plts	223	(150–400 thou/µL)	223	(150–400 × 10^9/L)
Retic	2.4 H	(0.5–1.5%)	2.4 H	(0.5–1.5%)

Table 10.3 Chemistry

			SI Units	
Glucose	84	(60–100 mg/dL)	4.7	(3.6–5.55 mmol/L)
BUN	9	(5–18 mg/dL)	3.2	(1.79–6.43 mmol/L)
Creatinine	0.7	(0.3–0.7 mg/dL)	61.9	(26.52–61.9 µmol/L)
Uric acid	5.3	(2.0–5.5 mg/dL)	0.32	(0.12–0.33 mmol/L)
Calcium	9.2	(8.8–10.8 mg/dL)	2.3	(2.2–2.7 mmol/L)
Protein	4.8 L	(6–8 g/dL)	48 L	(60–80 g/L)
Albumin	1.41 L	(3.8–5.4 g/dL)	14.1 L	(38–54 g/L)
Alk Phos	115	(60–270 U/L)	115	(60–270 U/L)
AST	242 H	(15–60 U/L)	242 H	(15–60 U/L)
Bilirubin	0.6	(0.3–1.2 mg/dL)	10.3	(5.13–20.5 µmol/L)

Table 10.4 Electrolytes

			SI Units	
Na	121 L	(138–145 mEq/L)	121 L	(138–145 mmol/L)
K	2.2 L	(3.4–4.7 mEq/L)	2.2 L	(3.4–4.7 mmol/L)
Cl	75 L	(98–107 mEq/L)	75 L	(98–107 mmol/L)
CO$_2$	40.8 H	(23–29 mEq/L)	40.8 H	(23–29 mmol/L)

Table 10.5 Arterial blood gases

			SI Units	
pH	7.48 H	(7.35–7.45)	7.48 H	(7.35–7.45)
PCO$_2$	46.5 H	(32–46 mmHg)	6.18 H	(4.26–6.13 kPa)
PO$_2$	86	(74–108 mmHg)	11.5	(9.9–14.4 kPa)
HCO$_3^-$	35.0 H	(19–24 mEq/L)	35.0 H	(19–24 mmol/L)

Table 10.6 Urinalysis

pH	5	(5.0–7.5)
Protein	2+ H	(Neg)
Glucose	Neg	(Neg)
Ketone	Neg	(Neg)
Color	Yellow	(Yellow)
Clarity	Clear	(Clear)
Sp. grav.	1.019	(1.010–1.035)
WBC	9 H	(0–5/HPF)
RBC	0	(0–2/HPF)
Casts	Neg	(Neg)
Bacteria	Neg	(Neg)

Table 10.7 Microbiology

Wound (ankle) culture	Pending

Table 10.8 Special hematology

			SI Units	
Iron	40 L	(50–120 μg/dL)	7.2 L	(8.96–21.5 μmol/L)
TIBC	275 L	(300–360 μg/dL)	49.2 L	(53.7–64.5 μmol/L)
Serum ferritin	145 H	(7–140 ng/mL)	145 H	(7–140 μg/L)

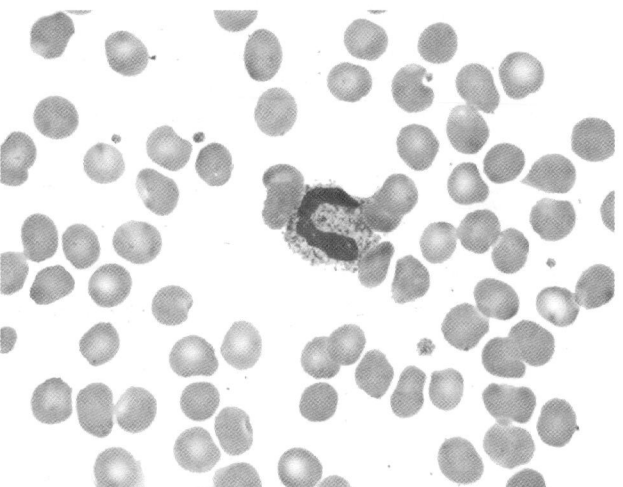

Figure 10.1 Peripheral blood smear (patient). Wright/Giemsa stain.

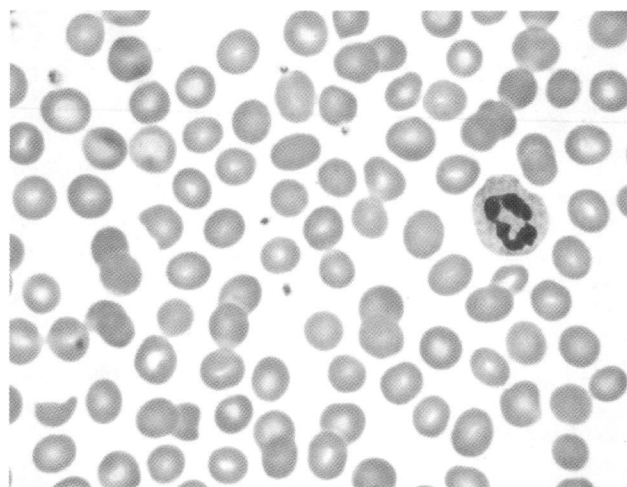

Figure 10.2 Peripheral blood smear (normal). Wright/Giemsa stain.

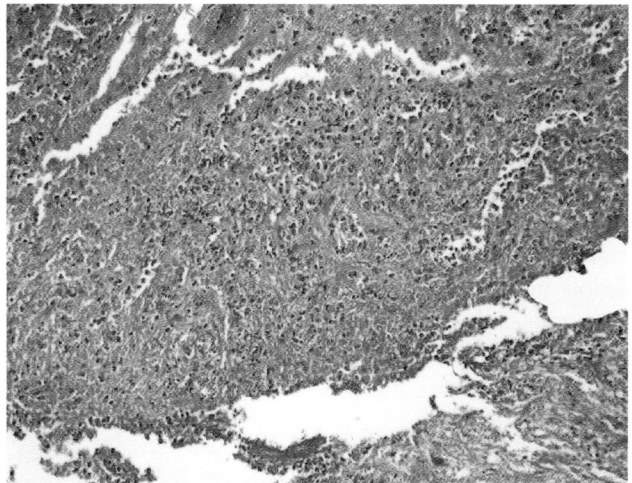

Figure 10.3 Debridement of the ankle wound (patient). Hematoxylin & eosin stain.

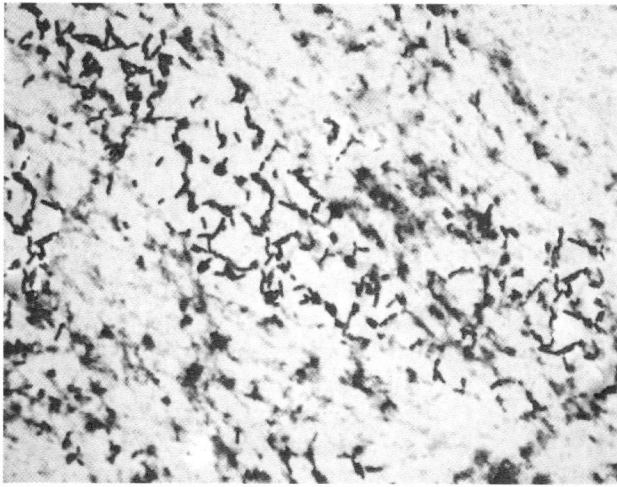

Figure 10.4 Culture from ankle wound (patient). Gram stain.

Questions

Based on the above information, you can best conclude the following:

INTERMEDIATE

1. The white blood cell count and differential in this patient reflect:

   a. increased numbers of myeloid precursors in the bone marrow
   b. a shortened myeloid maturation time
   c. increased granulocyte-macrophage colony-stimulating factor (GM-CSF) activity
   d. all of the above
   e. none of the above

INTERMEDIATE

2. All of the following statements concerning the type of anemia seen in this patient are correct EXCEPT:

   a. the bone marrow would show plentiful reticuloendothelial iron stores
   b. it is classified as a hypoproliferative anemia
   c. the bone marrow would show a marked increase in erythroid precursors
   d. it is related to the suppression of bone marrow progenitor cells by cytokines
   e. the serum iron level is usually decreased

ADVANCED

3. All of the following statements concerning the reticulocyte count, in general, are correct EXCEPT:

   a. it is a measure of effective erythropoiesis

   b. the normal absolute reticulocyte count is approximately 50×10^9/L
   c. the reticulocyte maturation time in the peripheral blood is 1 day in a non-anemic patient
   d. the value seen in our patient reflects increased erythropoiesis
   e. the degree of red cell production may vary with the degree of anemia

INTERMEDIATE

4. Which of the following factors is most likely contributing to this patient's hypokalemia?

   a. trauma resulting in rhabdomyolysis
   b. fever
   c. vomiting
   d. all of the above
   e. none of the above

ADVANCED

5. All of the following statements concerning this patient's acid–base status are correct EXCEPT:

   a. it is mainly due to the loss of fixed acids
   b. it is related to the patient's hypokalemia
   c. there has been an increased movement of H^+ from the extracellular fluid compartment to the intracellular fluid compartment
   d. there is probably renal loss of H^+
   e. it is primarily respiratory in etiology

Clinical course

The child was begun on potassium replacement, intravenous fluids, and antibiotic therapy. Because of his significant past medical history, additional laboratory studies were performed. On the third hospital day, he had a grand mal seizure with his temperature (rectal) rising to 106.5°F (41.4°C). Over the next several days his temperature ranged from 101°F to 104°F (38.3°C to 40°C), the wounds increased in size, and fluctuant areas developed over the left shoulder and left scalp. Surgical exploration of these areas was performed and purulent material was obtained and sent for culture. The patient became progressively more lethargic and developed additional seizures. Urine output decreased, and hypokalemia persisted despite replacement therapy. Additional lesions, requiring incision and drainage appeared on his face and extremities. An abdominal CT (not shown) revealed multiple lesions in the liver and spleen. The patient expired three weeks after admission and an autopsy was performed (Figs 10.5 and 10.6).

Table 10.9 Serum protein electrophoresis & immunoelectrophoresis (day 2)

			SI Units	
Albumin	1.41 L	(3.8–5.4 g/dL)	14.1 L	(38–54 g/L)
Alpha$_1$-globulin	0.64 H	(0.1–0.3 g/dL)	6.4 H	(1–3 g/L)
Alpha$_2$-globulin	0.97	(0.6–1.0 g/dL)	9.7	(6–10 g/L)
Beta-globulin	0.73	(0.7–1.1 g/dL)	7.3	(7–11 g/L)
Gamma-globulin	1.04	(0.8–1.6 g/dL)	10.4	(8–16 g/L)
IgG	875	(370–1500 mg/dL)	8750	(3700–15 000 mg/L)
IgA	90	(30–200 mg/dL)	900	(300–2000 mg/L)
IgM	40	(20–220 mg/dL)	400	(200–2200 mg/L)

Table 10.10 Special hematology (day 2)

	Patient	Control
Nitroblue tetrazolium (NBT) test	No blue precipitate in neutrophils	Blue precipitate in neutrophils

Table 10.11 Coagulation (day 2)

PT	13	(11–15 s)
aPTT	31	(<35 s)
INR	1.037	

Table 10.12 Microbiology

Wound (ankle) culture (admission)	*Enterobacter aerogenes*
Left shoulder culture (day 5)	*Enterobacter aerogenes*
Left scalp culture (day 5)	*Enterobacter aerogenes*

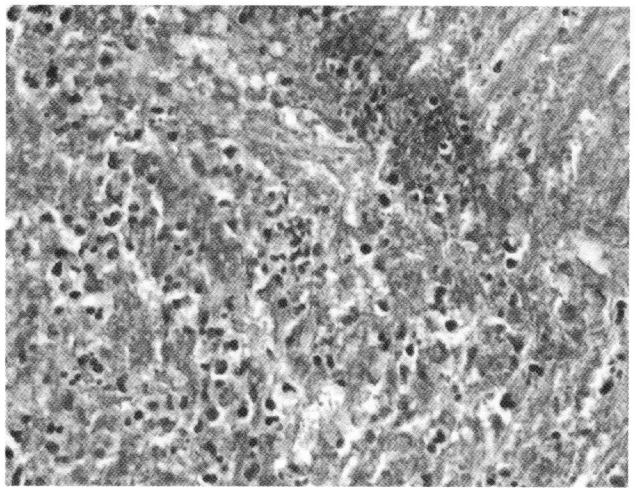

Figure 10.5 Portion of lung (patient's autopsy). Hematoxylin & eosin stain.

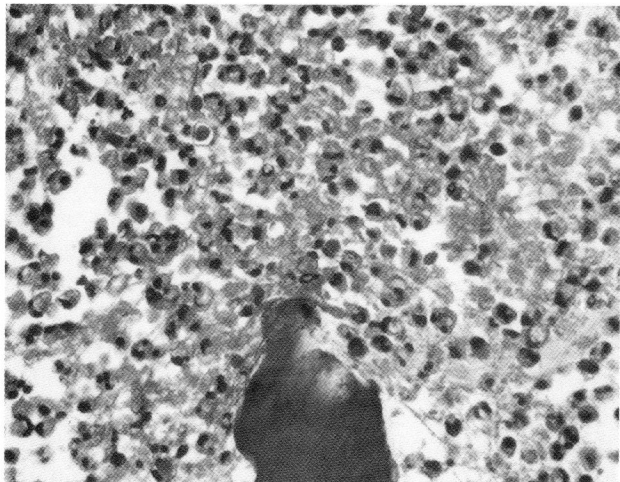

Figure 10.6 Portion of the left clavicle (patient's autopsy). Hematoxylin & eosin stain.

Questions

6. All of the following statements concerning the serum protein electrophoresis and immunoelectrophoresis data seen in Table 10.9 are correct EXCEPT:

   a. they are consistent with homozygous alpha$_1$-antitrypsin (AAT) deficiency
   b. they are consistent with infection
   c. they are consistent with a protein-losing state
   d. they are consistent with malnutrition
   e. they are consistent with severe liver disease

7. The results of the nitroblue tetrazolium (NBT) test in this patient indicate:

   a. inability of the patient's neutrophils to phagocytose bacteria
   b. a myeloperoxidase deficiency
   c. deficient production of superoxide (O_2^-) by the patient's neutrophils
   d. defective neutrophil degranulation
   e. impaired opsonization

8. Which of the following organisms would LEAST LIKELY cause disease in this patient?

   a. *Streptococcus pneumoniae*
   b. *Staphylococcus aureus*
   c. *Escherichia coli*
   d. *Pseudomonas cepacia* (*Burkholderia cepacia*)
   e. *Serratia marcescens*

9. All of the following statements concerning the underlying disorder in this patient are correct EXCEPT:

   a. it is an X-linked hereditary disorder
   b. neutrophil chemotaxis is deficient
   c. most patients with this disorder lack neutrophil cytochrome b_{558}
   d. the disease mainly presents in childhood
   e. respiratory burst activity is markedly decreased

ANSWERS AND FURTHER INFORMATION

Figure descriptions

Figure 10.1 Peripheral blood smear (patient). Wright/Giemsa stain.
The patient's peripheral blood smear shows a band with toxic granulations. The red blood cells are decreased in number, normal in size, and show mild aniso-poikilocytosis. Several platelets are also present.

Figure 10.2 Peripheral blood smear (normal). Wright/Giemsa stain.
This is a photomicrograph of a normal blood smear for comparison. The red blood cells' size is approximately two-thirds that of the neutrophil (present on the right side).

Figure 10.3 Debridement of the ankle wound (patient). Hematoxylin & eosin stain.
Section from the ankle wound. Debridement shows necrotic fibroconnective tissue with a marked neutrophilic infiltrate and abscess formation.

Figure 10.4 Culture from ankle wound (patient). Gram stain.
Gram stain of the cultured ankle wound shows large Gram-negative rods, which were identified as *Enterobacter aerogenes*.

Figure 10.5 Portion of lung (from patient's autopsy). Hematoxylin & eosin stain.
At autopsy the patient's lungs were consolidated, heavy, and with poor aeration. Numerous tan-yellow nodules were present within the lung parenchyma. This image shows the center of one of those nodules. It is composed of necrotic tissue with a marked acute inflammatory cell infiltrate. The intervening pulmonary parenchyma (not shown in this image), shows congestion and thickening of the alveolar septa.

Figure 10.6 Portion of the left clavicle (patient's autopsy). Hematoxylin & eosin stain.
Acute osteomyelitis: A marked neutrophilic infiltrate is seen in the marrow cavity. A fragment of dead bone is noted in the center of the lower edge of this photomicrograph.

Answers

1. D. All of the above listed responses are correct in this patient. The patient presents with signs of an active infection (fever, cellulitis, and purulent-draining wounds). This would lead to increased activity of GM-CSF, as well as other growth factors, resulting in increased numbers of myeloid precursors in the bone marrow. Myeloid development time (myelocyte to neutrophil development) would also be shortened. When needed (infection, stress, etc.), myeloid cells from the storage compartment (myelocytes, metamyelocytes, bands, and polymorphonuclear neutrophils) may be released prematurely into the circulation and one can see bands and even metamyelocytes, as in our patient.

2. C. The patient exhibits a normocytic normochromic anemia, which when looked at in the context of his long medical history represents an anemia of chronic disease. This is a hypoproliferative anemia and as such would not show a marked increase in bone marrow erythrocyte precursors. The bone marrow does not adequately adjust for the moderately reduced red blood cell survival time that is seen in this condition, and it is now thought that this is due in part to the suppression of bone marrow progenitor cells by cytokines. A reduced serum iron level is commonly seen in the anemia of chronic disease and is also suggested as being due to the effects of cytokines (interleukin-1 (IL-1) and tumor necrosis factor (TNF)) on white blood cells and lactoferrin release. The diversion of iron from hemoglobin synthesis to the reticuloendothelial storage pool results in increased bone marrow iron. In infectious states this may be beneficial to the patient, as iron is needed by most microorganisms for growth and reproduction, and decreased serum iron limits its availability to these pathogens.

3. D. As will be seen below, the percentage of reticulocytes in our patient, while elevated, does not reflect an increased erythropoiesis. Reticulocytes are immature red cells containing RNA that are present in the peripheral blood and appear gray in Wright/Giemsa preparations in contrast to the pink-staining mature erythrocytes. They mature (lose their RNA) within 1 day of entry into the peripheral circulation in a non-anemic patient and thus are a measure of effective erythropoiesis. The absolute reticulocyte count, which is normally about 50×10^9 reticulocytes per liter per day (1% of circulating erythrocytes), is more useful in evaluating red blood cell production than a simple percentage value. It is obtained by multiplying the reticulocyte percentage by the red blood cell count. In an anemic patient, two corrections are necessary in order to evaluate accurately the red blood cell production: (1) a correction for the anemia itself and (2) a correction for the increased maturation time of reticulocytes that are prematurely released (due to the effect of erythropoietin). In our patient this correction is made by dividing the reticulocyte percent (2.4%) by the normal percentage of reticulocytes (1%) and multiplying that number (2.4) by the quotient of our patient's hematocrit (0.27) divided by the normal hematocrit for our patient's age (0.38), which is 0.71. The result is 1.7, implying that he is producing 1.7 times as many reticulocytes as normal. This value has to be corrected for the increased maturation time of the reticulocytes, which at a hematocrit of 27% (0.27) is approximately 2 days (1.7/2 = 0.85). This means that reticulocyte release is only 85% of normal and therefore red blood cell production is less than normal even in the presence of an anemia. This again points to a hypoproliferative anemia.

4. C. Our patient presents with several episodes of vomiting. Gastrointestinal fluid loss, either by vomiting or diarrhea, is a major cause of decreased total body stores of potassium resulting in hypokalemia. The arterial blood gases are consistent with a metabolic alkalosis, which can also result in the renal loss of potassium and is another contributing factor to the patient's hypokalemia. Fever often occurs in conditions in which there is cellular damage with a resulting movement of potassium from the intracellular compartment to the extracellular compartment eventually leading to hyperkalemia. Rhabdomyolysis, the destruction of muscle fibers, would also result in the shift of potassium to the extracellular compartment and would cause hyperkalemia.

5. E. This patient has a metabolic alkalosis, which is not a primary respiratory problem. This is due to the loss of fixed acids (HCl) through prolonged vomiting and from the movement of H^+ into the intracellular compartment, due in part to the hypokalemia. The urine pH is 5.0, suggesting also some loss of H^+ into the urine. The respiratory component in metabolic alkalosis is a secondary compensatory increase in PCO_2.

Simple rules to help decide if the acid–base abnormality is respiratory or metabolic in origin (compensatory mechanisms may affect the HCO_3^- and PCO_2 levels):
1. If pH is less than 7.35, the patient is acidotic.
   - metabolic acidosis: HCO_3^- and PCO_2 both low
   - respiratory acidosis: HCO_3^- and PCO_2 both high
2. If pH is greater than 7.45, the patient is alkalotic.
   - metabolic alkalosis: HCO_3^- and PCO_2 both high
   - respiratory alkalosis: HCO_3^- and PCO_2 both low

6. A. The protein electrophoresis shows a decrease in the albumin fraction and low normal values for the remaining fractions except for the α_1-globulin fraction, which is elevated and contains several proteins including alpha$_1$-antitrypsin (AAT). In homozygous alpha$_1$-antitrypsin deficiency, the level of this proteinase inhibitor is 10–20% of normal; since it accounts for about 90% of the α_1-globulin fraction, this fraction would be markedly decreased in this condition. All of the other statements concerning the electrophoretic data are correct. Given our patient's clinical presentation and history, one would expect an acute-phase response (decreased albumin with increased α_1-globulin and α_2-globulin fractions)

along with signs of a chronic inflammatory state (polyclonal hypergammaglobulinemia). With reference to our case, the data are consistent with an acute-phase reaction due to an infection; the response, however, has been limited because of malnutrition, protein loss from the kidneys, and liver disease. This explains the lack of an increase in both the α_2-globulin fraction and the immunoglobulins (γ-globulin fraction).

7. C. In the nitroblue tetrazolium test, neutrophils from a drop of blood are incubated with a soluble yellow dye, nitroblue tetrazolium, which forms a complex with fibrinogen. The complex is phagocytosed by activated neutrophils and in a normal individual the dye is reduced to an insoluble blue precipitate (negative test), which is readily apparent under the light microscope. This reduction depends on the generation by the neutrophils of superoxide. The inability to produce this blue (formazan) precipitate indicates deficient superoxide production, the underlying pathogenesis of our patient's problem, which is chronic granulomatous disease. Neutrophil opsonization, phagocytosis, and degranulation are unaffected in this disorder. In myeloperoxidase deficiency, there is increased superoxide production.

8. A. *Streptococcus pneumoniae* is a frequent cause of disease in children but it does not cause significant illness in patients with chronic granulomatous disease. All of the other organisms are frequent pathogens in this disorder. The oxygen-dependent killing of microorganisms depends on the release of superoxide (O_2^-) radicals and hydrogen peroxide (H_2O_2) by a membrane-bound enzyme, found in neutrophils and monocytes, known as the respiratory burst oxidase. In order to explain why *Streptococcus pneumoniae* is killed by the neutrophils of these patients, one must remember that although hydrogen peroxide is a normal oxidative end-product of aerobic carbohydrate metabolism in most bacteria, it becomes toxic to the microbe when the organism is trapped in a phagosome and therefore most microbes possess the enzyme catalase to convert the peroxide into water and oxygen. *Streptococcus pneumoniae* lacks catalase but generates sufficient amounts of hydrogen peroxide so that the neutrophils in patients with chronic granulomatous disease can effectively kill these bacteria. All of the other listed organisms are catalase-positive and/or produce little hydrogen peroxide and thus are frequent infecting organisms in patients with this disease.

9. B. Several types of chronic granulomatous disease (CGD) exist, with the most common form being an X-linked inherited disorder in which the neutrophils lack the electron transporting oxidase, cytochrome b_{558}, an essential factor needed for the activation of the membrane-bound respiratory burst oxidase. As such, respiratory burst activity is markedly decreased following phagocytosis. Other forms of the disease exist in which the mode of inheritance is autosomal recessive and cytochrome b_{558} is present, but one of the other components needed for activation of the respiratory burst oxidase is absent. The essential defect in all forms of CGD is a markedly decreased respiratory burst activity; there is no deficiency in neutrophil chemotaxis, and mild forms of the disease may not present until adulthood, when it usually presents as idiopathic pulmonary fibrosis.

Final diagnosis and synopsis of the case

- Chronic granulomatous disease
- Multiple abscesses (*Enterobacter aerogenes*)
- Osteomyelitis (*Enterobacter aerogenes*)
- Bronchopneumonia
- Malnutrition
- Metabolic alkalosis
- Anemia of chronic disease

A 5-year-old boy with a significant past medical history presented with a fever, several episodes of vomiting over the past 24 hours, a draining wound on his right ankle, several red, indurated areas on the right leg, right-sided inguinal lymphadenopathy, decreased breath sounds bilaterally, hepatosplenomegaly, and limited motion of his head and left shoulder. Radiographic studies revealed lytic lesions of the skull, bone destruction of the right tibia, a pathological fracture of the humerus, and a pulmonary infiltrate. The effects of his chronic disease on his bone marrow were reflected in the hematological findings: a hypoproliferative anemia, in this case normocytic, normochromic, and a limited leukocyte response in the presence of a bacterial infection (normal total white blood cell count with a left shift). The serum protein electrophoresis and immunoelectrophoresis showed an acute-phase reaction pattern in conjunction with a chronic inflammatory state consistent with the decreased protein synthesis that can occur with malnutrition. Increased protein catabolism and renal loss may also have been playing a role in this patient. The patient also had a severe metabolic alkalosis, due to the loss of fixed acids from his vomiting and exacerbated by his hypokalemia. The positive nitroblue tetrazolium test indicated that the patient's neutrophils were unable to generate sufficient quantities of superoxide (O_2^-), a necessary component in the oxygen-dependent killing of many microorganisms, and confirmed the diagnosis of chronic granulomatous disease. In this, his final admission, he developed widespread abscesses due to *Enterobacter aerogenes* (Figs 10.3, 10.5 and 10.6), an organism whose killing depends on adequate superoxide production by the host. The autopsy also revealed granulomatous changes in his lung, a consequence of repeated past infections.

A 78-year-old pale woman with fever

CASE AND MCQS

Clinical history and presentation

A 78-year-old woman was admitted with a chief complaint of weakness, malaise, and fever. The patient also complained of dysuria and urinary frequency. She was recently discharged after a 2-week-long hospitalization for severe anemia. Physical examination revealed a weak and pale woman in moderate distress. Her temperature was 100.3°F (37.9°C), pulse rate was 104/min and regular, blood pressure was 125/45 mmHg, and her respiratory rate was 18/min. Her sclerae showed mild yellow discoloration. Except for suprapubic tenderness to palpation, the rest of the physical examination was unremarkable.

Admission data

Table 11.1 Hematology

			SI Units	
WBC	31.8 H	(3.3–11.0 thou/µL)	31.8 H	(3.3–11.0 × 10⁹/L)
Neut	93 H	(44–88%)	93 H	(44–88%)
Lymph	4 L	(12–43%)	4 L	(12–43%)
Mono	2	(2–11%)	2	(2–11%)
Eos	0.3	(0–5%)	0.3	(0–5%)
Baso	0.7	(0–2%)	0.7	(0–2%)
RBC	2.44 L	(3.9–5.0 mill/µL)	2.44 L	(3.9–5.0 × 10¹²/L)
HGB	7.3 L	(11.6–15.6 g/dL)	73 L	(116–156 g/L)
HCT	22.4 L	(37.0–47.0%)	0.224 L	(0.37–0.47)
MCV	91.7	(79.0–99.0 fL)	91.7	(79.0–99.0 fL)
MCH	29.9	(26.0–32.6 pg)	29.9	(26.0–32.6 pg)
MCHC	32.6	(31.0–36.0 g/dL)	326	(310–360 g/L)
Plts	310	(130–400 thou/µL)	310	(130–400 × 10⁹/L)
Retic	3.5 H	(0.1–2.0%)	3.5 H	(0.1–2.0%)

Table 11.2 Chemistry

			SI Units	
Glucose	110	(65–110 mg/dL)	6.11	(3.6–6.11 mmol/L)
BUN	56 H	(7–24 mg/dL)	20 H	(2.50–8.57 mmol/L)
Creatinine	1.7 H	(0.7–1.4 mg/dL)	150 H	(61.9–123.7 µmol/L)
Uric acid	5.6	(3.0–8.5 mg/dL)	0.33	(0.18–0.51 mmol/L)
Calcium	8.0 L	(8.5–10.5 mg/dL)	2.0 L	(2.13–2.63 mmol/L)
Protein	6.4	(6–8 g/dL)	64	(60–80 g/L)
Albumin	3.2 L	(3.7–5.0 g/dL)	32 L	(37–50 g/L)
Cholesterol	113	(150–200 mg/dL)	2.29	(3.88–5.17 mmol/L)
Alk Phos	74	(0–120 U/L)	74	(0–120 U/L)
GGTP	14	(0–50 U/L)	14	(0–50 U/L)
LDH	431 H	(100–250 U/L)	431 H	(100–250 U/L)
AST	34	(0–55 U/L)	34	(0–55 U/L)
Bilirubin	3.9 H	(0.0–1.5 mg/dL)	66.7 H	(0–25.7 µmol/L)
Bilirubin-direct	0.57 H	(0.02–0.18 mg/dL)	9.7 H	(0.34–3.08 µmol/L)

Table 11.3 Electrolytes

			SI Units	
Na	138	(134–143 mEq/L)	138	(134–143 mmol/L)
K	4.4	(3.5–4.9 mEq/L)	4.4	(3.5–4.9 mmol/L)
Cl	100	(95–108 mEq/L)	100	(95–108 mmol/L)
CO_2	26	(21–32 mEq/L)	26	(21–32 mmol/L)

Table 11.4 Special hematology

			SI Units	
Iron	100	(42–135 µg/dL)	17.9	(7.5–24.2 µmol/L)
TIBC	310	(280–400 µg/dL)	55	(50.1–71.6 µmol/L)
Transferrin sat.	40	(15–50%)	0.4	(0.15–0.50)

Table 11.5 Urinalysis

Sp. grav.	1.015	(1.010–1.035)
pH	6	(5.0–7.5)
Protein	Neg	(Neg)
Glucose	Neg	(Neg)
Bile	Neg	(Neg)
Ketone	Neg	(Neg)
Blood	2+ H	(Neg)
Color	Yellow	(Pale yellow)
Clarity	Clear	(Clear)
WBC	50 H	(0–5/HPF)
RBC	19 H	(0–2/HPF)
Casts	Neg	(Neg)
Bacteria	4+ H	(Neg)
Urobilinogen	2+ H	(Neg)
Hemosiderin	Neg	(Neg)

Table 11.6 Microbiology

Blood cultures	Pending
Urine culture	Pending

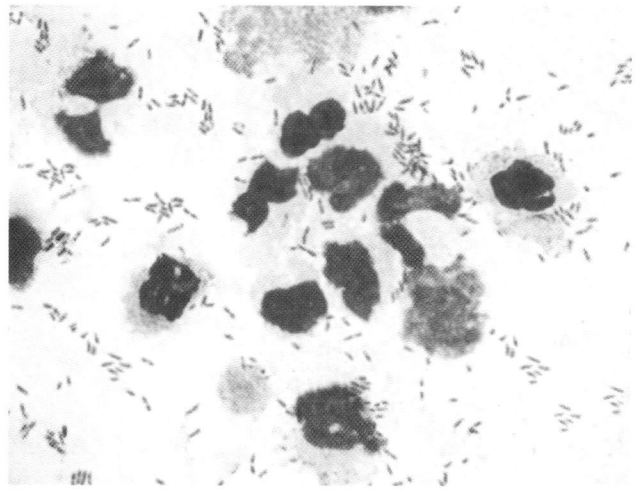

Figure 11.1 Urine sediment smear (patient). Giemsa stain.

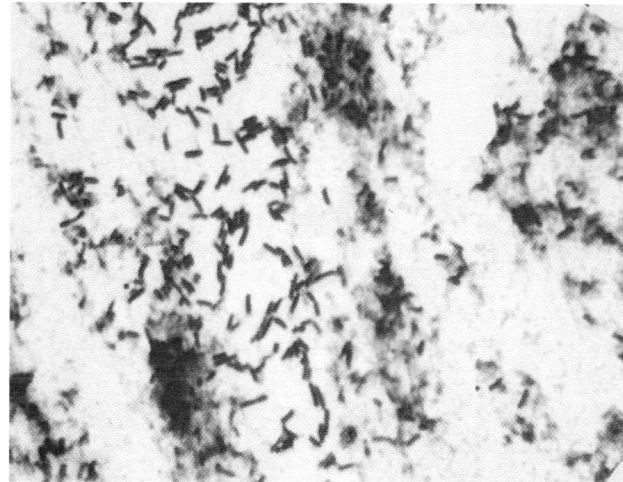

Figure 11.2 Blood culture smear (patient). Gram stain.

Questions

Based on the above information you can best conclude the following:

1. The patient's clinical presentation, admission laboratory data, urine sediment smear (Fig. 11.1) and blood culture smear (Fig. 11.2) are suggestive of:

   a. lower urinary tract infection
   b. Gram-positive bacteremia
   c. pyelonephritis
   d. macrocytic anemia

2. The most likely cause of this patient's hyperbilirubinemia is:

   a. biliary obstruction
   b. hemolytic anemia
   c. hepatic cirrhosis
   d. acute viral hepatitis
   e. none of the above

3. This patient's abnormal BUN and creatinine levels are most likely related to:

   a. acute pyelonephritis
   b. acute tubular necrosis
   c. hepato-renal syndrome
   d. none of the above

4. The increased percentage of reticulocytes in this patient is LEAST likely to indicate:

   a. functional bone marrow
   b. destruction of red blood cells
   c. recent episodes of bleeding
   d. early stage of iron deficiency
   e. anemia of chronic disease

5. This patient's increased level of serum lactate dehydrogenase (LDH) can be best related to:

   a. liver disease
   b. lung disease
   c. underlying occult malignant disease
   d. hemolysis
   e. myocardial infarction

Clinical course

The patient's urine and blood cultures were positive for *Escherichia coli*. Her fever, urinary tract symptoms, and WBC improved after a course of antibiotic therapy. The results of additional laboratory tests are shown below. The patient was transfused with packed red blood cells (PRBC) and she improved symptomatically. A few days later her anemia again worsened (CBC (FBC) results not shown) and she developed a dark-purple discoloration at the tips of her fingers and toes.

Table 11.7 Special hematology

			SI Units		
Retic	5.5 H	(1–2%)	5.5 H	(1–2%)
Haptoglobin	5 L	(40–270 mg/dL)	50 L	(400–2700 mg/L)

Table 11.8 Serology and immunology

Cold agglutinin	> 1:10 000 H	(1:32)
Cryoglobin	Neg	(Neg)

Table 11.9 Coombs' test (direct antiglobulin test – DAT)

Polyspecific, IgG & C3d	1+ H	(Neg)
Monospecific, IgG	Neg	(Neg)
Monospecific, C3d	3+ H	(Neg)

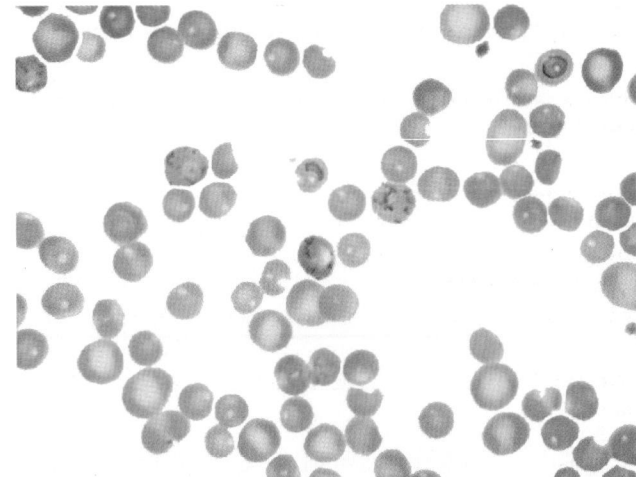

Figure 11.3 Peripheral blood smear (patient). New methylene blue stain.

Questions

ADVANCED

6. All of the following statements regarding this patient's anemia are correct EXCEPT:

   a. it is caused by an IgM autoantibody
   b. acrocyanosis is a feature of this disease
   c. RBC indices in themselves are diagnostic of this disease
   d. clinical symptoms are related to the ability of the cold agglutinin antibodies to activate complement

INTERMEDIATE

7. Based on the above clinical and laboratory findings, select the INCORRECT statement about this patient's condition:

   a. because of her age, splenectomy is the treatment of choice
   b. her elevated level of LDH and anemia are due to the same underlying condition
   c. the patient's azotemia is a reversible condition
   d. multiple blood transfusions are not advisable

8. Select the INCORRECT statement about the general features of anemias such as that diagnosed in this patient:

    a. the peak incidence is in the seventh and eighth decades

    b. automated red blood cell count and peripheral smear preparation are difficult to perform

    c. most patients with this disease require specific drug therapy

    d. red blood cells coated with complement fragment C3dg are protected from phagocytosis

9. In general, the serum haptoglobin level:

    a. decreases after massive blood transfusion

    b. decreases in acute inflammation

    c. increases in patients with hepatocellular diseases

    d. is a highly specific test for the diagnosis of hemolytic anemia

ANSWERS AND FURTHER INFORMATION

Figure descriptions

Figure 11.1 Urine sediment smear (patient). Giemsa stain.
This photomicrograph shows numerous aggregates of large rods, neutrophils, and necrotic debris.

Figure 11.2 Blood culture smear (patient). Gram stain.
Large Gram-negative rods morphologically consistent with Enterobacteriaceae such as *Escherichia coli* or *Klebsiella* species are seen in this photomicrograph. These rods were identified as *Escherichia coli*.

Figure 11.3 Peripheral blood smear (patient). New methylene blue stain.
For manual determination of the reticulocyte percentage, add 2 drops of supravital stain (new methylene blue stain) to 2 drops of anticoagulated venous blood and incubate for 15 minutes. New methylene blue stains the ribosomal ribonucleic acid (RNA). Cells that contain two or more blue-stained particles are counted as reticulocytes (immature RBCs). Three reticulocytes are noted in this photomicrograph.

Answers

1. A. This patient's WBC shows a marked leukocytosis; urinalysis reveals the presence of leukocytes, red blood cells, and bacteriuria. The blood culture and urine sediment smears show Gram-negative bacilli, which are consistent with Gram-negative bacteremia and bacteriuria. These findings combined with the patient's clinical presentation (dysuria and urinary frequency) are diagnostic of urinary tract infection and bacteremia. The absence of high-grade fever, chills, flank pain, vertebrocostal angle tenderness, and of urine casts makes the diagnosis of upper urinary tract infection (pyelonephritis) unlikely. This patient's CBC (FBC) suggests normocytic normochromic anemia.

2. B. This patient's hyperbilirubinemia is mainly due to an elevated level of unconjugated bilirubin (i.e. conjugated bilirubin accounts for only 14.6% of the total bilirubin). Predominantly unconjugated hyperbilirubinemia (conjugated bilirubin less than 20% of total bilirubin) is usually caused by RBC hemolysis or by rare hereditary diseases associated with impaired bilirubin conjugation or with reduced hepatic uptake of bilirubin. Biliary obstruction and hepatocellular damage, such as seen in hepatic cirrhosis and viral hepatitis, lead to conjugated hyperbilirubinemias and are also associated with abnormal liver function tests, which are not apparent in this patient.

3. D. The presence of elevated BUN and creatinine levels with a high BUN/creatinine ratio points to prerenal azotemia (i.e. impaired renal function, due to decreased renal blood flow, in the absence of organic renal disease). Hepato-renal syndrome is defined as a prerenal azotemia in patients with severe liver disease. Since this patient's liver function tests are within normal limits, a hepato-renal syndrome can be ruled out as the cause of this patient's abnormal renal function. In acute tubular necrosis (ATN), microscopic examination of the urine usually reveals renal epithelial cells and granular casts. In addition there would be a proportional increase of BUN and creatinine (normal BUN/creatinine ratio is 10–15:1). This patient did not show signs or symptoms of pyelonephritis (high-grade fever, chills, flank pain, vertebrocostal angle tenderness) and her urine did not exhibit leukocyte casts usually seen in upper urinary tract infection (acute pyelonephritis). Her prerenal azotemia could be best attributed to her febrile condition.

4. E. The increased percentage of reticulocytes indicates effective erythropoiesis. It is seen in patients after a blood loss, or an increased destruction of red blood cells, after the treatment of iron deficiency and of megaloblastic anemias. It is not seen in anemia of chronic disease.

5. D. This patient's laboratory data show anemia, increased percentage of reticulocytes, unconjugated hyperbilirubinemia, and an increased level of LDH. These findings suggest RBC hemolysis. There are no clinical or laboratory findings to support any of the other listed conditions (liver disease, lung disease, occult malignant disease, myocardial infarction), which are also known to cause an increased level of LDH.

6. C. This patient has cold agglutinin immune hemolytic anemia. This type of anemia is usually caused by IgM antibodies to red blood cells. Acrocyanosis (purplish-gray discoloration) is caused by agglutination of the RBCs leading to vascular obstruction in areas of the body that are exposed to cold. It usually involves the exposed distal extremities (toes, fingers), ear lobes, and nose. Complement is activated and may cause a direct intravascular hemolysis. More commonly, however, the complement fragments (especially C3b) bind to erythrocyte membrane and make it susceptible to phagocytosis by macrophages in the liver and spleen, thus leading to an extravascular hemolysis. RBC indices show a normocytic normochromic anemia. However, in themselves they are not diagnostic of this disease.

7. A. In patients with cold agglutinin immune hemolytic anemia, splenectomy is usually of no therapeutic value regardless of age. When treatment is indicated it is directed at avoiding the interaction of antibodies with RBCs or at reducing the serum concentration of antibodies. Both anemia and the elevated level of LDH in this patient are due to red blood cell hemolysis. This patient has a prerenal azotemia, which may be corrected by improving renal blood perfusion, e.g. by treatment of her infection. Multiple blood transfusions introduce to the body a large number of unprotected RBCs (RBCs not coated with C3b) and fresh complement components that may accelerate hemolysis in the presence of a high titer of cold agglutinin antibody, as occurred in this patient.

8. C. The majority of patients with this disease have mild chronic anemia that requires no specific therapy. Chronic idiopathic cold agglutinin immune hemolytic anemia has a peak incidence in the seventh and eighth decades. Other forms of this anemia, associated with infectious mononucleosis and *Mycoplasma pneumoniae* infections, are more common in children and young adults. In the presence of cold agglutinin antibodies, unless the blood is fresh and the equipment is preheated, automated red blood cell count and peripheral smear preparation are difficult to perform because of agglutination. The C3dg fragment of complement results from the degradation of C3b fragment. As RBCs in patient with cold agglutinin immune hemolytic anemia circulate to the periphery and the blood temperature drops, IgM antibodies bind to RBCs and fix complement. This may lead to intravascular hemolysis; erythrocytes that escape hemolysis loose the IgM cold agglutinin upon return to warm central areas, but the C3b remains bound to the red cell membrane. Such erythrocytes are left susceptible to phagocytosis by mononuclear phagocytes. The C3b opsonin, however, is degraded by C3 inactivator during the circulation to C3dg; this reduces the red blood cell ability to induce phagocytosis.

9. A. The serum haptoglobin is an alpha2 globulin with a long circulation time; it binds tightly to the globin protein in free hemoglobin; the hemoglobin–haptoglobin complex is rapidly cleared from the plasma by the reticuloendothelial system. The serum haptoglobin level is low or absent in both intravascular and extravascular hemolyses and following massive blood transfusions, as a result of hemolysis or destruction of senescent RBCs (increased free hemoglobin). It is an acute-phase reactant; its level increases 3 to 4-fold with inflammation or tissue necrosis. Haptoglobin synthesis is decreased in patients with hepatocellular diseases. The haptoglobin level is very sensitive but not specific for the diagnosis of hemolytic anemia, since its level may be normal in patients with hemolysis and co-existing inflammation.

Final diagnosis and synopsis of the case

- Lower urinary tract infection
- *Escherichia coli* bacteremia
- Chronic idiopathic cold agglutinin immune hemolytic anemia

An elderly woman presented with urinary tract infection caused by *E. coli*. These were also responsible for her prerenal azotemia. Incidentally she was also found to have severe normocytic normochromic anemia. The presence of an elevated LDH level, increased percentage of reticulocytes, and unconjugated hyperbilirubinemia pointed to hemolytic anemia. Additional work-up confirmed the diagnosis of cold agglutinin immune hemolytic anemia. The patient's anemia worsened after blood transfusion of PRBC and she developed acrocyanosis, which further confirmed the diagnosis. In her age category most cold agglutinin immune hemolytic anemias are idiopathic or secondary to a lymphoproliferative disease, not suspected in this patient. Upon her hospital discharge the patient was advised to protect extremities and acral parts against the cold.

Lab tips

The antihuman globulin test (Coombs' test)

Direct Coombs' test:

Detects the *in vivo* coating of red blood cells with antibody or complement (sensitization).

It is a one-step procedure, which is an essential part of the work-up of patients with hemolytic anemia such as autoimmune hemolytic anemia, drug-induced hemolytic anemia, and hemolytic disease of newborn. The patient's RBCs must be washed before adding antihuman globulin (AHG) to remove unbound globulins. "No agglutination" indicates that the patient's RBCs are not coated with antibodies (ABs) or complement. "Agglutination" indicates that the patient's RBCs are coated with antibodies (ABs) and/or complement.

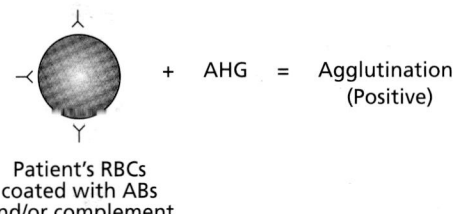

Figure 11.4 Positive direct Coombs' test: washed patient's RBCs + AHG → agglutination.

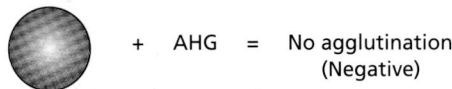

Figure 11.5 Negative direct Coombs' test: washed patient's RBCs + AHG → no agglutination.

Indirect Coombs' test:

Detects the presence of circulating antibodies against RBCs.

It is a two-step test procedure that is mainly used in blood banks for antibody detection, compatibility testing, and blood grouping. The patient's circulating antibodies can be detected by adding reagent red blood cells containing a known antigen. The patient's antibody will bind to the RBCs containing the specific antigen against which the antibody is directed (step 1). Adding AHG (an antibody against human globulin "antibodies") will agglutinate the reagent cells only if they are coated by the patient's antibody (step 2). "Agglutination" indicates that the patient's serum contains antibodies against test cells. (AHG: antihuman globulin; AB: antibody; ABs: antibodies; AG: antigen)

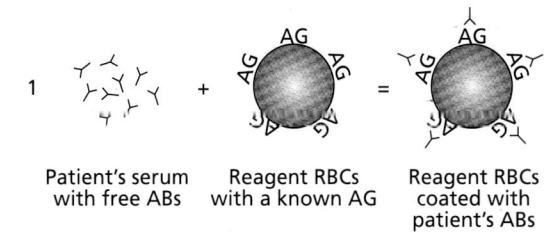

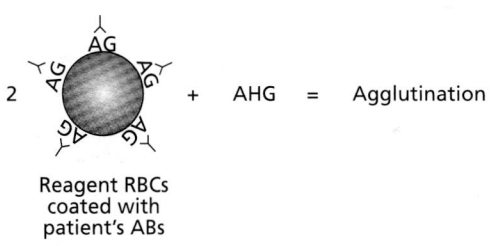

Figure 11.6 Positive indirect Coombs' test:
Step 1: patient's serum + reagent RBCs containing a known antigen → reagent RBCs coated with the patient's antibody.
Step 2: washed cells from step 1 + AHG → agglutination.

A 66-year-old retired truck driver with urinary frequency

CASE AND MCQS

Clinical history and presentation

The patient is a 66-year-old man who presented with urinary frequency and an elevated level of prostate specific antigen (PSA). His medical history includes hypertension and diabetes, for which he is being treated. He is a healthy-appearing man. He was afebrile, BP was 150/90 mmHg, pulse 76/min, and respirations 16/min. Physical examination of the chest revealed diffuse coarse breath sounds. The abdomen was soft, and no organomegaly was noted. Rectal examination revealed an enlarged asymmetric prostate, the right lobe being larger than the left.

Admission data

Table 12.1 Hematology

			SI Units	
WBC	10.1	(3.3–11.0 thou/µL)	10.1	(3.3–11.0 × 10⁹/L)
Neut	70	(44–88%)	70	(44–88%)
Band	0	(0–10%)	0	(0–10%)
Lymph	24	(12–43%)	24	(12–43%)
Mono	5	(2–11%)	5	(2–11%)
Eos	1	(0–5%)	1	(0–5%)
Baso	0	(0–2%)	0	(0–2%)
RBC	3.64 L	(3.9–5.0 mill/µL)	3.64 L	(3.9–5.0 × 10¹²/L)
HGB	12	(11.6–15.6 g/dL)	120	(116–156 g/L)
HCT	33.8 L	(37.0–47.0%)	0.338 L	(0.37–0.47)
MCV	92.9	(79.0–99.0 fL)	92.9	(79.0–99.0 fL)
MCH	33	(27.0–34.6 pg)	33	(27.0–34.6 pg)
MCHC	35.5	(31.0–37.1 g/dL)	355	(310–370 g/L)
Plts	191	(130–400 thou/µL)	191	(130–400 × 10⁹/L)

Table 12.2 Chemistry

			SI Units	
Glucose	128 H	(65–110 mg/dL)	7.11 H	(3.6–6.11 mmol/L)
Creatinine	1.2	(0.7–1.4 mg/dL)	106.1	(61.9–123.7 µmol/L)
BUN	22	(7–24 mg/dL)	7.9	(2.50–8.57 mmol/L)
Uric acid	6.5	(3.0–8.5 mg/dL)	0.37	(0.18–0.51 mmol/L)
Cholesterol	150	(150–200 mg/dL)	3.88	(3.88–5.17 mmol/L)
Protein	6.9	(6–8 g/dL)	69	(60–80 g/L)
Albumin	4.5	(3.7–5.0 g/dL)	45	(37–50 g/L)
LDH	194	(100–250 U/L)	194	(100–250 U/L)
Alk Phos	16	(0–120 U/L)	16	(0–120 U/L)
AST	20	(0–55 U/L)	20	(0–55 U/L)
ALT	16	(7–40 U/L)	16	(7–40 U/L)
GGTP	20	(0–50 U/L)	20	(0–50 U/L)
Bilirubin	1.0	(0.0–1.5 mg/dL)	17.1	(0–25.7 µmol/L)
Bilirubin-direct	0.10	(0.02–0.18 mg/dL)	1.7	(0.34–3.08 µmol/L)

Table 12.3 Electrolytes

		SI Units		
Na	136	(134–143 mEq/L)	136	(134–143 mmol/L)
K	4.5	(3.5–4.9 mEq/L)	4.5	(3.5–4.9 mmol/L)
Cl	102	(95–108 mEq/L)	102	(95–108 mmol/L)
CO_2	27	(21–32 mEq/L)	27	(21–32 mmol/L)

Table 12.4 Coagulation

PT	11.7	(11–14 s)
aPTT	24.0	(22–32 s)
INR	0.92	

Table 12.5 Tumor markers (serum)

			SI Units	
Prostate-specific antigen (PSA)	35 H	(0.1–4.0 ng/mL)	35 H	(0.1–4.0 µg/L)
Free PSA	14 L	(>25%)	14 L	(>25%)

Table 12.6 Urinalysis

pH	6	(5.0–7.5)
Protein	Neg	(Neg)
Glucose	Neg	(Neg)
Ketone	Neg	(Neg)
Color	Yellow	(Yellow)
Clarity	Clear	(Clear)
Sp. grav.	1.010	(1.010–1.035)
Blood	2+ H	(Neg)
WBC	3	(0–5/HPF)
RBC	6 H	(0–2/HPF)
Casts	Neg	(Neg)
Bacteria	Neg	(Neg)

Questions

Based on the above information, you can best conclude the following:

BASIC

1. The patient's hematological work-up shows:

   a. an absolute lymphocytosis
   b. evidence of chronic blood loss
   c. evidence of folate or vitamin B_{12} deficiency
   d. none of the above

INTERMEDIATE

2. The patient's urinalysis shows microscopic hematuria. Such a hematuria, in general, may be caused by:

   a. bladder tumor
   b. kidney disease
   c. sickle-cell anemia
   d. cystitis
   e. all of the above

INTERMEDIATE

3. The prostate-specific antigen (PSA) level in general:

   a. is a diagnostic test for prostate cancer
   b. is a highly sensitive and specific screening test for prostatic cancer
   c. is appropriate as a screening test for cancer recurrence
   d. is usually normal in benign prostatic hypertrophy
   e. all of the above

BASIC

4. The symptom of urinary frequency in general:

   a. is synonymous with polyuria
   b. is virtually diagnostic of an upper urinary tract infection
   c. reflects a decreased ability of the bladder to expand
   d. none of the above statements is correct

Clinical course

A transrectal ultrasound-guided needle biopsy of the prostate was performed (Figs 12.1–12.3 and Fig. 12.5). Treatment modalities were discussed with the patient and he elected surgical treatment. During the surgical procedure a frozen section of the pelvic lymph nodes was performed (Fig. 12.7). Based on the results, a further surgical procedure was performed.

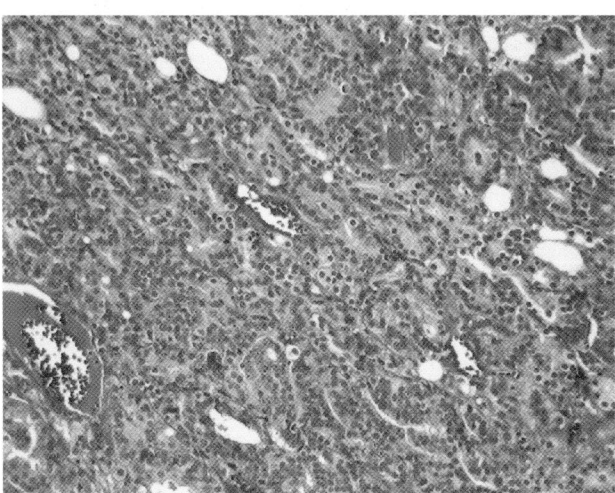

Figure 12.1 Prostate gland biopsy (patient). Hematoxylin & eosin stain.

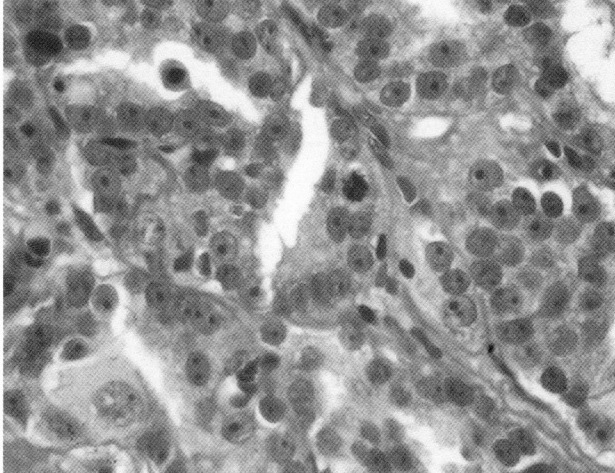

Figure 12.2 Prostate gland biopsy (patient). Hematoxylin & eosin stain.

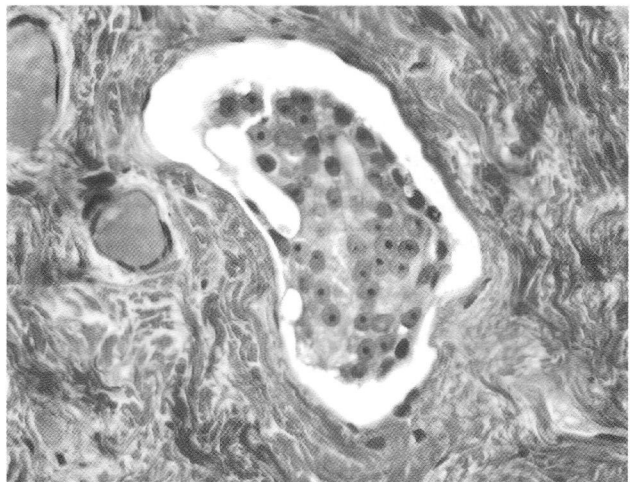

Figure 12.3 Prostate gland biopsy (patient). Hematoxylin & eosin stain.

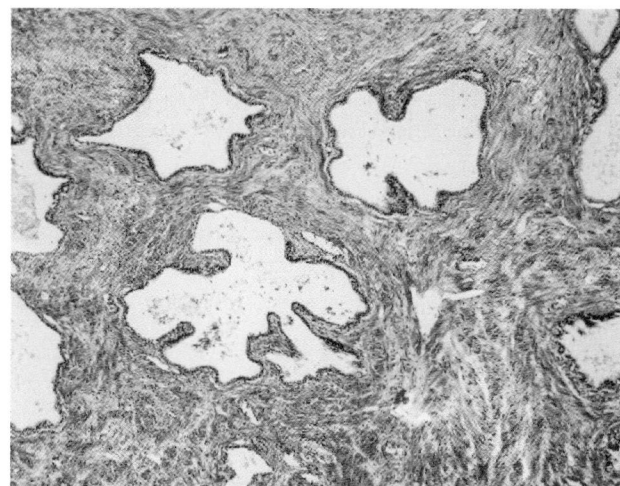

Figure 12.4 Prostate gland biopsy (normal). Hematoxylin & eosin stain.

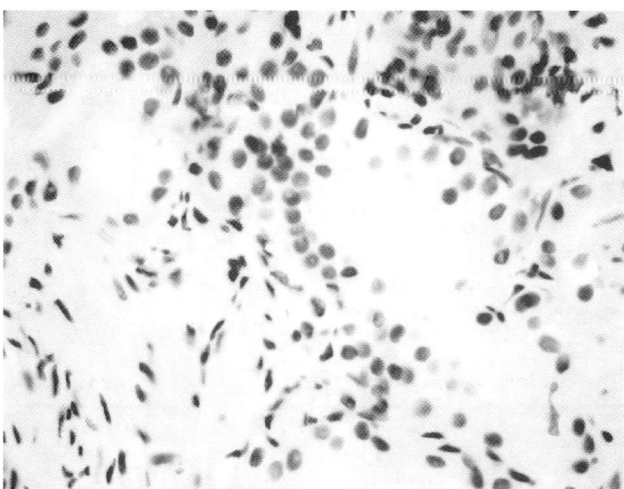

Figure 12.5 Prostate gland biopsy (patient). CK 903 stain.

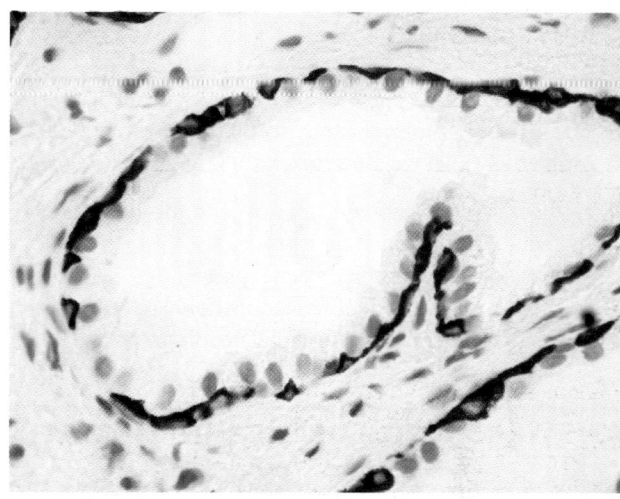

Figure 12.6 Prostate gland biopsy (normal). CK 903 stain.

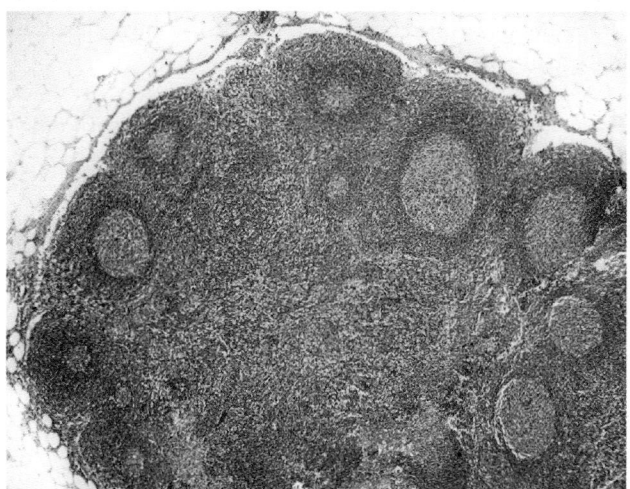

Figure 12.7 Right obturator lymph node (patient). Hematoxylin & eosin stain.

Questions

INTERMEDIATE

5. The biopsy specimen (Figs 12.1–12.3) of the prostate shows:

    a. acute prostatitis
    b. squamous metaplasia
    c. benign prostatic hypertrophy
    d. adenocarcinoma
    e. none of the above

INTERMEDIATE

6. The section of an excised pelvic lymph node (Fig. 12.7) shows:

    a. a metastatic carcinoma
    b. granulomatous changes
    c. a lymphoproliferative disorder
    d. a reactive lymph node

ADVANCED

7. The negative immunohistochemical staining for CK 903, a high molecular weight cytokeratin (Fig. 12.5), indicates:

    a. the lack of the basal cell layer of prostatic glands adjacent to the basement membrane
    b. the absence of an epithelial neoplasm
    c. the presence of a metastatic transitional cell carcinoma
    d. the presence of a mesenchymal neoplasm

INTERMEDIATE

8. In general, which of the following statements regarding the lesion depicted in Figs 12.1–12.3 is correct?

    a. it is associated with an elevated level of free PSA
    b. it is a disease that predominantly affects young men
    c. it is extremely common in Asian men
    d. all of the above statements are correct
    e. none of the above statements is correct

INTERMEDIATE

9. Which of the following statements about this patient's problems is correct?

    a. postoperative monitoring of the serum PSA level is valuable in assessing the response to therapy
    b. an elevated serum PSA level is virtually diagnostic of this prostatic lesion
    c. the histological findings in the pelvic lymph nodes indicate a worse prognosis for this prostatic disease
    d. all of the above statements are correct
    e. none of the above statements is correct

ANSWERS AND FURTHER INFORMATION

Figure descriptions

Figure 12.1 Prostate gland biopsy (patient). Hematoxylin & eosin stain.
Prostatic adenocarcinoma: Small glands with back-to-back arrangement are apparent in this image. Even at this magnification, the neoplastic glands appear to be lined by a single layer of low cuboidal epithelium.

Figure 12.2 Prostate gland biopsy (patient). Hematoxylin & eosin stain.
Prostatic adenocarcinoma: In this image the neoplastic prostatic glands are clearly lined by a single cell layer. The cells show hyperchromatic nuclei, an increased nuclear/cytoplasmic ratio, and prominent eosinophilic nucleoli. A mitotic figure is noted in this field.

Figure 12.3 Prostate gland biopsy (patient). Hematoxylin & eosin stain.
Prostatic adenocarcinoma: This photomicrograph shows a lymphatic space lined by endothelium, enclosing a cluster of malignant cells.

Figure 12.4 Prostate gland biopsy (normal). Hematoxylin & eosin stain.
This image shows a normal prostatic tissue with large irregular glands, lined by cuboidal to columnar epithelium, and surrounded by an intact flat basal layer (not apparent at this magnification).

Figure 12.5 Prostate gland biopsy (patient). CK 903 stain.
Prostatic adenocarcinoma: A section of the prostatic biopsy stained for CK 903, which is a high molecular weight cytokeratin, that would stain the basal cells. The negative staining in this section confirms the diagnosis of prostatic adenocarcinoma.

Figure 12.6 Prostate gland biopsy (normal). CK 903 stain.
A section of the normal prostatic tissue stained for CK 903. Normal prostatic glands have an intact basal layer and show positive staining with CK 903 antibodies.

Figure 12.7 Right obturator lymph node (patient).
Hematoxylin & eosin stain.
This image shows a normal reactive lymph node with intact and prominent lymphoid follicles, negative for metastatic carcinoma.

Answers

1. D. Absolute lymphocytosis is defined as a lymphocyte count of 4000 per µL (4×10^9/L) or more. Our patient has an absolute lymphocyte count of 2424 per µL (2.42×10^9/L). Chronic blood loss would lead to a microcytic hypochromic anemia. This patient has a mild normocytic normochromic anemia. Folate or vitamin B_{12} deficiency would be expected to cause a macrocytic anemia, which is not a finding here.

2. E. Hematuria may be caused by many disorders. The most common causes include tumors and inflammation of the urinary bladder, benign prostatic hypertrophy, kidney and bladder stones, kidney disease, and medications (e.g. quinine and phenytoin).

3. C. The sensitivity of the prostate-specific antigen (PSA) test for the diagnosis of prostatic carcinoma is about 80%, i.e. approximately 20% of patients with carcinoma of the prostate have PSA values within the "normal" range. It has a sensitivity of about 60% in the early stages of prostatic carcinoma. The test lacks specificity, since patients with benign prostatic hypertrophy have an increased PSA level in 50–60% of cases. The test is useful in monitoring for tumor recurrence.

4. C. Urinary frequency means voiding of small amounts of urine at frequent intervals. It does not have to be associated with polyuria, which is defined as the passing of more than 3 liters of urine per 24 hours. Urinary frequency not associated with polyuria is due to a sense of bladder fullness caused by an irritable, inflamed bladder.

5. D. Figs 12.1–12.3 show the growth of neoplastic glands invading the prostatic stroma. The sections show a moderately differentiated prostatic adenocarcinoma, composed of small to medium sized glands with irregular shape. The glands are packed together with little intervening stroma. The glands are lined by a single uniform layer of low columnar epithelium. The neoplastic cells exhibit large, vacuolated, and hyperchromatic nuclei with occasional large eosinophilic prominent nucleoli. Benign prostatic hypertrophy would show larger dilated glands with fibrous and muscular proliferation of the intervening stroma. The prostatic glands in benign prostatic hypertrophy are lined by two layers, an outer layer of flattened basal cells based on an intact basement membrane, and an inner cuboidal epithelium. Acute prostatitis would show prostatic gland lumina filled with acute inflammatory cells (neutrophils). Squamous metaplasia is not observed.

6. D. The lymph node (Fig. 12.7) shows a normal architecture with no evidence of metastatic carcinoma, lymphoproliferative disorder, or of granulomatous changes.

7. A. Cytokeratin 903 is a high-molecular-weight cytokeratin that identifies the prostatic basal cells. Negative immunohistochemical staining for CK 903 indicates a lack of prostatic basal cells and confirms the malignant nature of those glands.

8. E. The patient has an adenocarcinoma of the prostate, which, in general, is a disease of men over 50 years of age. Prostatic adenocarcinoma is extremely rare in Asians. Free PSA is the proportion of total PSA that circulates in the blood unbound to a protein carrier. Patients with elevated total PSA and an elevated level of free PSA (above 25%) usually have benign prostatic lesions.

9. A. The patient has an adenocarcinoma of the prostate. The pelvic lymph node shows a reactive pattern and is negative for carcinoma, which indicates a better prognosis for this patient. Elevated PSA level is not diagnostic of prostatic adenocarcinoma. Only about one-third of patients with PSA level between 4 and 10 ng/mL (µg/L) will show prostatic carcinoma. Postoperative monitoring of the serum PSA level is valuable in assessing the response to therapy and detecting recurrence and metastasis.

Final diagnosis and synopsis of the case

• Adenocarcinoma of the prostate

This 66-year-old patient has a prostatic adenocarcinoma. His original complaint, urinary frequency, combined with an increased circulating level of prostate specific antigen, led to the work-up of his prostatic problem, which was diagnosed as an adenocarcinoma of prostate. The exploration of pelvic lymph nodes for metastatic involvement (a staging procedure) revealed no evidence of metastatic carcinoma. The patient underwent radical prostatectomy and will be followed on an outpatient basis after his hospital discharge.

Lab tips

Tumor markers

Prostate-specific acid phosphatase (PSAP, PAP)

Prostate-specific acid phosphatase is one of several enzymes that hydrolyze phosphate esters in an acid environment. It can be measured in serum by hydrolysis of a substrate and subsequent determination of the reaction product spectrophotometrically. Since there are many non-prostatic sources of acid phosphatase, several different methodologies, utilizing different substrates and/or selective inhibitors, have been used to increase the specificity of this test and to exclude non-prostatic sources of acid phosphatase. Specific antibodies against PSAP are now available and immunohistochemical staining of tissue sections and cytological preparations is another method for the detection of PSAP. It is very useful in the differential diagnosis of poorly differentiated tumors involving the prostate gland, urinary bladder, and surrounding tissues.

Prostate-specific antigen (PSA)

Prostate-specific antigen is a protease present in prostatic duct cells. It is excreted in urine and seminal fluid. Serum levels reflect the total amount of prostatic tissue present.

CK 903

An antibody to CK 903, a high molecular weight cytokeratin, stains the basal cells. Negative staining in a prostatic biopsy indicates lack of the basal cell layer, which suggests a diagnosis of prostatic adenocarcinoma. The availability of such an antibody contributes to achieving a more definitive diagnosis of small foci of prostatic adenocarcinoma.

Table 12.7 Tartrate inhibition of serum acid phosphatases

Acid phosphatase	Sources	Comments
Tartrate-resistant acid phosphatase	Erythrocytes, osteoclasts, Gaucher cells, hairy cells	Acid phosphatase elevations in patients with cancers that have metastasized to bone and elevations in bone diseases are usually tartrate-resistant
Tartrate-sensitive acid phosphatase	Prostate gland, platelets, pancreas, granulocytes, lymphocytes	Significant acid phosphatase activity in vaginal specimens has been used to support the diagnosis of rape

Table 12.8 PSAP and PSA in patients with prostate cancer

	Usefulness	Caveats
Serum PSAP	Usually elevated in extension of tumor outside the gland. Usually normal in patients with tumor still confined to the gland	10–25% of patients with metastatic disease will have normal values. Methodology must exclude other sources of acid phosphatase. Elevated in benign prostatic hypertrophy, prostatic infarction, following prostatic biopsy or radiation therapy
Serum PSA	Increased sensitivity for diagnosis of prostatic carcinoma in patients with abnormal prostates or in elderly men. Useful in monitoring patients for residual or recurrent prostate cancer	Not useful as a screening test in the general population. Elevated in benign prostatic hypertrophy, prostatitis, urinary retention, and in some non-prostate tumors
PSAP/PSA (immunohistochemical staining)	Useful in the differential diagnosis of poorly differentiated tumors in the region of the prostate or in distant sites in which prostatic carcinoma is suspected	The tumor in question should always be stained for both as some prostate tumors are negative for PSAP and some are negative for PSA but very few are negative for both

A 30-year-old electrician with fever and vomiting

CASE AND MCQS

Clinical history and presentation

A 30-year-old electrician was rushed from a construction site by his friend to the emergency department complaining of intractable vomiting. He had been well until 36 hours ago when he developed fever, chills, malaise, and a burning sensation on urination. Over-the-counter analgesics offered some relief but for the past 12 hours he had had several episodes of vomiting watery fluid and had not been able to keep even clear liquids down. He denied recent travel or contact with persons having similar symptoms. His only other hospitalization was at the age of 8 for oral bleeding, when he was told that he had a β-thalassemia minor. He was born in Italy and has been in the United States for about 6 years. On physical examination he appeared thin and slightly dehydrated, with an oral temperature of 102.9°F (39.4°C), a blood pressure of 126/80 mmHg, a regular pulse rate of 110/min, and a respiratory rate of 20/min. Sclerae were non-icteric, conjunctivae were pink, and his mucous membranes were dry. His lungs were clear, the abdomen was soft without masses, tenderness, or organomegaly. Bowel sounds were present. Brown stool, which was guaiac negative, was present in the rectal ampulla. No peripheral lymphadenopathy was noted.

Admission data

Table 13.1 Hematology

			SI Units	
WBC	17.4 H	(3.3–11.0 thou/µL)	17.4 H	(3.3–11.0 × 10⁹/L)
Neut	86	(44–88%)	86	(44–88%)
Band	4	(0–10%)	4	(0–10%)
Lymph	7 L	(12–43%)	7 L	(12–43%)
Mono	3	(2–11%)	3	(2–11%)
Eos	0	(0–5%)	0	(0–5%)
Baso	0	(0–2%)	0	(0–2%)
RBC	6.69 H	(3.9–5.0 mill/µL)	6.69 H	(3.9–5.0 × 10¹²/L)
HGB	11.0 L	(11.6–15.6 g/dL)	110 L	(116–156 g/L)
HCT	40	(37.0–47.0%)	0.4	(0.37–0.47)
MCV	59.8 L	(79.0–99.0 fL)	59.8 L	(79.0–99.0 fL)
MCH	16.4 L	(26.0–32.6 pg)	16.4 L	(26.0–32.6 pg)
MCHC	27.5 L	(31.0–36.0 g/dL)	275 L	(310–360 g/L)
RDW	16.8 H	(11.50–14.50%)	16.8 H	(11.50–14.50%)
Plts	341	(130–400 thou/µL)	341	(130–400 × 10⁹/L)

Table 13.2 Chemistry

			SI Units	
Glucose	110	(65–110 mg/dL)	6.7	(3.6–6.11 mmol/L)
Creatinine	1.3	(0.7–1.4 mg/dL)	11.5	(61.9–123.76 µmol/L)
BUN	6 L	(7–24 mg/dL)	2.14 L	(2.50–8.57 mmol/L)
Uric acid	5.0	(3.0–8.5 mg/dL)	0.30	(0.18–0.51 mmol/L)
Cholesterol	157	(150–200 mg/dL)	4.1	(3.88–5.17 mmol/L)
Calcium	9.0	(8.5–10.5 mg/dL)	2.25	(2.13–2.63 mmol/L)
Protein	7.3	(6–8 g/dL)	73	(60–80 g/L)
Albumin	4.7	(3.7–5.0 g/dL)	47	(37–50 g/L)
LDH	156	(100–250 U/L)	156	(100–250 U/L)
Alk Phos	60	(0–120 U/L)	60	(0–120 U/L)
AST	6	(0–55 U/L)	6	(0–55 U/L)
GGTP	6	(0–50 U/L)	6	(0–50 U/L)
Bilirubin	3.3 H	(0.0–1.5 mg/dL)	56.4 H	(0–25.7 µmol/L)
Bilirubin-direct	0.32 H	(0.02–0.18 mg/dL)	5.47 H	(0.34–3.08 µmol/L)
Amylase	36	(13–85 U/L)	0.61	(0.22–1.45 µkat/L)

Table 13.3 Electrolytes

			SI Units	
Na	137	(134–143 mEq/L)	137	(134–143 mmol/L)
K	3.5	(3.5–4.9 mEq/L)	3.5	(3.5–4.9 mmol/L)
Cl	102	(95–108 mEq/L)	102	(95–108 mmol/L)
CO_2	26	(21–32 mEq/L)	26	(21–32 mmol/L)

Table 13.4 Urinalysis

pH	8.0 H	(5.0–7.5)
Protein	Neg	(Neg)
Glucose	Neg	(Neg)
Ketone	Neg	(Neg)
Blood	Neg	(Neg)
Color	Yellow	(Yellow)
Clarity	Cloudy	(Clear)
Sp. grav.	1.017	(1.010–1.035)
WBC	25 H	(0–5/HPF)
RBC	0	(0–2/HPF)
Urobilinogen	2+ H	(Neg)
Bacteria	3+ H	(Neg)

Table 13.5 Microbiology

Urine cultures	Pending
Stool cultures	Pending
Blood cultures	Pending

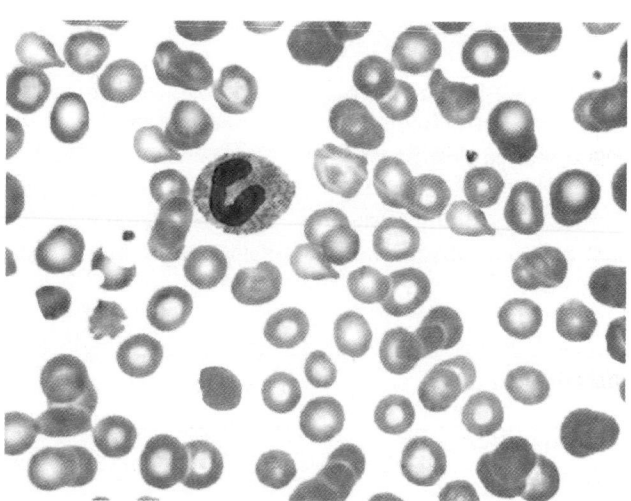

Figure 13.1 Peripheral blood smear. Wright/Giemsa stain.

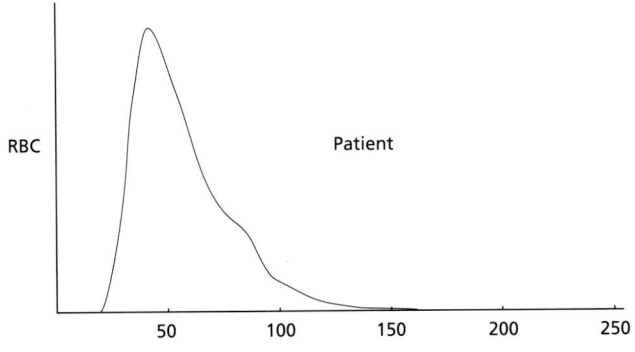

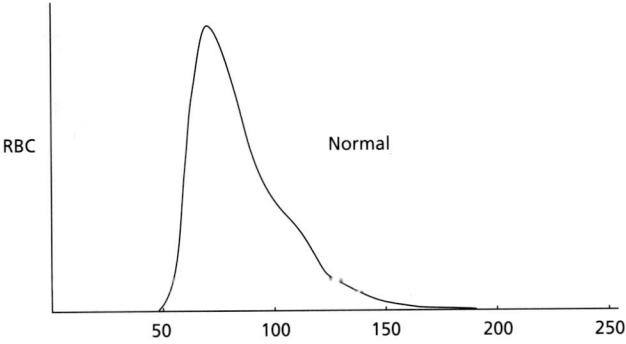

Figure 13.2 Red blood cell volume distribution histograms.

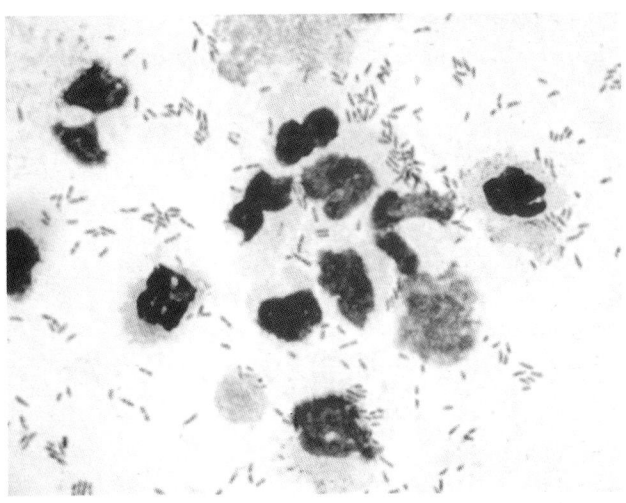

Figure 13.3 Urine sediment smear (patient). Giemsa stain.

Questions

On the basis of the preceding information, you can best conclude the following:

1. In general, a leukocyte count such as seen in this patient can be seen in which of the following conditions?

   a. intestinal obstruction
   b. acute appendicitis
   c. malaria
   d. urinary tract infection
   e. all of the above

2. This patient's admission hematological findings, including the peripheral blood smear (Fig. 13.1), are most consistent with:

   a. malaria due to *Plasmodium vivax*
   b. hemolytic anemia secondary to chemical poisoning
   c. pernicious anemia
   d. hemoglobin C disease
   e. none of the above

3. Which of the following statements concerning the red cell distribution width (RDW) in general, is correct?

   a. it is elevated in vitamin B_{12} deficiency
   b. it is elevated in iron deficiency anemia
   c. it reflects the degree of anisocytosis
   d. it may be elevated in thalassemia minor
   e. all of the above

4. Which of the following conditions is the most likely cause of this patient's elevated bilirubin?

   a. acute viral hepatitis
   b. alcoholic cirrhosis
   c. acute cholecystitis with cholelithiasis
   d. carcinoma of the head of the pancreas
   e. none of the above

5. A low blood urea nitrogen (BUN) can usually be seen in all of the following conditions EXCEPT:

  a. severe liver disease
  b. pregnancy
  c. low protein diet
  d. gastrointestinal hemorrhage
  e. inappropriate vasopressin (AVP) secretion

6. Which of the following statements concerning the admission urinalysis or the urine sediment smear seen in Fig. 13.3 is correct?

  a. a majority of WBCs seen in Fig. 13.3 are neutrophils
  b. the patient has pyuria
  c. the increased urinary leukocytes reflect a urinary tract infection
  d. the increase in urinary urobilinogen may be due to fever
  e. all of the above

Clinical course

The patient was started on intravenous hydration, and placed on appropriate medication. A surgical consultation ruled out an acute surgical problem. By the second day he had improved markedly and was able to take clear liquids without vomiting. Mild scleral icterus was noted at this time. That night he was started on a BRAT (bananas, rice, apple-sauce, and tea toast) diet, which he tolerated without vomiting. Additional laboratory tests are shown below. The patient was instructed about his problems and was discharged.

Table 13.6 Special hematology

			SI Units	
Retic	1.8	(0.1–2.0%)	1.8	(0.1–2.0%)
Iron	65	(42–135 µg/dL)	11.6	(7.5–24.2 µmol/L)
TIBC	295	(280–400 µg/dL)	52.8	(50.1–71.6 µmol/L)
Transferrin sat.	22	(15–50%)	0.22	(0.15–0.50)
Serum ferritin	245	(7–350 ng/mL)	245	(7–350 µg/L)
Serum haptoglobin	265	(60–270 mg/dL)	2650	(600–2700 mg/L)

Table 13.7 Chemistry (day 2)

			SI Units	
Glucose	101	(65–110 mg/dL)	5.61	(3.6–6.11 mmol/L)
Creatinine	1.1	(0.7–1.4 mg/dL)	97.2	(61.9–123.76 µmol/L)
BUN	6 L	(7–24 mg/dL)	2.14 L	(2.50–8.57 mmol/L)
Uric acid	3.9	(3.0–8.5 mg/dL)	0.23	(0.18–0.51 mmol/L)
Cholesterol	150	(150–200 mg/dL)	3.88	(3.88–5.17 mmol/L)
Calcium	8.5	(8.5–10.5 mg/dL)	2.3	(2.13–2.63 mmol/L)
Protein	6.5	(6–8 g/dL)	65	(60–80 g/L)
Albumin	4.0	(3.7–5.0 g/dL)	40	(37–50 g/L)
LDH	154	(100–250 U/L)	154	(100–250 U/L)
Alk Phos	55	(0–120 U/L)	55	(0–120 U/L)
AST	10	(0–55 U/L)	10	(0–55 U/L)
GGTP	17	(0–50 U/L)	17	(0–50 U/L)
Bilirubin	4.0 H	(0.0–1.5 mg/dL)	68.4 H	(0–25.7 µmol/L)
Bilirubin-direct	0.36 H	(0.02–0.18 mg/dL)	4.16 H	(0.34–3.08 µmol/L)

Table 13.8 Microbiology

Urine cultures	>100 000 colonies/mL *Proteus mirabilis*
Stool cultures	No enteric pathogens isolated
Blood cultures	Negative

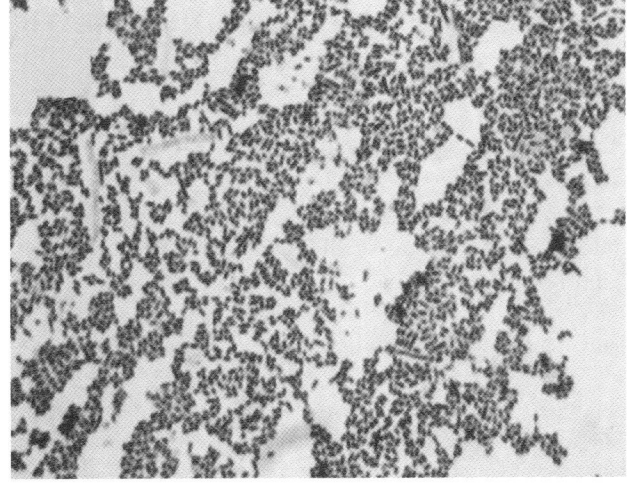

Figure 13.4 Urine culture (patient). Gram stain.

Questions

7. The most likely mechanism of this patient's bilirubin disorder is:

    a. partial deficiency of bilirubin glucuronosyl transferase

    b. familial defect in hepatic excretion of bilirubin

    c. extrahepatic biliary obstruction

    d. hepatocellular disease

    e. none of the above

8. The underlying disorder causing this patient's abnormal bilirubin level:

    a. is a common benign liver disorder

    b. is associated with normal liver aminotransferases

    c. does not require treatment

    d. is most likely a hereditary disorder

    e. all the above statements are correct

9. Which of the following statements concerning the liver problem such as this patient has is NOT correct?

    a. jaundice appears with serum bilirubin level above 2 mg/dL (34.2 μmol/L)

    b. the serum level of bilirubin fluctuates

    c. the primarily increased type of bilirubin is readily excreted into urine

    d. the primarily increased type of bilirubin is bound to serum albumin and transported to the liver

10. All of the following statements concerning this patient's hematological disease are true EXCEPT:

    a. it is characterized by decreased production of ß-globins

    b. Hgb F is elevated in about 30% of patients with this disease

    c. there is increased formation of α_2,δ_2-globin dimers

    d. the patient will eventually develop hypersplenism

    e. the disease has a broad geographic distribution

11. All of the following statements concerning the patient's urinary tract problem are correct EXCEPT:

    a. the organism isolated from his urine and depicted in Fig. 13.4 has been associated with the formation of renal stones

    b. the organism isolated from his urine has been associated with enteritis

    c. the patient's urinary tract problem is not frequently seen in otherwise healthy young men

    d. the patient's bilirubin abnormality is associated with an increased frequency of his urinary tract problem

    e. the patient's hematological abnormality played no role in his urinary tract problem

ANSWERS AND FURTHER INFORMATION

Figure descriptions

Figure 13.1 Peripheral blood smear (patient). Wright/Giemsa stain.
Microcytic hypochromic anemia: The red blood cells show mild to moderate aniso-poikilocytosis. Multiple teardrop, hypochromatic red blood cell, bite cells, schistocytes, target cells, and spherocytes are seen in this image. Also seen are a band neutrophil and a number of platelets.

Figure 13.2 Red blood cell volume distribution histogram.
The upper image shows the distribution histogram of the patient's red blood cell volume. The patient's MCV (mean corpuscular volume) lies closer to 50 fL than to the 100 fL mark (actual MCV = 59.8 fL). The red cell distribution width (RDW) is an index of the variation in red blood cell volume. RDW = (standard deviation of red cell volume ÷ mean cell volume) × 100. The lower image shows the distribution histogram of another patient with normal red blood cell mean corpuscular volume (MCV) for comparison.

Figure 13.3 Urine sediment smear (patient). Giemsa stain.
This photomicrograph shows numerous aggregates of short rods, neutrophils, and necrotic debris.

Figure 13.4 Urine culture (patient). Gram stain.
This is a photomicrograph of a Gram stain of the organism recovered from the urine culture. It shows numerous small, Gram-negative, pleomorphic rods, which biochemically were proven to be *Proteus mirabilis*.

Answers

1. E. This patient has a leukocytosis, which is an increase in the total (absolute) number of white blood cells. It is, as is seen here, usually due to an absolute increase in the number of neutrophils (neutrophilia). Because the white blood cell differential count gives only the gross relative frequency of each white blood cell type and since each white blood cell type has its own control mechanisms, it is sometimes useful to determine the absolute number of the various types of white blood cells rather than their percentage. All of the listed conditions can produce a leukocytosis. Although patients with malaria usually develop leukopenia and neutropenia, borderline leukocytosis may be present during acute attacks, and frank leukocytosis may develop in overwhelmingly severe disease. Leukocytosis may be seen in intestinal obstruction and frequently shows a left shift when strangulation is present. One of the criteria used for the diagnosis of acute appendicitis is

an elevated white blood cell count with increased numbers of band neutrophils. Acute gastrointestinal hemorrhage is frequently accompanied by an elevated white blood cell count, and there may also be a "left shift" (an increase in the proportion of circulating immature myeloid cells). The etiology of most urinary tract infections is bacterial and they may be accompanied by a leukocytosis (especially with upper urinary tract infections).

2. E. None of the listed conditions is consistent with the admission complete blood count and peripheral blood smear morphology. The hematological data define a microcytic (decreased MCV), hypochromic (decreased MCH) anemia (decreased HGB). On the peripheral blood smear the red blood cells are small, hypochromic, and show mild anisocytosis and poikilocytosis. A teardrop-shaped erythrocyte (dacryocyte) containing a number of bluish, irregularly shaped granules of different size is present. This is an example of basophilic stippling. The granules are composed of aggregates of ribosomes, and although they can be seen in pernicious anemia, the anemia would then be macrocytic and not microcytic in nature. Basophilic stippling can also be found in lead poisoning, thalassemia, and refractory anemia. It should not be confused with Shuffner's granules, which are much smaller, purplish-red granules found in the erythrocytes of patients with *Plasmodium vivax* malaria, an example of an acquired hemolytic anemia, which usually is normocytic, normochromic in nature. In hemolytic anemias due to chemical poisonings, again usually normocytic and normochromic in nature, precipitates of denatured hemoglobin (Heinz bodies) may occur, but they are not visible with the Wright/Giemsa stain. These are single or multiple, refractile irregular bodies that can be demonstrated by the use of a supravital dye such as new methylene blue. In hemoglobin C disease, erythrocyte morphology is markedly abnormal with prominent target erythrocytes. One can also usually find red blood cells distorted by hemoglobin C crystals. These features are not seen in Fig. 13.1.

3. E. The RDW, which is minimally elevated in this patient, is the coefficient of variation of the red cell volume distribution (the red cell volume histogram, Fig. 13.2) and is a measure of the heterogeneity of the distribution of red cell size. Thus, it reflects the degree of anisocytosis of the red blood cell population seen on the patient's peripheral blood smear (Fig. 13.1). It is almost always elevated in anemias due to a nutritional deficiency (i.e. vitamin B_{12}, folate, or iron) and is slightly elevated in thalassemia minor when anemia is present. It is usually normal in the anemia of chronic disease and other hypoproliferative anemias.

4. E. The patient has a small elevation in total bilirubin. While part of that is due to an increase in direct bilirubin, the bulk of the elevation appears to be due to unconjugated bilirubin. All of the listed conditions would most likely be associated with significant increases in bilirubin and/or liver enzyme elevations, but our patient's liver enzymes are normal. The cholestasis seen in acute cholecystitis with cholelithiasis and carcinoma of the head of the pancreas is that of extrahepatic biliary obstruction and results in significant elevations in both conjugated bilirubin and serum alkaline phosphatase. Acute viral hepatitis results in hepatocellular damage with elevations in both conjugated and unconjugated bilirubin as well as marked elevations in aspartate amino transferase (AST) and lactate dehydrogenase (LDH). Although the serum bilirubin may only be minimally elevated in cirrhosis, there is usually elevation of the liver enzymes, mainly gamma glutamyl transferase (GGTP), AST, and alkaline phosphatase.

5. D. The blood urea nitrogen (BUN) is usually elevated in significant gastrointestinal hemorrhage due to hypovolemia and increased protein catabolism. All of the other listed conditions (severe liver disease, pregnancy, low protein diet, inappropriate vasopressin (AVP) secretion) usually result in a decreased BUN. In severe liver disease, urea synthesis is decreased due to impairment of the urea cycle. In pregnancy there is often a temporary increase in the glomerular filtration rate, and since urea is freely filtered by the glomeruli, this often leads to increased excretion of urea and a decreased BUN. Decreased urea synthesis may also be seen in patients on a low protein diet. Vasopressin, synthesized in the anterior hypothalamus, acts on the distal tubular epithelium to concentrate urine resulting in the plasma dilution of a number of analytes, including urea nitrogen.

6. E. All of the listed options are correct. The majority of the cells seen in Fig. 13.3 are neutrophils. Pyuria is defined as an increased number of leukocytes in urine to more than 20 leukocytes per high-power field. Increased number of urinary leukocytes can be seen in almost any urinary tract disease and even after strenuous exercise, but our patient's history and presentation point toward an acute urinary tract infection. Urinary urobilinogen is often increased in patients with fever, presumably due to dehydration and a more concentrated urine.

7. A. This patient has Gilbert's syndrome, a hereditary condition characterized by mild (often unnoticed by the patient), unconjugated hyperbilirubinemia that is slightly increased by fasting and in infections. Liver enzymes are typically normal and a liver biopsy, which is usually not necessary in this disease, shows essentially normal histology. The mild elevation in the patient's serum bilirubin, which was mainly due to the unconjugated fraction, the normal liver enzymes, and the increased serum bilirubin are all consistent with this diagnosis. Although the disease is usually due to a partial deficiency of bilirubin glucuronosyl transferase, some patients exhibit a decreased hepatic uptake of bilirubin. Defects in the hepatic excretion of bilirubin (Dubin–Johnson syndrome, drug-induced cholestasis, obstruction of the biliary system by tumor, gallstones, etc.) are usually accompanied by elevations of both conjugated and unconjugated bilirubin, the presence of bilirubin in the urine, and the finding of pigment deposition or inflammation in the liver biopsy. In hepatocellular disease (viral or chemical hepatitis, cirrhosis), the elevated serum bilirubin is mainly due to the conjugated fraction, the liver biopsy is distinctly abnormal, and urine bilirubin may or may not be present depending on the stage of the disease.

8. E. This patient has Gilbert's syndrome. Gilbert's syndrome is a common benign hereditary liver disorder due to a partial deficiency of bilirubin glucuronosyl transferase. Gilbert's syndrome rarely requires any treatment.

9. C. Clinically evident jaundice is expected with an increase of serum bilirubin level over 2 mg/dL (34.2 μmol/L). In Gilbert's syndrome, the hyperbilirubinemia is usually mild and is fluctuating. There is a hereditary reduction in the hepatic bilirubin glucuronidating activity to about one-third of that of normal people. This leads to increase of unconjugated bilirubin, which is tightly bound to serum albumin and cannot be excreted in the urine.

10. D. The findings in this patient of a mild anemia with a decreased MCV, red blood cells showing basophilic stippling, and an increased red blood cell count are strongly suggestive of ß-thalassemia minor or ß-thalassemia trait. The elevated Hgb A_2, which is composed of α_2,δ_2-globin dimers, reflects the decreased production of ß-globins and confirms the diagnosis. About one-third of patients with ß-thalassemia minor will also have a slightly elevated Hgb F. The disease has a wide distribution extending from the countries surrounding the Mediterranean Sea (Greece, Italy, Northern Africa) through the Middle East and into Southeast Asia. The ß-thalassemias are a heterogeneous group of disorders that can be essentially asymptomatic when there is reduced or absent expression of one ß gene (ß-thalassemia minor or trait) or they can present with severe anemia when there is reduced expression or absence of both ß genes (ß-thalassemia major). Hypersplenism develops in most patients with ß-thalassemia major but is usually not seen in ß-thalassemia minor.

11. D. Our patient has an acute bacterial urinary tract infection, caused by the Gram-negative bacterium *Proteus mirabilis*. This organism is a frequent cause of urinary tract infections and has been associated with enteritis. It is a strong urease producer, converting urea to carbon dioxide and ammonia, raising the urine pH, which in turn facilitates the formation of struvite stones. Acute bacterial urinary tract infections are far more common in young women than in young men, and when seen in young men may indicate a structural voiding problem, or some underlying condition associated with increased susceptibility to infection such as diabetes mellitus, malignancy, or AIDS. Since none of these conditions exists in this patient, this case illustrates the fact that acute urinary tract infections can sometimes occur in otherwise healthy young men. The patient's bilirubin abnormality is due to Gilbert's syndrome and his hematological abnormality is due to ß-thalassemia minor, neither of which played a role in his urinary tract infection.

Final diagnosis and synopsis of the case

- Acute urinary tract infection (*Proteus mirabilis*)
- Gastroenteritis (etiology undetermined)
- β-Thalassemia minor with microcytic hypochromic anemia
- Gilbert's syndrome

A 30-year-old male with a past history of ß-thalassemia minor, presented with fever, leukocytosis, and intractable vomiting of 12 hours' duration. For the past 2 days he had been complaining of dysuria. When <100 000 colonies/ml of *Proteus mirabilis* were found on the admission urine culture, the diagnosis of acute bacterial urinary tract infection, most likely cystitis, was confirmed. He was given an appropriate antibiotic and started on intravenous hydration. It was felt that the vomiting was most likely due to gastroenteritis, but an etiologic agent was not identified. *Proteus mirabilis* is known to be associated with enteritis and may have been the etiologic agent. Also noted on admission was a mild microcytic, hypochromic anemia with an elevated red blood cell count, and basophilic stippled red cells in the peripheral smear, consistent with the patient's history of ß-thalassemia minor. The diagnosis of ß-thalassemia minor was later confirmed by the finding of an elevated hemoglobin A$_2$ level on hemoglobin electrophoresis (not shown here). The patient's mild hyperbilirubinemia (mainly unconjugated), which increased during his illness (with fever and fasting), the presence of normal liver enzymes, and the lack of significant evidence of hemolysis (normal LDH, normal haptoglobin, normal reticulocyte count) rule out most of the possible causes of hyperbilirubinemia. While it is true that the thalassemias are hemolytic anemias, most patients with ß-thalassemia minor do not show signs of hemolysis. The increased urinary urobilinogen was most likely due to his fever because of the dehydration and concentrated urine that tend to be seen with an elevated temperature. By exclusion we are left with a diagnosis of Gilbert's syndrome, a hereditary condition mainly due to a partial deficiency of bilirubin glucuronosyl transferase. Counseling on discharge reassured him that his anemia is mild and unlikely to result in any significant complications, and that his hyperbilirubinemia might increase slightly during periods of fasting and should not be a cause for concern.

Lab tips

Bilirubin

The majority of bilirubin is derived from the breakdown of hemoglobin. At the end of their life span, red blood cells are removed from the circulation by the reticuloendothelial system, and the hemoglobin contained within them is broken down to heme and globin. The heme part is split into biliverdin and iron. Biliverdin will then be converted to bilirubin.

Bilirubin formed outside the liver is bound to serum albumin (unconjugated bilirubin) and transported to the liver.

Bilirubin arriving at the liver is lipid soluble. In the hepatocytes the bilirubin will be conjugated with glucuronic acid. Conjugated bilirubin (water soluble and non-toxic) is excreted into bile. Conjugated bilirubin is deconjugated and degraded to colorless urobilinogens by bacterial beta-glucuronidases in the gastrointestinal tract. A large proportion of urobilinogens and the remaining intact bile pigments are excreted in the stool. Some (20%) urobilinogens and pigments are reabsorbed from the gastrointestinal tract and returned to the liver (enterohepatic circulation).

A small amount of urobilinogens and the residue of intact pigments that escapes removal from the blood by the liver and re-excretion into bile reaches the kidney through the systemic circulation and is excreted in the urine.

The liver also secretes bile acids into bile. Ten to twenty percent of those acids are deconjugated by bacterial action in the gastrointestinal tract. Almost all conjugated and deconjugated bile acids are reabsorbed, mainly in the ileum, and returned to the liver (enterohepatic circulation).

Laboratory findings in jaundice

Hepatic jaundice (intrahepatic obstruction):
- Increased circulating conjugated bilirubin
- Increased bilirubin in urine (dark urine)
- Decreased bilirubin, urobilinogens, and bile pigments in stool (clay-colored stool)

Obstructive jaundice (no bile reaches the gastrointestinal tract):
- Increased circulating conjugated bilirubin
- Increased bilirubin in urine
- Decreased urobilinogen in urine
- Markedly decreased bilirubin, urobilinogens, and bile pigments in stool (clay-colored stool)
- No bile salts (fatty stool, deficiency of fat-soluble vitamins)

Hemolytic jaundice:
- Increased mainly unconjugated bilirubin in blood
- Increased urobilinogen in urine
- No bile pigment in urine (acholuric jaundice)
- Dark stool (increased bile pigments)

A 30-year-old singer who could not open his mouth

CASE AND MCQS

Clinical history and presentation

A 30-year-old man presented with the complaint of severe pain and swelling of his right cheek, which was preventing him from eating, talking, and singing. His medical history includes a long-standing seasonal sinusitis and a 6-month history of episodic burning pain in his feet, which is usually relieved by cold compresses. This burning sensation was associated with redness and a mottled appearance of the affected foot. The patient is a heavy smoker and admits to excessive alcohol consumption for at least 10 years. At present he is not employed. The family history is non-contributory. Physical examination revealed a disheveled man in acute distress due to his cheek pain. He answered questions with a visible effort. The vital signs were: temperature 101.2°F (38.4°C), blood pressure 130/88 mmHg, pulse 84/min and regular. Pertinent findings included: a red, warm, and swollen right cheek, extremely tender to palpation. Examination of the oral cavity revealed dental caries and poor oral hygiene. The chest was clear, the abdomen was soft with no organomegaly present. The rectal examination revealed a guaiac-positive stool. The examination of extremities did not reveal any abnormalities; peripheral pulses were normal.

Admission data

Table 14.1 Hematology

			SI Units	
WBC	18.6 H	(3.3–11.0 thou/μL)	18.6 H	(3.3–11.0 × 10⁹/L)
Neut	66	(44–88%)	66	(44–88%)
Band	15 H	(0–10%)	15 H	(0–10%)
Lymph	11.7 L	(12–43%)	11.7 L	(12–43%)
Mono	4	(2–11%)	4	(2–11%)
Eos	2.3	(0–5%)	2.3	(0–5%)
Baso	0	(0–2%)	0	(0–2%)
RBC	3.77 L	(3.9–5.0 mill/μL)	3.77 L	(3.9–5.0 × 10¹²/L)
HGB	10.6 L	(11.6–15.6 g/dL)	106 L	(116–156 g/L)
HCT	31.1 L	(37.0–47.0%)	0.311 L	(0.37–0.47)
MCV	82.5	(79.0–99.0 fL)	82.5	(79.0–99.0 fL)
MCH	28	(26.0–32.6 pg)	28	(26.0–32.6 pg)
MCHC	33.9	(31.0–36.0 g/dL)	339	(310–360 g/L)
Plts	1529 H	(130–400 thou/μL)	1529 H	(130–400 × 10⁹/L)

Table 14.2 Chemistry

			SI Units	
Glucose	90	(65–110 mg/dL)	5	(3.6–6.11 mmol/L)
Creatinine	0.7	(0.7–1.4 mg/dL)	61.9	(61.9–123.76 µmol/L)
BUN	9	(7–24 mg/dL)	3.21	(2.50–8.57 mmol/L)
Uric acid	5.1	(3.0–8.5 mg/dL)	0.30	(0.18–0.51 mmol/L)
Cholesterol	185	(150–200 mg/dL)	4.08	(3.88–5.17 mmol/L)
Calcium	8.9	(8.5–10.5 mg/dL)	2.23	(2.13–2.63 mmol/L)
Protein	6.2	(6–8 g/dL)	62	(60–80 g/L)
Albumin	3.7	(3.7–5.0 g/dL)	37	(37–50 g/L)
LDH	138	(100–250 U/L)	138	(100–250 U/L)
Alk Phos	115	(0–120 U/L)	115	(0–120 U/L)
AST	7	(0–55 U/L)	7	(0–55 U/L)
GGTP	49	(0–50 U/L)	49	(0–50 U/L)
Bilirubin	0.3	(0.0–1.5 mg/dL)	5.1	(0–25.7 µmol/L)
Bilirubin-direct	0.02	(0.02–0.18 mg/dL)	0.34	(0.34–3.08 µmol/L)
Amylase	30	(13–85 U/L)	0.51	(0.22–1.45 µkat/L)

Table 14.3 Electrolytes

			SI Units	
Na	143	(134–143 mEq/L)	143	(134–143 mmol/L)
K	4.3	(3.5–4.9 mEq/L)	4.3	(3.5–4.9 mmol/L)
Cl	102	(95–108 mEq/L)	102	(95–108 mmol/L)
CO_2	28	(21–32 mEq/L)	28	(21–32 mmol/L)

Table 14.4 Urinalysis

pH	6	(5.0–7.5)
Protein	Neg	(Neg)
Glucose	Neg	(Neg)
Ketone	Neg	(Neg)
Color	Yellow	(Yellow)
Clarity	Turbid	(Clear)
Sp. grav.	1.027	(1.010–1.035)
WBC	0	(0–5/HPF)
RBC	0	(0–2/HPF)
Casts	Neg	(Neg)
Bacteria	Neg	(Neg)

Table 14.5 Chest X-ray

Normal

Table 14.6 X-ray of sinuses

Right maxillary sinus: opacification and air fluid level
Left maxillary sinus: mucosal thickening

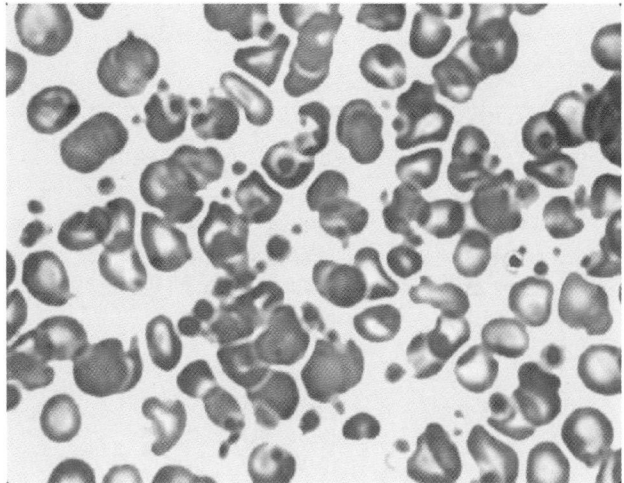

Figure 14.1 Peripheral blood smear (patient). Wright/Giemsa stain.

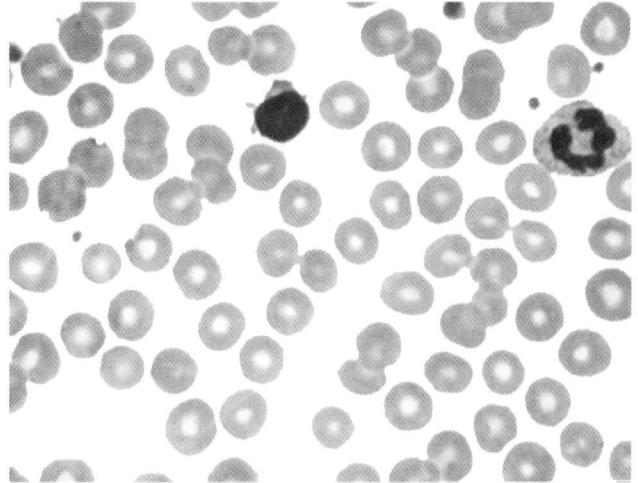

Figure 14.2 Peripheral blood smear (normal). Wright/Giemsa stain.

Questions

Based on the above information you can best conclude the following:

INTERMEDIATE

1. A painful facial problem such as this patient has:

    a. is most likely of bacterial origin
    b. is often preceded by rhinitis
    c. suggests an impairment of the sinus drainage
    d. can originate from a periapical infection
    e. all of the above statements are correct

ADVANCED

2. The burning foot pain in this patient:

    a. is likely to be related to his facial problem
    b. is likely to be related to his increased WBC count
    c. is likely to be related to his relative lymphopenia
    d. is likely to be related to his increased platelet count
    e. in general, none of the above conditions is known to be associated with this type of pain

INTERMEDIATE

3. The finding of occult blood in the patient's stool:

    a. may be related to the increased platelet count
    b. may be due to a yet unidentified intestinal inflammatory disease
    c. may be related to the patient's alcoholic abuse
    d. may be related to any of the above

INTERMEDIATE

4. Which of the following statements about the peripheral blood smear and/or the CBC (FBC) findings of this patient is correct?

    a. the WBC count most likely reflects bacterial infection
    b. the platelet distribution width (PDW) will be increased
    c. a flow cytometric lymphocyte analysis is not indicated at this time
    d. iron studies are indicated
    e. all of the above

INTERMEDIATE

5. Identify the INCORRECT statement about an increased platelet count in general:

    a. it can be caused by a myeloproliferative disorder
    b. it is one of the most common hematologic manifestations of AIDS
    c. it can be associated with inflammatory bowel disease
    d. it is seen in patients with malignancies
    e. it is commonly seen in chronic infections

Clinical course

A needle aspiration of the right maxillary sinus was performed, and the contents were sent for bacterial culture, which was positive for *Staphylococcus aureus*. Maxillary sinus content is shown in Figure 14.6. Blood cultures were negative. The patient was started on antibiotic treatment; the sinus, however, had to be surgically drained 2 days later. Repeated CBC (FBC) showed the WBC count to be decreasing, but the platelet numbers remained high (ranges from 1300 to 1500 thou cells/μL ($\times 10^9$/L)). Following the resolution of his acute facial problem, additional work-up was scheduled. A bone marrow biopsy was done, and the results are shown in Figs 14.3 and 14.4. Additional laboratory tests were performed (Tables 14.8–14.11). A work-up of his gastrointestinal bleeding was scheduled.

Table 14.7 Erythrocyte sedimentation rate

ESR	34 H	(0–20 mm/hr)

Table 14.8 Special hematology

			SI Units	
Retic	1.5	(0.1–2.0%)	1.5	(0.1–2.0%)
Iron	70	(42–135 μg/dL)	14.0	(7.5–24.2 μmol/L)
TIBC	320	(280–400 μg/dL)	57.3	(50.1–71.6 μmol/L)
Transferrin sat.	23	(15–50%)	0.23	(0.15–0.50)
Ferritin	305 H	(7–250 ng/mL)	305 H	(7–250 μg/L)
Haptoglobin	146	(38–270 mg/dL)	1460	(380–2700 mg/L)

Table 14.9 Bleeding time

Bleeding Time	8	(2–9 min)

Table 14.10 Platelet count

Plts	1530 H	(130–400 thou/μL)

Table 14.11 Platelet aggregation studies

Unresponsive to epinephrine; others within normal range

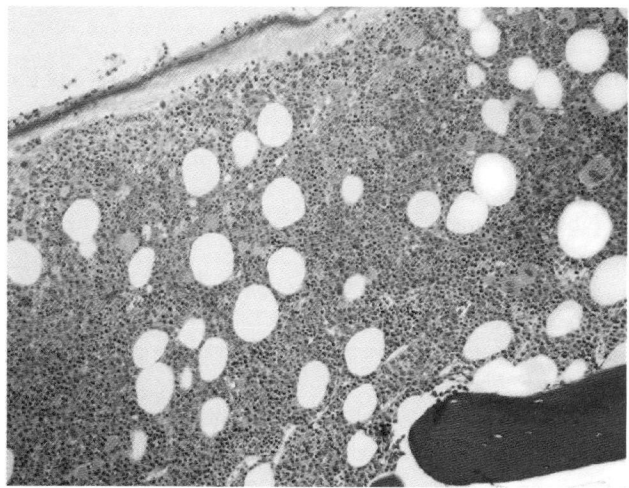

Figure 14.3 Bone marrow biopsy (patient). Hematoxylin & eosin stain.

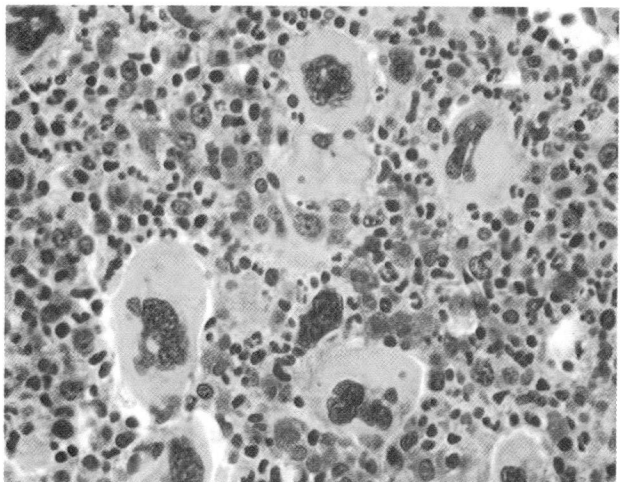

Figure 14.4 Bone marrow biopsy (patient). Hematoxylin & eosin stain.

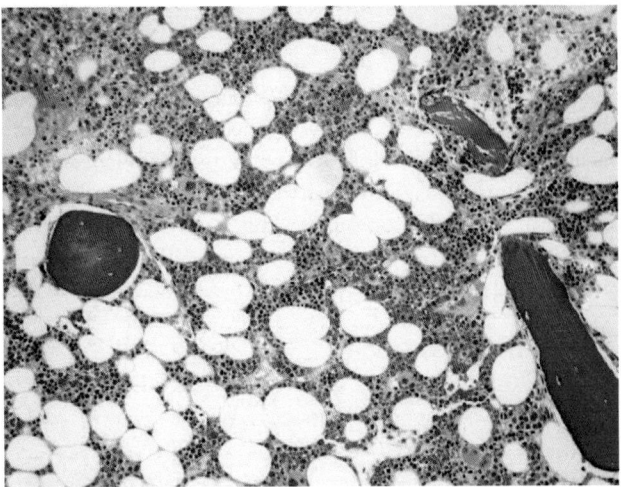

Figure 14.5 Bone marrow biopsy (normal). Hematoxylin & eosin stain.

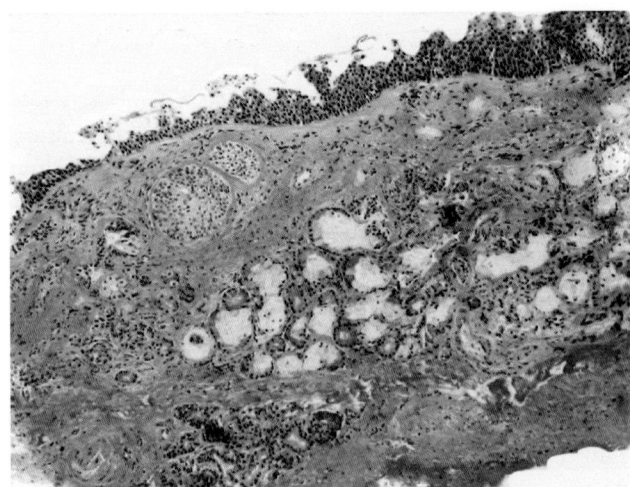

Figure 14.6 Maxillary sinus content (patient). Hematoxylin & eosin stain.

Questions

INTERMEDIATE

6. The bone marrow appearance (Figs 14.3 and 14.4) is consistent with:

a. aplastic anemia
b. acute lymphoblastic leukemia
c. myelofibrosis
d. granulomatous process involving bone marrow
e. none of the above

INTERMEDIATE

7. The major complications of the condition leading to a high platelet count such as is seen in this patient include all of the following EXCEPT:

a. transformation to acute leukemia
b. thrombosis
c. hemorrhage
d. hypertension
e. microvascular ischemia

INTERMEDIATE

8. Identify the INCORRECT statement about this platelet disorder:

a. this disorder typically affects patients between the ages of 50 and 70
b. it is best characterized as a clonal disorder
c. a loss of *in vitro* platelet aggregation response to epinephrine is a frequent finding in this disorder
d. the bone marrow characteristically shows myelofibrosis
e. iron deficiency is not a feature of this disorder

ADVANCED

9. Identify an INCORRECT statement about platelets in general:

a. in a healthy individual, approximately 20% of platelets circulate, while 80% are in the spleen
b. the platelets circulate for about 10 days
c. ineffective thrombocytopoiesis is characterized by an increased number of megakaryocytes in the bone marrow and by a reduction of the number of circulating platelets
d. patients with thrombocytosis may show a serum hyperkalemia
e. both thrombocytopenia and thrombocythemia may lead to hemorrhages

INTERMEDIATE

10. Based on this patient's history and findings, which of the following statements is correct?

a. this patient is predisposed to peripheral vascular insufficiency
b. this patient is predisposed to gastrointestinal hemorrhage
c. this patient is at increased risk of developing lung cancer
d. this patient is at increased risk of developing cerebrovascular ischemia
e. all of the above statements are correct

ANSWERS AND FURTHER INFORMATION

Figure descriptions

Figure 14.1 Peripheral blood smear (patient). Wright/Giemsa stain.

The patient's peripheral blood smear shows a marked increase in the number of platelets. The platelets' size and shape are variable, with several giant platelets.

Figure 14.2 Peripheral blood smear (normal). Wright/Giemsa stain.

Normal peripheral blood smear with much fewer platelets compared with Figure 14.1. The red blood cells are normal in size and shape and show normal center pallor. A normal lymphocyte and a normal neutrophil are seen in this image.

Figure 14.3 Bone marrow biopsy (patient). Hematoxylin & eosin stain.

Hypercellular bone marrow biopsy consistent with thrombocythemia: The bone marrow is hypercellular (85–90% hematopoietic cellularity) for the patient's age. Even at this low magnification numerous atypical megakaryocytes can be seen.

Figure 14.4 Bone marrow biopsy (patient). Hematoxylin & eosin stain.

Hypercellular bone marrow biopsy consistent with thrombocythemia: A higher magnification showing trilineage hematopoietic hyperplasia and a cluster of atypical megakaryocytes.

Figure 14.5 Bone marrow biopsy (normal). Hematoxylin & eosin stain.

Normal bone marrow biopsy: This is a normal bone marrow biopsy from another patient of a similar age. The hematopoietic bone cellularity is approximately 70%. The bone marrow shows trilineage hematopoiesis and no abnormal megakaryocyte clusters.

Figure 14.6 Maxillary sinus content (patient). Hematoxylin & eosin stain.

Acute sinusitis: Upper respiratory tract mucosa lined by pseudostratified columnar epithelium showing acute and chronic inflammatory cell infiltrate and hemorrhage.

Answers

1. E. The painful facial problem this patient presented with was diagnosed as an acute sinusitis (maxillary). It is likely to be of bacterial etiology, and it is the cause of fever, pain, and leukocytosis. An infectious etiology is also supported by the finding of an air-fluid level, which is usually not present in allergic sinusitis. Acute sinusitis is commonly preceded by acute or chronic rhinitis, but it can also arise by extension of a periapical infection. An inflammatory mucosal edema contributes to the process by impairment of sinus drainage, thus facilitating infection of the sinus.

2. D. The burning foot pain described by the patient, which is relieved by exposure to cold and associated with a mottled redness of the affected parts, is known as erythromelalgia and accompanies or sometimes precedes essential thrombocythemia, a myeloproliferative disorder. It is not related to sinusitis, leukocytosis, or relative lymphopenia. This pain is thought to be due to arteriolar inflammation and thrombotic occlusions.

3. D. The patient was repeatedly found to have guaiac-positive stools, which, after exclusion of dietary factors, etc., is indicative of gastrointestinal (GI) bleeding. The GI bleed could be associated with the patient's history of alcohol abuse (gastritis). An increased platelet count (reactive thrombocytosis) is known to be associated with gastrointestinal inflammatory diseases causing GI bleeding. It can also be a manifestation of essential thrombocythemia, a clonal disorder of the hematopoietic stem cells, in which hemorrhages are common complications.

4. E. The CBC (FBC) shows an increase of WBC count, an increased number of platelets, and anemia (normocytic). The peripheral blood smear (Fig. 14.1) shows abnormal platelet morphology (see Fig. 14.1 description). The leukocytosis is due to bacterial sinusitis, which was the presenting problem of this patient. The platelet distribution width (PDW) is increased due to abnormal platelet morphology. Evaluation of the anemia is necessary, and iron studies are part of this evaluation. There is no reason to perform flow cytometric analysis of lymphocytes, since there is no indication of a lymphocytic disorder.

5. B. An increase in the number of circulating platelets is seen in many conditions; in general it can be of a reactive origin (thrombocytosis), accompanying inflammatory conditions, or chronic infections; it is also seen in patients with malignancies or as one of a group of chronic myeloproliferative disorders (thrombocythemia). Patients with AIDS, however, often suffer from thrombocytopenia, a decrease in platelet numbers.

6. E. The bone marrow in this patient (Figs 14.3 and 14.4) shows a cellular marrow and an increased proportion of megakaryocytes; these findings are not consistent with the diagnoses of aplastic anemia, acute lymphoblastic leukemia, myelofibrosis, or with a granulomatous process.

7. D. This patient has essential thrombocythemia, a clonal disorder of hematopoietic stem cells leading to the over-production of platelets. Thrombosis and hemorrhage are common complications of this disorder, as is microvascular ischemia, sometimes leading to gangrene and necrosis of digits, especially toes. The risk of developing an acute leukemia is well recognized; hypertension, however, is not recognized as a major complication of this disease.

8. D. The patient has essential thrombocythemia, a clonal disorder of the multipotential hematopoietic stem cell. This disorder most commonly affects persons older than 50 years of age, but it is now seen with increasing frequency in a younger population. This disorder should be differentiated from the reactive thrombocytosis and from thrombocytosis associated with other chronic myeloproliferative disorders. The bone marrow typically shows normal or increased hematopoietic cellularity with a markedly increased number of giant and immature megakaryocytes, which are found dispersed diffusely and also in clusters. The marrow should show a stainable iron, since iron deficiency is not a feature in the pathogenesis of essential thrombocythemia. Myelofibrosis is not present. Another typical laboratory finding is loss of the *in vitro* aggregation response to epinephrine (Table 14.11).

9. A. Approximately 70% of platelets are circulating and 30% are in the spleen in a normal individual. In a hypersplenic patient, however, about 90% of platelets may be pooled in the spleen. The normal circulating life of a platelet is about 10 days. In states of an ineffective thrombocytopoiesis (such as in vitamin B_{12} deficiency, Wiscott–Aldrich syndrome, etc.) the bone marrow shows an increased number of megakaryocytes, but ineffective platelet production, leading to a reduced number of circulating platelets. An increased number of platelets, known as thrombocytosis (when physiologic or reactive) or thrombocythemia (if primary or independent of normal regulatory processes), sometimes gives rise to spurious laboratory values for constituents normally present in platelets. Potassium is one of these and is released into serum upon clotting. The potassium level, however, would be normal in plasma. Both thrombocytopenia and thrombocythemia cause hemorrhages.

10. E. This patient has a history of smoking and alcohol abuse, and he has been diagnosed as having essential thrombocythemia (ET). He is clearly predisposed to peripheral vascular insufficiency (smoking, ET). The predisposition to gastrointestinal hemorrhage is due to his history of alcoholism and also due to ET. The increased risk of lung cancer is associated with the smoking history, and the increased risk of developing cerebrovascular ischemia is due to ET.

Final diagnosis and synopsis of the case

- Acute bacterial sinusitis
- Acute gastritis
- Essential thrombocytosis (thrombocythemia)
- Erythromelalgia

A young man presented with a severe right-sided facial pain and swelling accompanied by fever and leukocytosis. In addition, the patient complained of episodic burning pain in his feet and of red discoloration of the affected parts, which was relieved by exposure to the cold. He was diagnosed as having an acute maxillary sinusitis of staphylococcal origin. The treatment required surgical drainage of the sinus in addition to antibiotic therapy. The initial work-up also revealed a marked thrombocytosis, anemia, and occult blood in the stool. After the symptoms of his sinusitis subsided, the patient underwent a work-up of his persistent thrombocytosis. This included a bone marrow biopsy, tests of platelet function, and a variety of tests to exclude the known causes of reactive thrombocytosis. The gastrointestinal work-up revealed the presence of an acute gastritis, which was the likely cause of the patient's guaiac-positive stools and was probably due to his abuse of alcohol. Based on all findings present (persistent, markedly elevated platelet count, *in vitro* platelet non-responsiveness to epinephrine, megakaryocytic hyperplasia of the bone marrow, and the characteristic discoloration and pain in the extremities – called erythromelalgia), it was concluded that the patient has essential thrombocythemia, which is a clonal disorder of the multipotential hematopoietic cell. The patient will be closely monitored and treated, if necessary.

Lab tips

Bleeding time test:
A useful test to screen for abnormalities of platelet function; it measures the time it takes for bleeding to cease after a small skin wound is made under standardized conditions.

Method:
A blood pressure cuff is placed around the patient's upper arm and inflated to 40 mmHg. A standardized cut is made on the volar surface of the forearm and the resulting blood is blotted with filter paper (paper must not touch wound edge). The time from the making of the cut to the cessation of bleeding is the bleeding time, and is usually around 8 min.

Comments:
1. Aspirin ingestion is the most common cause of an abnormal bleeding time test as the test can be prolonged for up to 7 days following the ingestion of as little as 650 mg of the drug. Many people do not consider aspirin a drug and are not aware of the large number of proprietary products of which it is a component.
2. The bleeding time is increased in patients with uremia and in about one-third of all patients with von Willebrand's disease.
3. The test is not recommended as a routine preoperative screening measure to assess hemorrhagic risk in an asymptomatic patient.

Table 14.12 Bleeding time test

Platelets – qualitative function	Platelet – quantity	Results of bleeding time test
Normal	$<80\,000/\mu L$ ($80 \times 10^9/L$)	Bleeding time becomes prolonged
	$<40\,000/\mu L$ ($40 \times 10^9/L$)	Bleeding time is significantly prolonged and should not be performed
Abnormal	Can be within normal range	Bleeding time may be prolonged

A 68-year-old cashier with a loss of appetite

CASE AND MCQS

Clinical history and presentation

A 68-year-old woman was brought to the emergency room by her son. She complained of an increasing weakness and a loss of appetite in the last 2 weeks. She noticed vaginal bleeding 3 weeks ago and complained of abdominal distension and discomfort. She denied hematemesis, melena, or hematuria. She has had no fever or chills. She has gained 3 pounds over the last few days. Her past medical history was unremarkable. She was on no medication, only vitamins on a daily basis. She has three children. Physical examination revealed an alert and oriented but noticeably weak woman. Her blood pressure was 170/86 mmHg, pulse 78 beats/min and regular. She was afebrile. The lungs were clear to auscultation. The abdomen was grossly distended and diffusely tender to palpation. Bowel sounds were absent. Rectal and vaginal examination had to be deferred because of the patient's extreme discomfort. X-rays of the chest and abdomen (Figs 15.2 and 15.3) were obtained and the patient was admitted to the hospital.

Admission data

Table 15.1 Hematology

			SI Units	
WBC	7.6	(3.3–11.0 thou/μL)	7.6	(3.3–11.0 × 10⁹/L)
Neut	72	(44–88%)	72	(44–88%)
Band	5	(0–10%)	5	(0–10%)
Lymph	16	(12–43%)	16	(12–43%)
Mono	3	(2–11%)	3	(2–11%)
Eos	3	(0–5%)	3	(0–5%)
Baso	1	(0–2%)	1	(0–2%)
RBC	3.2 L	(3.9–5.0 mill/μL)	3.2 L	(3.9–5.0 × 10¹²/L)
HGB	9.6 L	(11.6–15.6 g/dL)	96 L	(116–156 g/L)
HCT	31.3 L	(37.0–47.0%)	31.3 L	(0.37–0.47)
MCV	97.8	(79.0–99.0 fL)	97.8	(79.0–99.0 fL)
MCH	30.0	(26.0–32.6 pg)	30.0	(26.0–32.6 pg)
MCHC	32.6	(31.0–36.0 g/dL)	326	(310–360 g/L)
Plts	500 H	(130–400 thou/μL)	500 H	(130–400 × 10⁹/L)

Table 15.2 Chemistry

			SI Units	
Glucose	103	(65–110 mg/dL)	5.7	(3.6–6.11 mmol/L)
Creatinine	1.1	(0.7–1.4 mg/dL)	97.2	(61.9–123.76 µmol/L)
BUN	14	(7–24 mg/dL)	5.0	(2.50–8.57 mmol/L)
Uric acid	7.0	(3.0–8.5 mg/dL)	0.24	(0.18–0.51 mmol/L)
Cholesterol	180	(150–200 mg/dL)	4.65	(3.88–5.17 mmol/L)
Calcium	8.0 L	(8.5–10.5 mg/dL)	1.25 L	(2.13–2.63 mmol/L)
Protein	6.5	(6–8 g/dL)	65	(60–80 g/L)
Albumin	3.7	(3.7–5.0 g/dL)	37	(37–50 g/L)
LDH	415 H	(100–250 U/L)	415 H	(100–250 U/L)
Alk Phos	120	(0–120 U/L)	120	(0–120 U/L)
AST	38	(0–55 U/L)	38	(0–55 U/L)
ALT	27	(7–40 U/L)	27	(7–40 U/L)
GGTP	23	(0–50 U/L)	23	(0–50 U/L)
Bilirubin	0.5	(0.0–1.5 mg/dL)	8.6	(0–25.7 µmol/L)
Bilirubin-direct	0.12	(0.02–0.18 mg/dL)	2.05	(0.34–3.08 µmol/L)
Amylase	41	(13–85 U/L)	0.70	(0.22–1.45 µkat/L)

Table 15.3 Electrolytes

			SI Units	
Na	141	(134–143 mEq/L)	141	(134–143 mmol/L)
K	3.8	(3.5–4.9 mEq/L)	3.8	(3.5–4.9 mmol/L)
Cl	99	(95–108 mEq/L)	99	(95–108 mmol/L)
CO_2	31	(21–32 mEq/L)	31	(21–32 mmol/L)

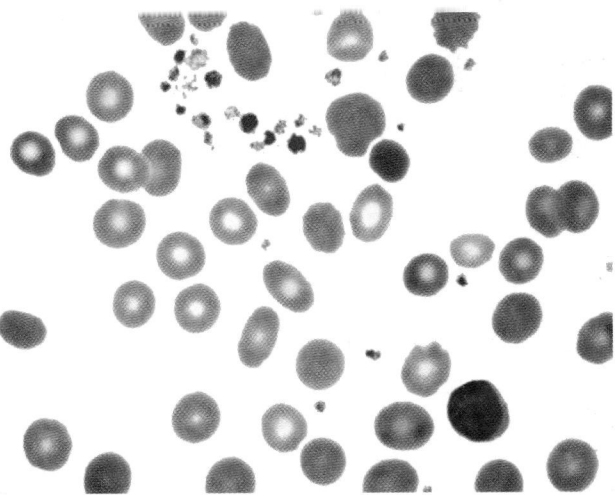

Figure 15.1 Peripheral blood smear (patient). Wright/Giemsa stain.

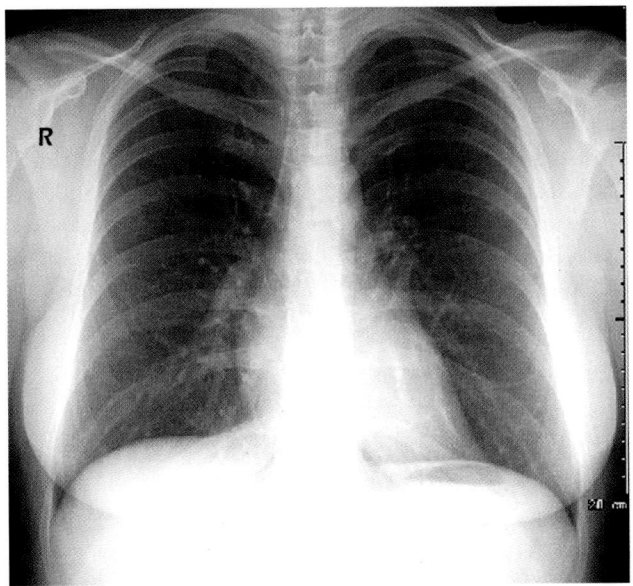

Figure 15.2 Chest X-ray, A-P view on admission (patient).

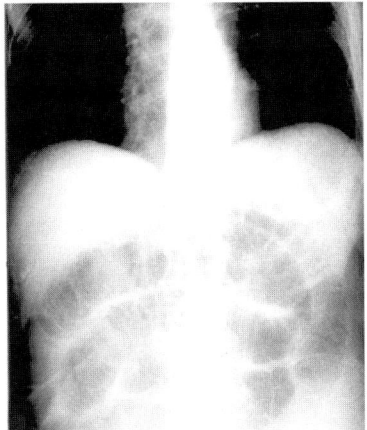

Figure 15.3 Flat plate of abdomen (patient).

Questions

Based on the above information you can best conclude the following:

BASIC

1. What would be the LEAST likely cause of post-menopausal vaginal bleeding?

a. uterine prolapse
b. cervical cancer
c. endometrial cancer
d. administration of estrogen without adding progesterone.
e. endometrial polyps

INTERMEDIATE

2. What would be the most likely cause of an increased platelet count in this patient?

a. the patient has an essential thrombocytosis
b. it is secondary to iron deficiency anemia
c. it is secondary to chronic inflammatory disorder
d. it is secondary to an underlying malignancy
e. it is due to severe dehydration

INTERMEDIATE

3. An X-ray of the patient's chest (Fig.15.2) shows:

a. pleural effusion
b. pneumonia
c. pneumothorax
d. lung mass
e. none of the above

INTERMEDIATE

4. Figure 15.3 shows an X-ray of the patient's abdomen. Which of the following problems can you identify?

a. dilated small intestine
b. an aortic aneurysm
c. free air in the peritoneal cavity
d. all of the above
e. none of the above

INTERMEDIATE

5. This patient has an increase in the serum level of lactate dehydrogenase (LDH). Which of the following conditions would most likely account for this increase?

a. liver cirrhosis
b. viral hepatitis
c. hemolytic anemia
d. malignancy
e. all of the above

Clinical course

A vaginal examination was performed followed by a CT scan of the abdomen and pelvis. The pelvic CT showed an enlarged uterus with a hypodense center, suspicious for an endometrial mass. A cytological specimen from the abdominal paracentesis is shown in Fig. 15.4. The patient underwent surgery. A hysterectomy and bilateral salpingo-oophorectomy were performed, and a tissue sample from the omentum was obtained. The histological findings are depicted in Figs 15.5–15.9. Based on these findings, special tests were ordered. The patient was started on a specific therapy, but soon became increasingly lethargic, and expired.

Table 15.4 Tumor markers

			SI Units	
CA-125	29	(0–35 AU/mL)	29	(0–35 kAU/L)
CEA	0.8	(0–3.0 µg/L)	0.8	(0–3.0 µg/L)

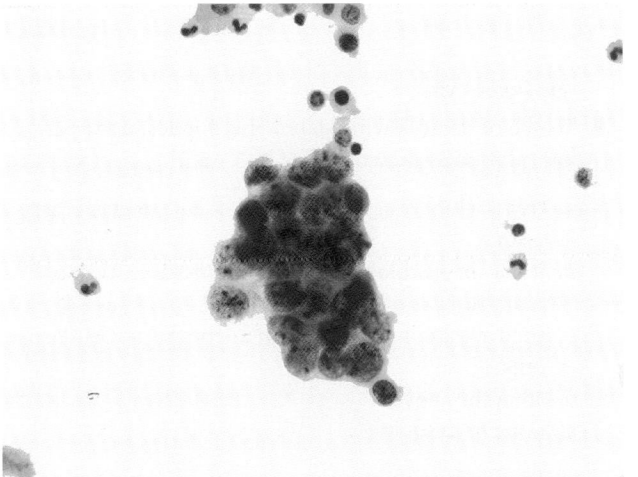

Figure 15.4 Peritoneal fluid cytology (patient). Papanicolaou stain.

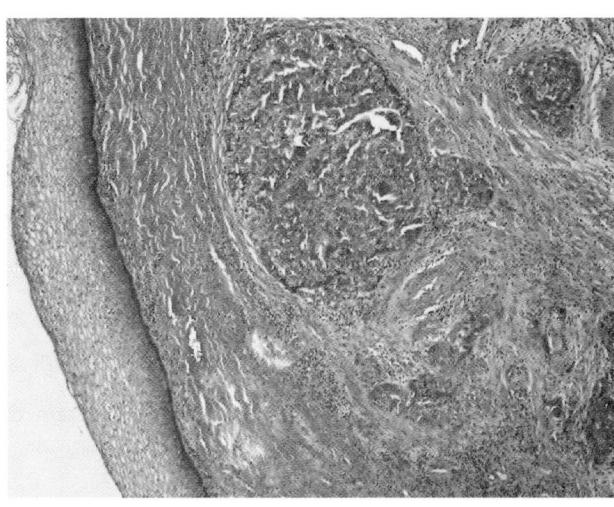

Figure 15.5 Uterine cervix (patient). Hematoxylin & eosin stain.

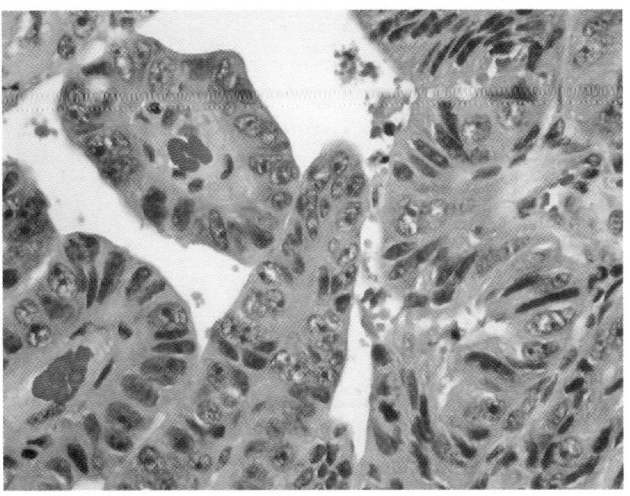

Figure 15.6 Uterine body (patient). Hematoxylin & eosin stain.

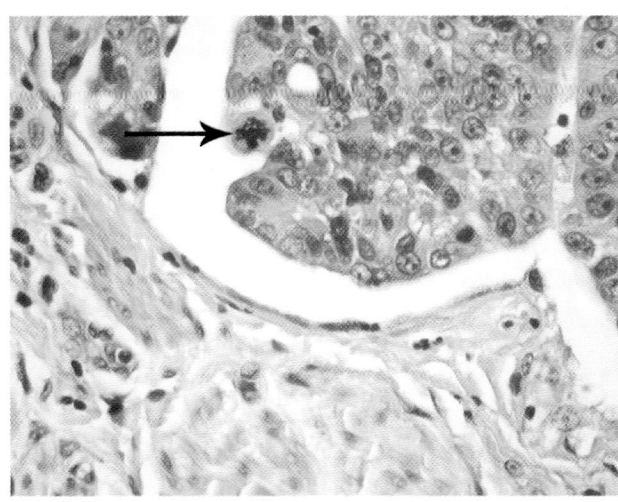

Figure 15.7 Uterine body (patient). Hematoxylin & eosin stain.

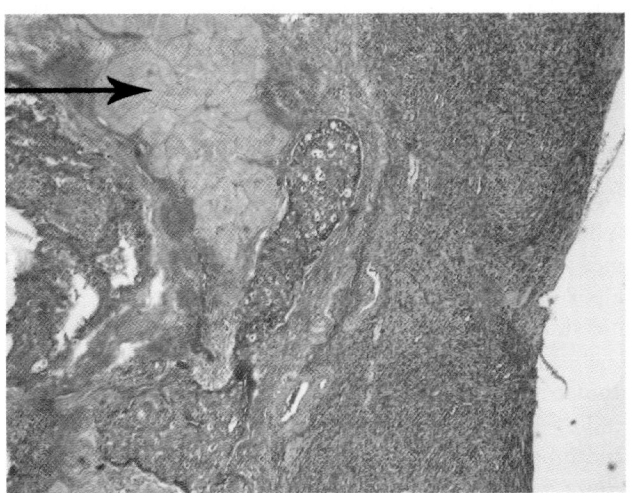

Figure 15.8 Left ovary (patient). Hematoxylin & eosin stain.

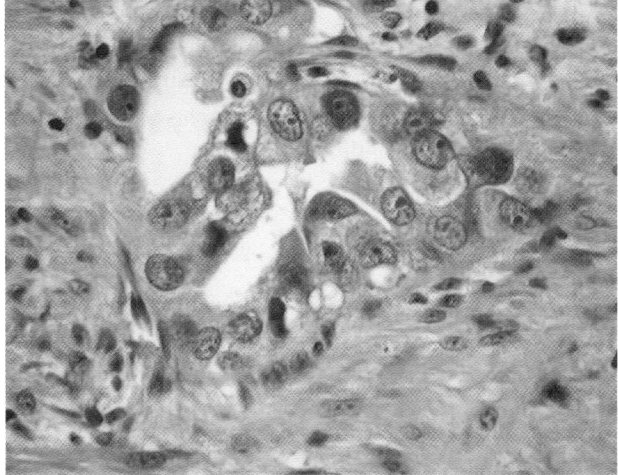

Figure 15.9 Omental biopsy (patient). Hematoxylin & eosin stain.

Questions

ADVANCED

6. The cytological preparation from the patient's paracentesis (Fig. 15.4) shows which of the following?

    a. the presence of a purely suppurative process
    b. the presence of a malignant process
    c. evidence of a deep mycosis
    d. none of the above

INTERMEDIATE

7. Figures 15.5–15.9 show the appearance of H & E stained sections of tissue from the omentum, ovary, and from uterus. The most likely diagnosis is:

    a. squamous cell carcinoma
    b. leiomyosarcoma
    c. lymphoma
    d. adenocarcinoma

INTERMEDIATE

8. Based on the histological findings seen in Figs 15.5–15.9 you can conclude that there is:

    a. an invasion of a lymphatic channel by abnormal cells
    b. cervical involvement by this disease process
    c. ovarian metastasis
    d. all of the above
    e. none of the above

INTERMEDIATE

9. Which of the following statements applies to the pathological process shown in Figs 15.5–15.9?

    a. this is a highly aggressive form of endometrial carcinoma
    b. it may be histologically indistinguishable from primary tumors of the fallopian tube
    c. such a lesion may arise from uncommitted Müllerian cells
    d. all of the above
    e. none of the above

INTERMEDIATE

10. The pathological process depicted in Figs 15.5–15.9:

    a. has the highest incidence in women of childbearing age
    b. is associated with human papilloma virus (HPV)
    c. is relatively frequent in woman with ovarian agenesis or in ovariectomized women
    d. all of the above statements are correct
    e. none of the above statements is correct

ANSWERS AND FURTHER INFORMATION

Figure descriptions

Figure 15.1 Peripheral blood smear (patient). Wright/Giemsa stain.
Normocytic normochromic anemia with thrombocytosis: The red blood cells show mild aniso-poikilocytosis. The platelet count is increased. A normal lymphocyte is present at the lower right corner of this image.

Figure 15.2 Chest X-ray, A-P view on admission (patient).
This X-ray shows a normal frontal radiograph of the chest in a female patient.

Figure 15.3 Flat plate of abdomen (patient).
This frontal radiograph of the abdomen demonstrates multiple loops of dilated small bowel. Little, if any, air is seen in the colon or rectum. These findings are consistent with a small bowel obstruction. No free air is present.

Figure 15.4 Peritoneal fluid cytology (patient). Papanicolaou stain.
This photomicrograph shows a cluster of malignant cells. The cells are pleomorphic with hyperchromatic enlarged nuclei and prominent nucleoli. These cells are suggestive of an adenocarcinoma; however, the primary origin cannot be determined with certainty from this cytological specimen.

Figures 15.5–15.9
A hysterectomy with bilateral salpingo-oophorectomy specimen was submitted for pathological examination. In addition a portion of the omentum was also submitted. The uterus measured $13 \times 8 \times 6$ cm and weighed 307 g. The endometrial cavity was asymmetrical and was lined by a thick endometrium. A hard nodule was identified extending from the endometrium to the serosal surface of the uterus. Both ovaries and tubes appear grossly normal. The omentum measured $20 \times 8 \times 4$ cm and shows multiple hard tan nodules measur-

ing up to 1.9 cm. Sections from the cervix are shown in Fig. 15.5, from uterine body in Fig. 15.6, from the deep portion of the myometrium in Fig. 15.7, from the left ovary in Fig. 15.8, and from the omentum in Fig. 15.9.

Figure 15.5 Uterine cervix (patient). Hematoxylin & eosin stain.
Endometrial adenocarcinoma: Section from the uterine cervix showing a normal squamous epithelium from the ectocervix on the left. The cervical stroma is infiltrated by clusters of adenocarcinoma cells. At this magnification the cellular details are not apparent.

Figure 15.6 Uterine body (patient). Hematoxylin & eosin stain.
Endometrial adenocarcinoma: Section from the uterine body showing adenocarcinoma with papillary projections. The papillary projections are lined by stratified disorganized epithelium, and contain fibrous stroma. The neoplastic cells exhibit nuclear pleomorphism, large hyperchromatic nuclei with occasional prominent nucleoli. These morphological features are those of serous papillary adenocarcinoma. Serous papillary adenocarcinoma is an aggressive variant of endometrial adenocarcinoma.

Figure 15.7 Uterine body (patient). Hematoxylin & eosin stain.
Endometrial adenocarcinoma with lymphatic invasion: A dilated lymphatic channel with a solid cluster of malignant cells. A mitotic figure is clearly seen in this image (arrow).

Figure 15.8 Left ovary (patient). Hematoxylin & eosin stain.
Section of the left ovary showing metastatic adenocarcinoma involving the ovarian parenchyma. Both normal ovarian stroma and a corpus albicans (arrow) are seen in this image.

Figure 15.9 Omental biopsy (patient). Hematoxylin & eosin stain.
Endometrial adenocarcinoma: Section from the omentum showing a malignant gland, consistent with a moderately differentiated adenocarcinoma, an inflammatory cell infiltrate and a desmoplastic response (a stromal response to tumor invasion that results in extensive fibrosis with scarring).

Answers

1. A. In postmenopausal women, the common causes of vaginal bleeding are carcinoma of the endometrium, polyps, and cervical cancer. Uterine prolapse is not a cause of postmenopausal bleeding.

2. D. The patient's platelet count is increased. Severe dehydration as a possible cause is not validated by any of the clinical or laboratory findings. The patient does not have an iron deficiency anemia (microcytic, hypochromic) or a history of a chronic inflammatory disorder (such as rheumatoid arthritis, ulcerative colitis, etc.) known to be associated with an increased platelet count. Essential thrombocytosis is a stem cell disorder, leading to proliferation of the megakaryocytic elements, in which the peripheral platelet count usually exceeds 600 000 per mm^3, and the peripheral blood smear usually shows abnormally large platelets, not seen in Fig. 15.1. A malignant neoplasm is often accompanied by an increase in the platelet count.

3. E. The chest X-ray (Fig. 15.2) is within normal limits. There is no evidence of pleural effusion, pneumonia, pneumothorax, or of a lung mass.

4. A. This patient's abdominal X-ray shows a distended small intestine, an appearance almost pathognomonic of adynamic ileus. Adynamic ileus is mediated by the autonomic nervous system. It may occur after any peritoneal insult; in this case the most likely insult was carcinomatosis of the peritoneum. Adynamic ileus occurs for a few days after any abdominal operation. The presence of gas in the large intestine would make the diagnosis of adynamic ileus less likely. The presence of fluid in the abdomen was not noted in this case, but this single view does not rule it out. Its presence would be indicated by a haziness of the X-ray image. There is no evidence of an aortic aneurysm or of air in the peritoneal cavity.

5. D. In viral hepatitis or liver cirrhosis, the other liver enzymes (aspartate amino transferase (AST), alkaline phosphatase (Alk Phos), alanine amino transferase (ALT), gamma glutamyl transferase (GGTP)) and bilirubin levels would also be abnormal. None of these findings is present in this patient. Hemolytic anemia, if present, would lead to an increase in lactate dehydrogenase (LDH) and in the serum bilirubin (mostly unconjugated) levels. There is, also, no evidence of hemolysis noted on this patient's blood smear (Fig. 15.1). In about 50% of patients with cancer the LDH serum level is increased and the isoenzyme pattern is non-specific.

6. B. The cytological preparation shown in Fig. 15.4 exhibits a cluster of highly atypical cells consistent with a diagnosis of adenocarcinoma.

7. D. Figures 15.5–15.9 show an endometrial adenocarcinoma involving the ectocervix (Fig. 15.5), the left ovary (Fig. 15.8), and omentum (Fig. 15.9). The tumor invades lymphatics (Fig. 15.6). There is no evidence of squamous cell carcinoma, leiomyosarcoma, or lymphoma seen on these images.

8. D. The histology of this tumor is that of a serous papillary adenocarcinoma, affecting and evidently originating in the endometrium. It is composed of papillary and solid areas of poorly differentiated cells of tubal type. It is quite distinct from the weaving pattern of fusiform smooth muscle cells of a leiomyoma, and from any of the varieties of lymphoma.

9. D. All the statements are correct. Papillary serous carcinomas of the endometrium are highly aggressive tumors, which mimic the histology of primary tumors of the fallopian tube. This similarity of endometrial to tubal tumors has been explained by postulating their origin from foci of tubal metaplasia of the endometrium, or from uncommitted Müllerian cells.

10. E. None of the choices is correct; the lesion does not have the highest incidence in woman of childbearing age, is not associated with HPV and is not relatively frequent in women with ovarian agenesis or ovariectomized women. The peak incidence of endometrial carcinoma is in women of 50 to 70 years of age, and there is an increased incidence in women who have been exposed to unopposed estrogen in the past.

Final diagnosis and synopsis of the case

- Papillary serous adenocarcinoma of the endometrium
- Carcinomatosis
- Bowel obstruction

An 68-year-old woman was admitted to the hospital with increasing weakness, loss of appetite, nausea, and abdominal distention and discomfort. A diagnosis was made of adynamic ileus. Her work-up, which included a CT scan of the abdomen and pelvis, revealed ascites and multiple omental lesions. Aspirated peritoneal fluid was found to contain malignant cells. Laparotomy revealed carcinomatosis of the peritoneum; sections from omentum, peritoneal metastases, an implant on the ovary, and endometrial curettings were diagnosed as papillary serous adenocarcinoma originating in the endometrium. The patient ultimately underwent bilateral salpingo-oophorectomy with lysis of adhesions. The patient was started on a regimen of cancer chemotherapy, and was to be considered for possible radiotherapy. However, the patient became extremely weak and lethargic. The family refused further surgery for bowel obstruction, and the patient expired on the 32nd hospital day.

A 41-year-old teacher with pruritic rash

CASE AND MCQS

Clinical history and presentation

A 41-year-old man presented to his primary care physician with a pruritic rash on his thigh, forearm, and neck, which he noticed several weeks ago. There was some improvement initially, after treatment with topical steroids, but later the rash worsened and about a week ago it extended to his anterior neck. The patient denies any significant medical or surgical history, and he claims not to be allergic or to have a family history of allergic problems. He has been afebrile, his appetite is good, and his activity level (he is a physical education teacher) has been normal. He denies contact with pets, and he has not noticed a tick bite. Physical examination showed a healthy appearing male. His vital signs were normal. Examination of the skin revealed a scaly erythematous rash (about 5 cm in diameter) on the anterior neck and similar but larger lesions on his left anterior thigh and left forearm. The lesions were flat with irregular borders. There was no lymphadenopathy; the examination of the chest was normal, the abdomen was soft and no organomegaly was appreciated. The neurological examination was entirely normal. The patient was referred to a dermatologist. The results of the work-up are shown below.

Admission data

Table 16.1 Hematology

			SI Units	
WBC	5.3	(3.3–11.0 thou/μL)	5.3	(3.3–11.0 × 10⁹/L)
Neut	68	(44–88%)	68	(44–88%)
Band	0	(0–10%)	0	(0–10%)
Lymph	27	(12–43%)	27	(12–43%)
Mono	3	(2–11%)	3	(2–11%)
Eos	1	(0–5%)	1	(0–5%)
Baso	1	(0–2%)	1	(0–2%)
RBC	4.74	(3.9–5.0 mill/μL)	4.74	(3.9–5.0 × 10¹²/L)
HGB	15.6	(11.6–15.6 g/dL)	156	(116–156 g/L)
HCT	44.2	(37.0–47.0%)	0.442	(0.37–0.47)
MCV	93	(79.0–99.0 fL)	93	(79.0–99.0 fL)
MCH	32.9	(26.0–35.6 pg)	32.9	(26.0–35.6 pg)
MCHC	35.3	(31.0–36.0 g/dL)	353	(310–360 g/L)
Plts	150	(130–400 thou/μL)	150	(130–400 × 10⁹/L)
RDW	12.9	(12–16.2%)	12.9	(12–16.2%)

Table 16.2 Chemistry

			SI Units	
Glucose	89	(65–110 mg/dL)	4.94	(3.6–6.11 mmol/L)
Creatinine	1.2	(0.7–1.4 mg/dL)	106	(61.9–123.76 µmol/L)
BUN	14	(7–24 mg/dL)	5.0	(2.50–8.57 mmol/L)
Uric acid	5.1	(3.0–8.5 mg/dL)	0.3	(0.18–0.51 mmol/L)
Cholesterol	202 H	(150–200 mg/dL)	5.22 H	(3.88–5.17 mmol/L)
Calcium	9.9	(8.5–10.5 mg/dL)	2.5	(2.13–2.63 mmol/L)
Protein	7.1	(6–8 g/dL)	71	(60–80 g/L)
Albumin	4.7	(3.7–5.0 g/dL)	47	(37–50 g/L)
LDH	162	(100–250 U/L)	162	(100–250 U/L)
Alk Phos	101	(0–120 U/L)	101	(0–120 U/L)
AST	28	(0–55 U/L)	28	(0–55 U/L)
GGTP	25	(0–50 U/L)	25	(0–50 U/L)
Bilirubin	0.89	(0.0–1.5 mg/dL)	15.2	(0–25.7 µmol/L)
Bilirubin-direct	0.02	(0.02–0.18 mg/dL)	0.34	(0.34–3.08 µmol/L)

Table 16.3 Electrolytes

			SI Units	
Na	140	(134–143 mEq/L)	140	(134–143 mmol/L)
K	4.6	(3.5–4.9 mEq/L)	4.6	(3.5–4.9 mmol/L)
Cl	104	(95–108 mEq/L)	104	(95–108 mmol/L)
CO_2	26	(21–32 mEq/L)	26	(21–32 mmol/L)

Table 16.4 CT scan of chest, abdomen, and pelvis

Normal

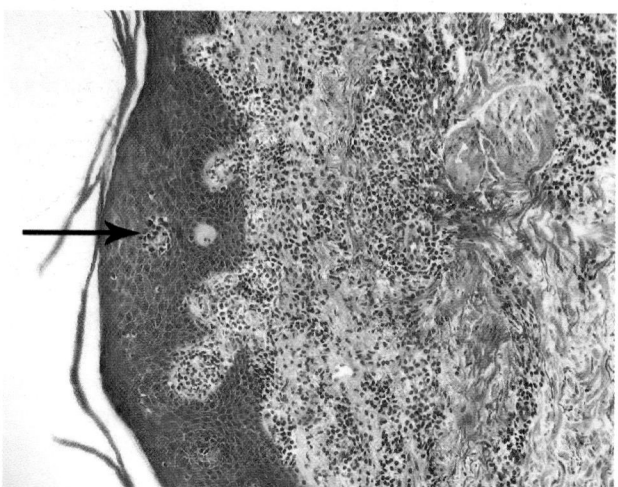

Figure 16.1 Skin biopsy (patient). Hematoxylin & eosin stain.

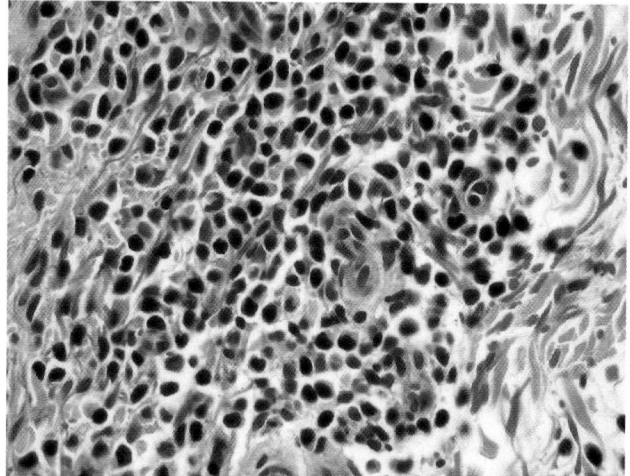

Figure 16.2 Skin biopsy (patient). Hematoxylin & eosin stain.

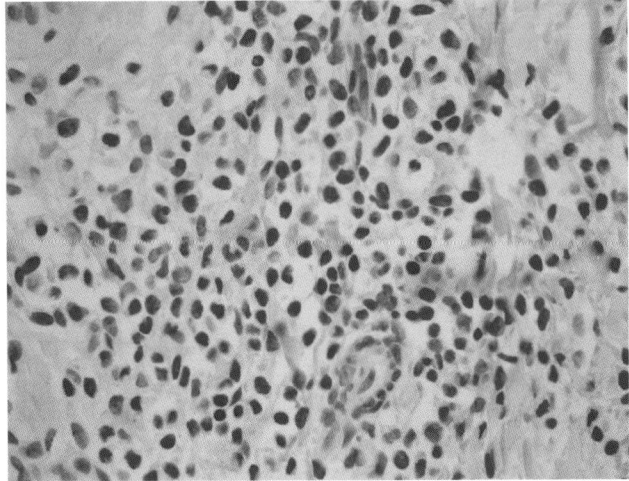

Figure 16.3 Skin biopsy (patient). Immunohistochemical staining with anti-CD20 antibodies.

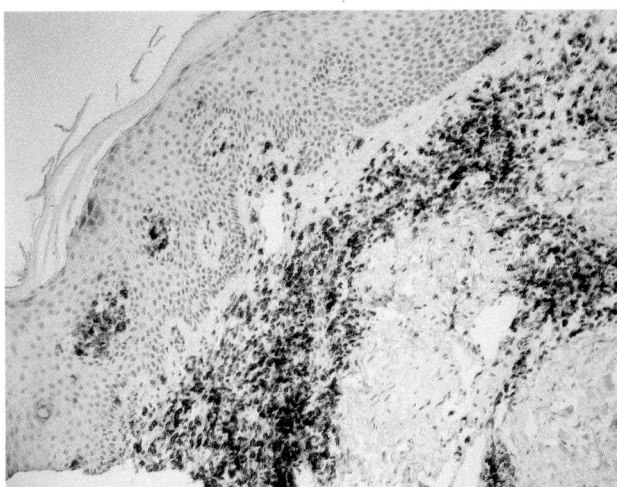

Figure 16.4 Skin biopsy (patient). Immunohistochemical staining with anti-CD4 antibodies.

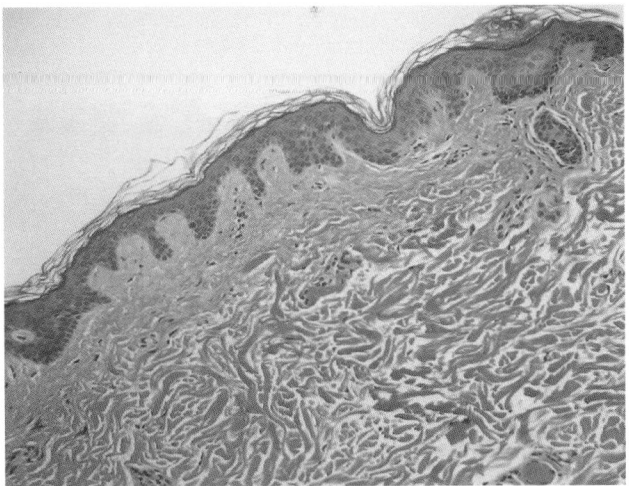

Figure 16.5 Skin biopsy (normal). Hematoxylin & eosin stain.

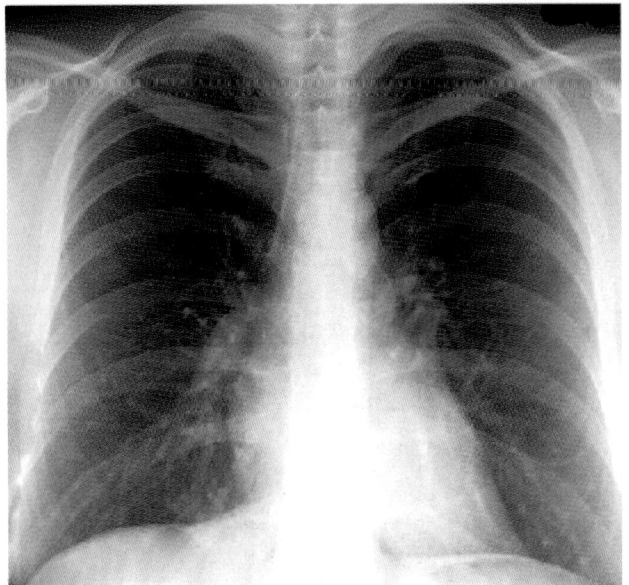

Figure 16.6 Chest X-ray, A-P view (patient).

Questions

Based on the above information, you can best conclude the following:

1. In general, which of the following skin conditions does NOT typically present as erythematous, flat, and scaly patches?

  a. psoriasis
  b. seborrhoeic dermatitis
  c. molluscum contagiosum
  d. candidiasis

2. The itching, in general, is NOT a feature of which of the following skin conditions?

  a. erythema multiforme
  b. candidiasis
  c. seborrhoeic dermatitis
  d. psoriasis
  e. atopic dermatitis

INTERMEDIATE

3. The microscopic appearance of the skin lesion (Figs 16.1 and 16.2) shows:

    a. a lymphoid infiltrate of dermis
    b. the presence of atypical lymphocytes in the dermis
    c. the presence of atypical lymphocytes in the epidermis
    d. all of the above
    e. none of the above

INTERMEDIATE

4. In general, the predominance of T lymphocytes in a lymphocytic infiltrate in a skin biopsy may be seen in:

    a. T cell lymphomas
    b. B cell lymphomas
    c. inflammatory conditions
    d. all of the above
    e. none of the above

Clinical course

The patient was referred to a specialist and started on a specific therapy to which he has responded well. His skin lesions regressed and there was no additional complication. About 4 months after the completion of this therapy, he started to notice new skin lesions on his face, chest, both arms, and legs. He also developed a palpable mass in the groin. Physical examination at this time revealed raised, indurated, reddish, plaque-like skin lesions and an enlarged lymph node in the left groin region. The rest of the physical examination was normal. The results of some additional evaluation and testing are shown below. The repeated CT scan of chest, abdomen, and pelvis remained unchanged from the previous examinations.

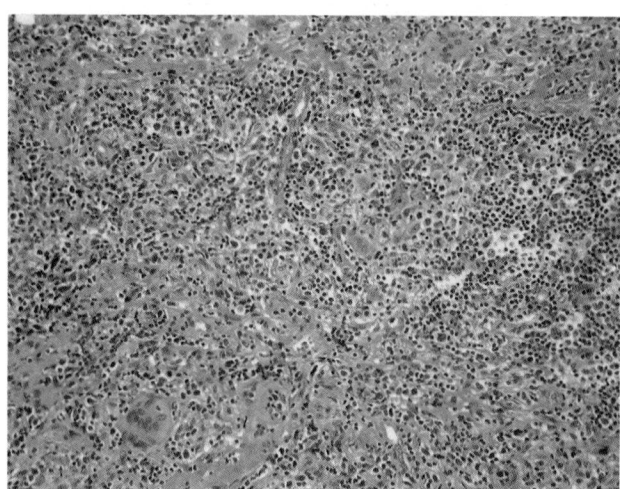

Figure 16.7 Lymph node biopsy (patient). Hematoxylin & eosin stain.

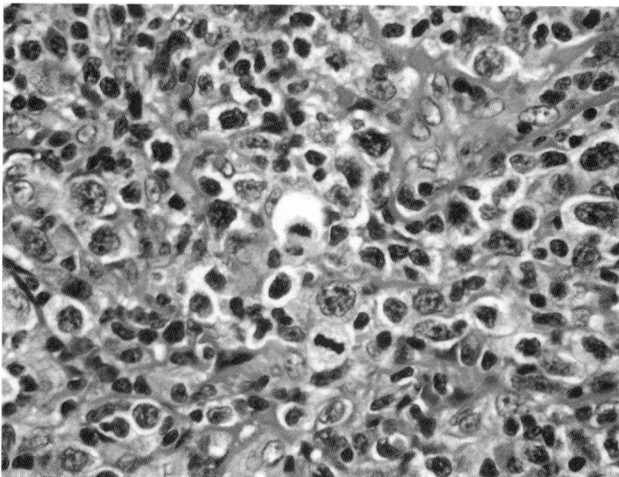

Figure 16.8 Lymph node biopsy (patient). Hematoxylin & eosin stain.

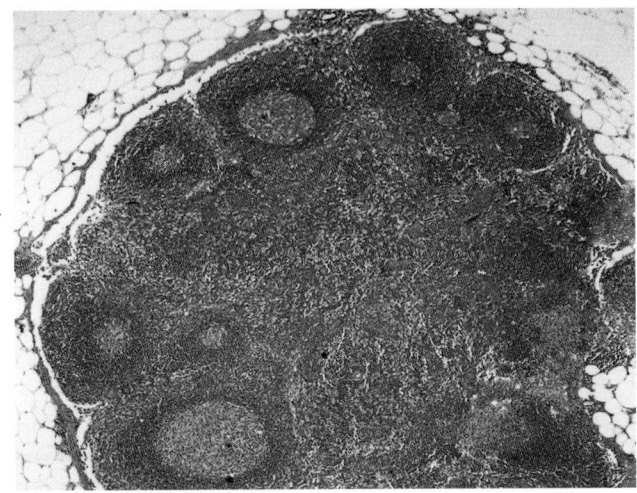

Figure 16.9 Lymph node (normal). Hematoxylin & eosin stain.

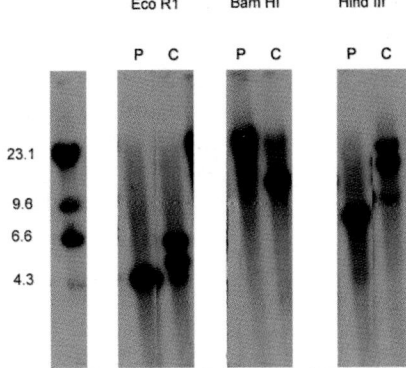

T-cell Receptor, beta chain, joining region 2

Eco R1   Bam HI   Hind III

P   C   P   C   P   C

23.1

9.6

6.6

4.3

Figure 16.10 Lymph node (patient) immunogenotyping (gene rearrangement).

Table 16.5 Flow cytometric analysis of the lymph node

Cluster designation	(Reactivity)	% of positive cells lymphoid gate
CD45	(Pan-leukocytic)	93.4
CD14	(Mo2; monocytic)	0.3
CD2	(Pan-T-Cell)	84.6
CD3	(T-cell; receptor)	81.8
CD4	(T-cell; helper)	76.6
CD8	(T-cell; suppressor)	3.1
CD5	(T-cell; B CLL)	60.0
CD7	(T-cell)	5.8
CD19	(Pan-B-cell)	6.2
CD20	(B-cell)	5.1
CD10	(Early B cell)	1.3
Kappa	(Mature B cell)	4.5
Lambda	(Mature B cell)	2.1
HLA-DR	(Diverse)	30.0

Questions

ADVANCED

5. Identify the INCORRECT statement about the special examination of the lymph node (flow cytometric immunophenotyping, Table 16.5, and immunogenotyping, Fig. 16.10):

   a. it shows changes consistent with a chronic inflammatory disorder

   b. it shows changes consistent with the extension of the patient's skin problem

   c. it shows changes that have negative prognostic implications

   d. it shows changes that represent the most common complication of the original skin problem

INTERMEDIATE

6. Which of the following statements about the immunophenotypic flow cytometric analysis (Table 16.5) of this patient's lymph node is correct?

   a. the significant increase in the percentage of CD4-positive cells (T helper cells) is diagnostic of the patient's underlying condition

   b. the expression of CD7 (pan-T cell) antigen on T cells is within the normal range

   c. B lymphocytes are immature

   d. T cells show a post-thymic stage of development

   e. all of the above statements are correct

7. All of the following statements about this patient's condition are correct EXCEPT:

a. the disorder classically presents in the skin

b. the disorder is known to involve the peripheral blood in some patients

c. once this disorder is established, the morphological appearance of abnormal cells remains unchanged

d. this disorder is not usually associated with HTLV-I infection

e. the immunophenotype of abnormal cells in this disorder may differ at different sites involved

8. Identify the correct statement about this disorder:

a. it occurs more commonly in men than women

b. it tends to affect young people (second and third decades of life)

c. most patients with this disorder die within a year of diagnosis

d. the incidence of infections in patients with this disorder is no higher than that in normal populations of the same age

e. all of the above statements are correct

ANSWERS AND FURTHER INFORMATION

Figure descriptions

Figure 16.1 Skin biopsy (patient). Hematoxylin & eosin stain.
Mycosis fungoides: There is epidermal hyperplasia with a mononuclear (neoplastic) cell infiltrate of the superficial and reticular dermis. The neoplastic cells infiltrate the epidermis and form occasional Pautrier's microabscesses (arrow).

Figure 16.2 Skin biopsy (patient). Hematoxylin & eosin stain.
Mycosis fungoides: A higher magnification showing the cytological details of the neoplastic cells. The neoplastic cells are composed of small lymphocytes, and occasional large convoluted cells.

Figure 16.3 Skin biopsy (patient). Immunohistochemical staining with anti-CD20 antibodies.
Mycosis fungoides: This section of skin is immunohistochemically stained with CD20 (B-cell) antibodies. The neoplastic cells appear to lack the CD20 antigen, i.e. they are not B lymphocytes.

Figure 16.4 Skin biopsy (patient). Immunohistochemical staining with anti-CD4 antibodies.
Mycosis fungoides: This section of skin immunohistochemically stained for CD4 (helper T-cell). The neoplastic cells appear to be CD4-positive T-lymphocytes.

Figure 16.5 Skin biopsy (normal). Hematoxylin & eosin stain.
Normal skin: This image shows normal skin with no epidermal hyperplasia. There is no abnormal cellular infiltrate of the papillary or the reticular dermis.

Figure 16.6 Chest X-ray A-P view (patient).
A normal frontal radiograph of the chest in a male patient.

Figure 16.7 Lymph node biopsy (patient). Hematoxylin & eosin stain.
T-cell lymphoma: This is an image from an expanded paracortical "T-cell zone" area of an enlarged left groin lymph node. The paracortical area is widened and contains small and large lymphocytes.

Figure 16.8 Lymph node biopsy (patient). Hematoxylin & eosin stain.
T-cell lymphoma: At this higher magnification, the cytological details of the neoplastic lymphocytes are apparent. Small lymphocytes, lymphoblasts, and large cells with convoluted "cerebriform" nuclei are seen.

Figure 16.9 Lymph node (normal). Hematoxylin & eosin stain.
Normal lymph node: Normal lymph node with preserved nodal architecture. Several lymphoid follicles with a prominent mantle zone are seen in this image.

Figure 16.10 Lymph node (patient) immunogenotyping (gene rearrangement).
DNA was extracted from the patient's lymph node, digested with *Eco*R1, *Bam*H1, and *Hind*III restriction endonucleases, electrophoresed, and developed by the Southern blot technique using the relevant probes. Rearrangements are seen in all three digests (patient "P", control "C"). This pattern shows restricted clonality of the beta chain of the T-cell receptor gene.

Answers

1. C. Psoriasis, candidiasis, and seborrhoeic dermatitis all may present as a flat, scaly erythema. Molluscum contagiosum, however, presents typically as papules or nodules.

2. A. Erythema multiforme is not associated with itching. All other conditions listed (candidiasis, seborrhoeic dermatitis, psoriasis, and atopic dermatitis) cause itching of varying degrees.

3. D. All of the features mentioned (lymphoid infiltrate of the dermis with atypical lymphoid cell and clusters of atypical lymphocytes in the epidermis) are obvious from Figs 16.1 and 16.2 (also see figure descriptions).

4. D. The predominance of T lymphocytes (without additional specification, whether the cells are morphologically normal or abnormal and without complete analysis of T cell surface markers) is a normal finding in both peripheral blood and in the tissues. It is seen in inflammatory conditions, but also in T cell lymphoproliferative disorders and sometimes in a B cell lymphoma (in some cases of cutaneous B cell lymphoma, there is a heavy inflammatory T cell infiltrate that may obscure the neoplastic B cell population – "pseudo-T cell lymphoma").

5. A. The patient has mycosis fungoides (a cutaneous T cell lymphoma). The morphologic appearance of the lymph node, together with the immunophenotyping and immunogenotyping, is consistent with the extension of the mycosis fungoides into the lymph node. This is the most common extracutaneous site for this type of lymphoma, and such extension is associated with a poorer prognosis than disease limited to the skin. The lymph node evaluation is consistent with the diagnosis of lymphoma, not with the diagnosis of a chronic inflammatory disorder.

6. D. This patient has a cutaneous lymphoma, known as mycosis fungoides, which has extended to his lymph node. This tumor is a malignant proliferation of T lymphocytes of the CD4+ (T helper) phenotype. The T cells are of a post-thymic phenotype, i.e., they express CD2, CD3, and CD4

antigen, but they do not co-express CD8 antigen, as is seen in the less mature stage of T cell development in the thymus. The significant increase in the percentage of CD4-positive T cells is seen also in T cell leukemia and lymphoma other than mycosis fungoides, therefore it is not by itself diagnostic of mycosis fungoides. An increase in CD4-positive cells is also seen in non-malignant conditions; the normal ratio of CD4- over CD8-positive cells ranges from 1 to 5:1. The CD7 antigen is normally expressed on about 85% of normal T cells. The absence of this antigen's expression, as observed in this lymph node, is an abnormal finding. B lymphocytes in this specimen are mature, since they express surface immunoglobulin (kappa or lambda light chains). Immature B cells lack surface immunoglobulin expression, and express some antigens (such as CD10 or CD34) that are typically found in early developmental stages of B cells.

7. C. Mycosis fungoides is a cutaneous T cell lymphoma in most cases not associated with HTLV-I infection. The initial presentation is usually in the skin and begins with an erythematous stage, which progresses through an infiltrative plaque stage to the tumor stage. Extracutaneous involvement is most common in the peripheral lymph nodes, but leukemic involvement of the peripheral blood is not uncommon. The immunophenotype of tumor cells may differ depending on the site of involvement. The CD7 antigen is often missing on mycosis fungoides cells in the skin, but it is usually present on the circulating tumor cells (Sézary cells). Mycosis fungoides may transform into a large cell lymphoma with different morphologic and immunophenotypic features.

8. A. Mycosis fungoides occurs more commonly in men than in women (ratio is 2:1). The median age at diagnosis is 55 years, and the median survival after the diagnosis is about 10 years. The most common causes of death are infections, especially those resulting from cutaneous lesions, but pneumonia and sepsis are also common.

Final diagnosis and synopsis of the case

- Mycosis fungoides

A previously healthy 41-year-old male presents with skin lesions, which have been spreading in spite of treatment with topical steroids. Biopsy and immunophenotyping identify the lesions as an early stage of cutaneous T cell lymphoma, known as mycosis fungoides. This is an uncommon malignancy of T helper (CD4-positive) cells, presenting primarily with cutaneous disease. Extracutaneous involvement occurs most commonly in the peripheral lymph nodes. Leukemic

involvement and the visceral involvement (spleen, lungs, and liver) occur especially in late stages of the disease. The patient is referred to a specialized clinic for treatment. After what appears to be a short remission the patient relapses and develops more extensive skin lesions, characteristic of a later stage of the disease, and involvement of the peripheral lymph node, which carries a negative prognosis. No visceral or peripheral blood involvement is detected by CT scan or by examination of the peripheral blood smear.

A 70-year-old gardener with backache

CASE AND MCQS

Clinical history and presentation

A 70-year-old man with a history of osteoarthritis developed a severe backache while working in the garden about 2 weeks ago. His family physician prescribed acetaminophen (paracetamol) with codeine for his pain and a muscle relaxant. Several days later the patient developed a dry cough, a rash on his arms, and fever. He also complained of night sweats and of weakness. His family history is unremarkable. The patient used to be a heavy smoker, but quit smoking 15 years ago; he drinks socially, and there was no history of recent travel outside of his home town in New Jersey. Physical examination revealed a well-developed and well-nourished male in no acute distress. His temperature was 100.6°F (38.1°C), pulse 114/min and regular, respirations 20/min. Blood pressure was 128/76 mmHg. The pertinent findings included decreased breath sounds at the left lung base, and several erythematous, slightly raised, round lesions on the arms and legs, some of which appeared like small target type lesions. Rectal examination revealed an enlarged prostate. The rest of the physical examination was normal. A chest X-ray was performed (Table 17.8).

Admission data

Table 17.1 Hematology

			SI units	
WBC	12.1 H	(3.6–11.2 thou/μL)	12.1 H	(3.6–11.2 × 10⁹/L)
Neut	60.2	(44–88%)	60.2	(44–88%)
Band	0	(0–10%)	0	(0–10%)
Lymph	14.1	(12–43%)	14.1	(12–43%)
Mono	3.2	(2–11%)	3.2	(2–11%)
Eos	19.7 H	(0–5%)	19.7 H	(0–5%)
Baso	3 H	(0–2%)	3 H	(0–2%)
RBC	3.5 L	(4.0–5.6 mill/μL)	3.5 L	(4.0–5.6 × 10¹²/L)
HGB	10.5 L	(12.6–17 g/dL)	10.5 L	(126–170 g/L)
HCT	31.7 L	(37.2–50.4%)	31.7 L	(0.37–0.50)
MCV	90.5	(80.5–102.1 fL)	90.5	(80.5–102.1 fL)
MCH	29.9	(27.0–35.0 pg)	29.9	(27.0–35 pg)
MCHC	33	(30.7–36.7 g/dL)	330	(307–367 g/L)
Plts	220	(130–400 thou/μL)	220	(130–400 × 10⁹/L)

Table 17.2 Chemistry

			SI Units		
Glucose	108	(65–110 mg/dL)	6.0	(3.6–6.11 mmol/L)
Creatinine	1.3	(0.7–1.4 mg/dL)	115	(61.9–123.76 µmol/L)
BUN	17	(7–24 mg/dL)	6.1	(2.50–8.57 mmol/L)
Uric acid	5.2	(3.0–8.5 mg/dL)	0.31	(0.18–0.51 mmol/L)
Cholesterol	120 L	(150–200 mg/dL)	3.1 L	(3.88–5.17 mmol/L)
Calcium	8.5	(8.5–10.5 mg/dL)	2.13	(2.13–2.63 mmol/L)
Protein	9.1 H	(6–8 g/dL)	91 H	(60–80 g/L)
Albumin	2.9 L	(3.7–5.0 g/dL)	29 L	(37–50 g/L)
LDH	203	(100–250 U/L)	203	(100–250 U/L)
Alk Phos	115	(0–120 U/L)	115	(0–120 U/L)
AST	35	(0–55 U/L)	35	(0–55 U/L)
GGTP	55 H	(0–50 U/L)	55 H	(0–50 U/L)
Bilirubin	0.6	(0.0–1.5 mg/dL)	10.3	(0–25.7 µmol/L)
Bilirubin-direct	0.12	(0.02–0.18 mg/dL)	2.05	(0.34–3.08 µmol/L)

Table 17.3 Electrolytes

		SI units		
Na	136	(134–143 mEq/L)	136	(134–143 mmol/L)
K	4.5	(3.5–4.9 mEq/L)	4.5	(3.5–4.9 mmol/L)
Cl	99	(95–108 mEq/L)	99	(95–108 mmol/L)
CO_2	28	(21–32 mEq/L)	28	(21–32 mmol/L)

Table 17.4 Coagulation

PT	12	(11–14 s)
aPTT	22	(22–32 s)
INR	0.98	

Table 17.5 Erythrocyte sedimentation rate (ESR)

ESR	128 H	(0–15 mm/hr)

Table 17.6 Urinalysis

pH	5	(5.0–7.5)
Protein	Neg	(Neg)
Glucose	Neg	(Neg)
Ketone	Neg	(Neg)
Color	Yellow	(Yellow)
Clarity	Clear	(Clear)
Sp. grav.	1.020	(1.010–1.035)
WBC	2	(0–5/HPF)
RBC	1	(0–2/HPF)
Mucus	1+	(Neg)
Bacteria	2+	(Neg)

Table 17.7 Microbiology

Blood culture	Pending
Sputum culture	Not done, no sputum available
Stool culture, ova, and parasites	Pending

Table 17.8 Chest X-ray

Left lower lobe infiltrate with pleural effusion

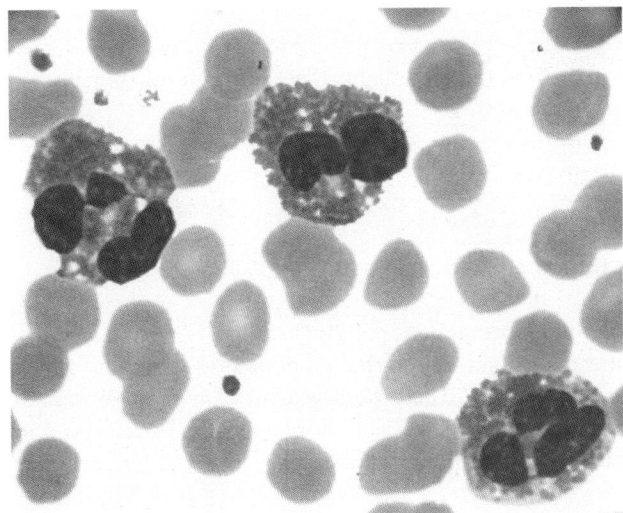

Figure 17.1 Peripheral blood smear (patient). Wright/Giemsa stain.

Questions

Based on the above information, you can best conclude the following:

INTERMEDIATE

1. The markedly elevated erythrocyte sedimentation rate (ESR) in this patient is LEAST likely caused by:

   a. the presence of an acute infection
   b. presumed osteoarthritis
   c. a possible connective tissue disease
   d. a possible underlying malignancy
   e. the presence of possible chronic inflammation

INTERMEDIATE

2. Eosinophilia in this patient would NOT be related to:

   a. his rash
   b. his pulmonary problem
   c. his presumed osteoarthritis
   d. the medication he used
   e. a yet undetected underlying malignant process

INTERMEDIATE

3. The total serum protein level in this patient is elevated while the serum albumin level is reduced. Which of the following statements is INCORRECT?

   a. serum protein electrophoresis is indicated
   b. a protein-losing nephropathy is a likely cause of this patient's hypoalbuminemia
   c. these findings are not due to dehydration
   d. these findings might reflect a chronic inflammatory process
   e. these findings might reflect a collagen vascular disease

ADVANCED

4. The distribution and the character of the skin lesions in this patient are rather characteristic of a self-limited disorder, known to be:

   a. associated with certain infections
   b. associated with collagen-vascular disorders
   c. associated with the use of certain medications
   d. associated with carcinomas and lymphomas
   e. associated with any of the above

INTERMEDIATE

5. The patient's cholesterol level is decreased. In general, all of the following conditions are known to lead to decreased cholesterol levels EXCEPT:

   a. infection and sepsis
   b. liver disease
   c. stress
   d. nephrotic syndrome
   e. malabsorption

INTERMEDIATE

6. At this stage, you would consider which of the following possible causes of this patient's problems?

   a. a drug reaction
   b. infection
   c. an unidentified collagen vascular disease
   d. an unidentified malignancy
   e. any of the above

Clinical course

Both medications prescribed for backache were discontinued, and the patient was started on antibiotic treatment, which had to be modified because the patient's clinical status was not improving. Additional laboratory tests were performed, and their results are shown in Tables 17.9–17.15. All cultures came back as negative, and no ova or parasites were identified in the stool. A bone marrow biopsy was performed and is depicted in Figs 17.2 and 17.3. A CT scan of the chest, abdomen, and pelvis was, with the exception of an enlarged prostate, normal. Several days later the patient improved symptomatically, his skin lesions resolved, and a repeated chest X-ray was normal. He was discharged and will be followed as an outpatient.

Table 17.9 Hematology (Days 3, 5, 7)

	Reference (SI Units)	Day 3	Day 5	Day 7
WBC	3.6–11.2 thou/µL (3.6–11.2 × 10⁹/L)	12.35 H	17.46 H	9.2
Neut	44–88%	56.2	45.8	42.7
Lymph	12–43%	12.0	15.1	21.5
Mono	2–11%	3.5	3.1	5.0
Eosin	0–5%	27.3 H	34.5 H	28.1 H
Baso	0–2%	0.6	1.1	2.3
RBC	4.0–5.6 mill/µL (4.0–5.6 × 10¹²/L)	3.49 L	3.74 L	3.98 L
HGB	12.6–17.0 g/dL (126–170 g/L)	10.5 (105) L	11.5 (115) L	12.3 (123) L
HCT	37.2–50.4% (0.37–0.50)	31.5 (0.315) L	34.7 (0.347) L	36.4 (0.364) L
MCV	80.5–102.1 fL	90.3	92.9	91.3
MCH	27.0–35.0 pg	30.2	30.8	31.0
MCHC	30.7–36.7 g/dL (307–367 g/L)	33.5 (335)	33.2 (332)	33.9 (339)
Plts	130–400 thou/µL (130–400 × 10⁹/L)	230	342	363

Table 17.10 Special hematology (Day 2)

			SI units		
Iron	107	(42–135 µg/dL)	19.2	(7.5–24.2 µmol/L)	
TIBC	163 L	(280–400 µg/dL)	29.2 L	(50.1–71.6 µmol/L)	
Transferrin sat.	66 H	(15–50%)	0.66 H	(0.15–0.50)	
Ferritin	625 H	(7–350 ng/mL)	625 H	(7–350 µg/L)	
Retic.	3.5 H	(0.1–2.0%)	3.5 H	(0.1–2.0%)	

Table 17.11 Erythrocyte sedimentation rate (ESR) (Days 3, 5, 7)

Reference	Day 3	Day 5	Day 7
0–15 mm/hr	130 H	115 H	130 H

Table 17.12 Serology (Day 3)

Cold aggl.	1:32 H	(Neg)
RA Test	20	(0–40 IU/mL)
RPR	Non-reactive	(Non-reactive)
Mycoplasma	Neg	(Neg)
Lyme	Neg	(Neg)
ANA	Neg	(Neg)
Legionella	Neg	(Neg)

Table 17.13 Prostate-specific antigen (PSA)

			SI Units	
PSA	1.84	(0–4.0 ng/mL)	1.84	(0–4.0 µg/L)

Table 17.14 Serum protein electrophoresis

			SI Units	
Tot. prot.	8.6 H	(6.0–8.2 g/dL)	86 H	(60–82 g/L)
Albumin	3.5 L	(3.6–5.4 g/dL)	35 L	(36–54 g/L)
Alpha-1 globulin	0.4 H	(0.1–0.3 g/dL)	4 H	(1–3 g/L)
Alpha-2 globulin	0.9	(0.4–0.9 g/dL)	9	(4–9 g/L)
Beta globulin	0.9	(0.5–1.1 g/dL)	9	(5–11 g/L)
Gamma globulin	2.9 H	(0.6–1.6 g/dL)	29 H	(6–16 g/L)

Table 17.15 IgE level

			SI Units	
IgE	0.02	(<0.025 mg/dL)	0.2	(<0.25 mg/L)

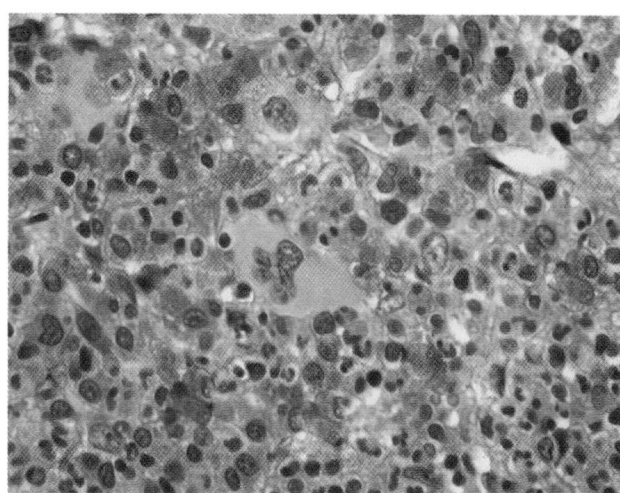

Figure 17.2 Bone marrow biopsy (patient). Hematoxylin & eosin stain.

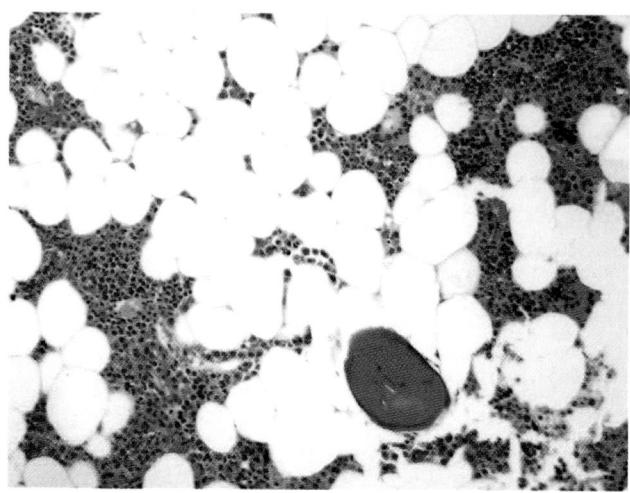

Figure 17.3 Bone marrow biopsy (normal). Hematoxylin & eosin stain.

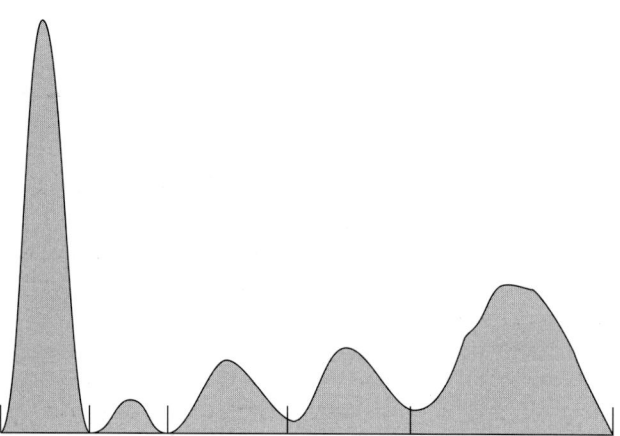

Figure 17.4 Serum protein electrophoresis (SPE) (patient).

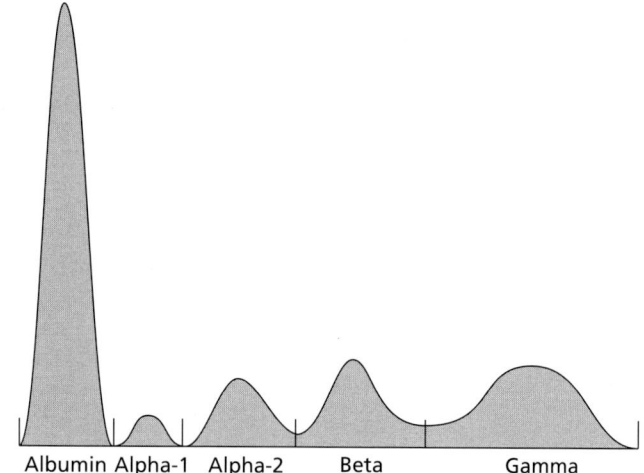

Albumin Alpha-1 Alpha-2   Beta   Gamma

Figure 17.5 Serum protein electrophoresis (SPE) (normal).

Questions

7. Which of the following statements about this patient is correct?

   a. the increase in serum ferritin is best explained as due to an iron storage overload
   b. a low TIBC reflects a low transferrin level
   c. the anemia in this patient is due to iron deficiency
   d. none of the above statements is correct

8. Serum protein electrophoresis shows an increase in the gamma globulin region and a small increase in the alpha-1 globulin region. Identify the INCORRECT statement about these findings:

   a. the gamma region is predominantly composed of antibodies of the IgG type
   b. the gamma region is elevated in chronic infectious conditions
   c. the gamma region may be elevated in hematologic malignancies
   d. transferrin is the predominant protein of the alpha-1 globulin region
   e. the alpha-1 globulin region may be elevated in the acute-phase reaction protein pattern

9. An increased titer of cold agglutinins is found in:

   a. influenza
   b. infectious mononucleosis
   c. infection with *Mycoplasma pneumoniae*
   d. lymphoma
   e. all of the above

10. Identify the INCORRECT statement about this patient's symptoms and findings:

   a. pneumonia caused by *Mycoplasma pneumoniae* should be considered
   b. the persistent increase in the erythrocyte sedimentation rate and the eosinophilia could be due to an as yet unidentified malignant process
   c. the increased number of eosinophils (Figs 17.1 and 17.2) is likely to be of reactive character
   d. the serum protein electrophoresis does not reflect an acute infectious process
   e. the available data rule out the diagnosis of idiopathic hypereosinophilic syndrome

ANSWERS AND FURTHER INFORMATION

Figure descriptions

Figure 17.1 Peripheral blood smear (patient). Wright/Giemsa stain.
This photomicrograph of the patient's peripheral blood smear shows three eosinophils. The red blood cells show mild aniso-poikilocytosis and mild normocytic normochromic anemia. Several normal-appearing platelets are present.

Figure 17.2 Bone marrow biopsy (patient). Hematoxylin & eosin stain.
Hypercellular bone marrow for the patient's age (80% hematopoietic cellularity), with prominent eosinophils. One can see numerous eosinophils (cells with red-staining cytoplasmic granules) even at this magnification. The heterogeneity of this bone marrow is apparent. Multiple megakaryocytes, normoblasts, myeloid precursors, and mature neutrophils are seen.

Figure 17.3 Bone marrow biopsy (normal). Hematoxylin & eosin stain.
This is a normal bone marrow from another patient of the same age. It shows 30% hematopoietic cellularity and trilineage heterocellular hematopoietic tissue.

Figure 17.4 Serum protein electrophoresis (SPE) (patient).
This serum protein electrophoresis from the patient shows a wide elevation in the γ-globulin region. This pattern is consistent with polyclonal gammopathy.

Figure 17.5 Serum protein electrophoresis (SPE) (normal).
Normal serum electrophoresis. No abnormal peak or elevation is seen.

Answers

1. B. Osteoarthritis does not cause a marked elevation of erythrocyte sedimentation rate (ESR). All other causes (acute and chronic infection, connective tissue diseases, or underlying malignancy) are known to cause a higher ESR.

2. C. Osteoarthritis is a degenerative process, and it does not cause an increase in circulating eosinophils. The patient's rash, as well as his pulmonary infiltrate, may be of allergic origin, and both could be associated with eosinophilia. Many drugs (including those used by the patient), as well as underlying malignant processes, are known to cause eosinophilia.

3. B. This patient has no symptoms or signs of protein-losing nephropathy (his BUN and serum creatinine are within the normal range, and there is no protein detectable in the urine). Serum protein electrophoresis is indicated because of the increase in total serum protein. Based on the electrophoretic separation one will be able to visualize the protein distribution pattern and estimate the content of different serum protein components. The finding of an increased total serum protein and of a decreased serum albumin level is seen in chronic inflammatory processes, collagen vascular diseases, etc. This patient does not appear to be dehydrated, and his BUN (expected to be increased in dehydration) is normal.

4. E. The skin lesions represent a self-limited disorder, known as erythema multiforme. Such lesions tend to involve most commonly the extremities and include macules, papules, vesicles, and a typical target lesion represented by red papule or macule with a pale center. The lesions are considered to be a hypersensitivity response to drugs and infections and are also found in patients with collagen vascular diseases and with malignancies.

5. D. Most patients with a nephrotic syndrome have increased levels of serum cholesterol, triglycerides, and very low density lipoprotein (VLDL). These abnormalities appear to be caused by increased synthesis of lipoproteins combined with decreased catabolism and abnormal transport of lipid particles in the circulation. All other conditions listed lead to a decrease in cholesterol levels, due to impaired absorption from the gastrointestinal tract, liver cell injury, or malnutrition.

6. E. This patient presents with a plethora of findings: back pain followed by constitutional symptoms, a dry cough, night sweats, and skin lesions characteristic of erythema multiforme. Laboratory findings show eosinophilia, abnormal levels of serum protein and albumin, low cholesterol, and a markedly increased erythrocyte sedimentation rate. The chest X-ray showed a left lower lobe infiltrate and a small pleural effusion, which explains the decreased breath sounds on the left side. The prostate is enlarged. All the suggested options concerning the causes and relationships of these abnormalities should be considered and explored.

7. B. Serum total iron binding capacity (TIBC) is an approximate estimate of serum transferrin. Transferrin decreases in both acute and chronic diseases and is considered to be a "negative" acute-phase reactant. The increase in serum ferritin level reflects an acute-phase response; in this case it does not represent an iron storage overload (in which the serum iron would also be increased). The patient's anemia is not likely due to iron deficiency (the ferritin level is much increased, serum iron is within the normal range, and there is an increase in the transferrin saturation with iron).

8. D. Transferrin is not a predominant protein of alpha-1 globulin region; it is a component of a beta-globulin region. The major component of alpha-1 globulin region is alpha-1 antitrypsin. The alpha-1 globulin region is sometimes elevated during an acute-phase response. The gamma region is composed predominantly of antibodies of the IgG type, which may be elevated in many conditions, such as infections, collagen vascular diseases, and lymphoproliferative disorders.

9. E. Cold agglutinins are antibodies that occur spontaneously, or in the course of diseases such as influenza, infectious mononucleosis, infection with *Mycoplasma pneumoniae*, and in the course of lymphoproliferative diseases. They also occur in patients with collagen vascular diseases. They are of IgM type; they have the ability to agglutinate red blood cells in cooler parts of the body circulation and through complement fixation cause hemolysis.

10. E. The cause of eosinophilia in this patient remains unclear. Based on the bone marrow examination and on the appearance of the peripheral blood smear, his eosinophilia appears to be of the reactive type and not of neoplastic origin. The pulmonary infiltrate could have been due to *Mycoplasma pneumoniae* infection, despite the lack of direct evidence; the patient's symptoms and findings of an increased titer of cold agglutinins and the presence of erythema multiforme lesions are compatible with mycoplasmal pneumonia. Eosinophilia, however, is not a typical finding in mycoplasmal pneumonia. The diagnosis of the hypereosinophilic syndrome has not been ruled out. In fact, many of the symptoms and findings in this patient are consistent with this syndrome, which is a chronic and progressive disorder. The persistent eosinophilia and markedly increased erythrocyte sedimentation rate are worrisome findings and warrant a follow-up of the patient for possible malignancy, collagen vascular diseases, and other possible causes.

Final diagnosis and synopsis of the case

- Pneumonia
- Erythema multiforme
- Eosinophilia
- Polyclonal hypergammaglobulinemia

An elderly, physically active man was treated for his back pain, presumed to be caused by an osteoarthritis, and subsequently developed fever, dry cough, night sweats, and general malaise. He also showed skin lesions characteristic of erythema multiforme. Physical examination and the chest X-ray were suggestive of pneumonia, for which he was treated with antibiotics. All cultures and specific serology tests to identify an etiologic agent were negative except for an increased titer of cold agglutinins. Based on these findings, combined with the presence of erythema multiforme, persistent dry cough, and lack of response to the original antibiotic regimen, the patient was considered to have mycoplasmal pneumonia. He was started on erythromycin, after which his symptoms, erythema multiforme, and his chest X-ray, rapidly cleared. His elevated serum ferritin and decreased transferrin level were considered to be due to an acute-phase reaction to his pneumonia. A decreased serum cholesterol level was attributed to the same cause. In addition the patient was found to have a significant eosinophilia, polyclonal hypergammaglobulinemia, and a markedly increased erythrocyte sedimentation rate (ESR). The work-up to identify the causes of these findings consisted of: a bone marrow biopsy and aspiration, which showed reactive changes; stool examination for ova and parasites, which was negative; CT scans of chest, abdomen, and pelvis, which were negative for neoplasm or lymphadenopathy; and a work-up for collagen vascular diseases (RA, etc.), which was also negative. Prostatic enlargement was thought to reflect benign prostate hyperplasia (note a normal level of prostate-specific antigen). A drug reaction was briefly considered as a cause of eosinophilia, but was soon disregarded owing to the persistence of eosinophilia after the medications were discontinued and because of the other persisting abnormalities. The patient was discharged, and his eosinophilia, ESR, and hyperproteinemia will be monitored on an outpatient basis. If the eosinophilia, raised ESR, and hyperproteinemia persist, the patient will undergo additional evaluation for possible causes of these abnormalities.

Lab tips

Peroxidase (myeloperoxidase) scattergram (automated hematology analyzer)

Several different automated hematology analyzers are currently available for measuring the components of peripheral blood, and they have been very useful in analyzing red cell disorders, white cell distributions, and some platelet abnormalities. Here we will examine the distribution of white blood cells in the peripheral smear of the patient in this case, by flow cytometry using cell size and cell content of the enzyme myeloperoxidase.

Thousands of cells are measured as to their size (y-axis) and their myeloperoxidase activity (x-axis) by moving the cells, one at a time, past a pair of detectors in a specified period of time. A scattergram is produced that can define five groups of leukocytes: neutrophils, lymphocytes, monocytes, eosinophils, and "large unstained cells," which are often blasts.

The intensity of the groups on the histogram depends on the number of dots (i.e. cells), which reflects the total white cell count.

The diameter and volume of WBCs are as follows:
- neutrophils measure 10–15 μm in diameter and 120–250 fL in volume
- monocytes measure 11–16 μm in diameter and 80–140 fL in volume
- basophils measure 9–14 μm in diameter and 60–120 fL in volume
- eosinophils measure 11–16 μm in diameter and 70–130 fL in volume
- lymphocytes measure 7–12 μm in diameter and 30–80 fL in volume

Two scattergrams from our patient (Fig. 17.6) and a normal adult patient (Fig. 17.7) are shown here.

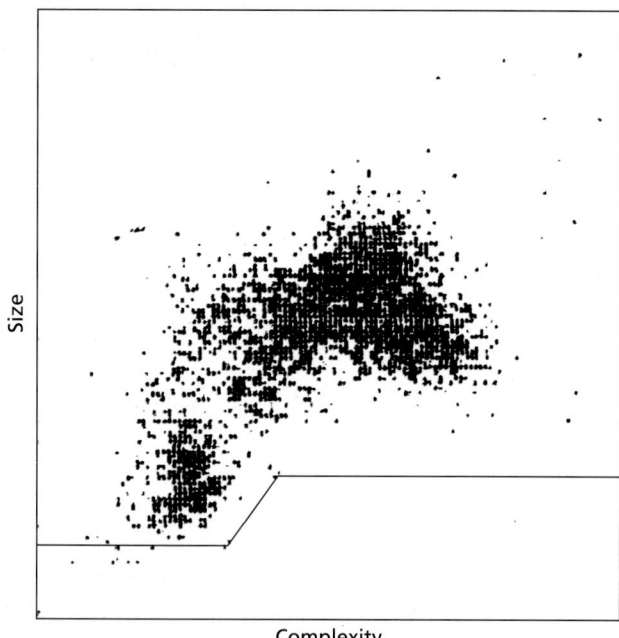

Figure 17.6 White blood cells scattergram (automated hematology analyzer) (patient).

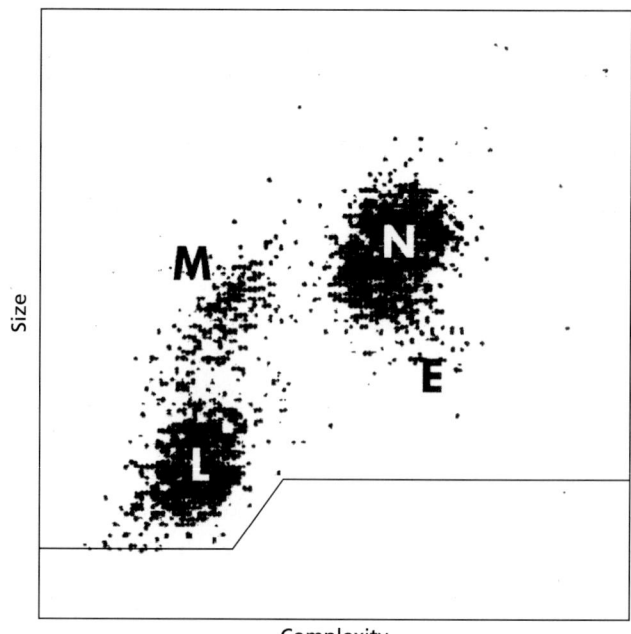

Figure 17.7 White blood cells scattergram (automated hematology analyzer) (normal).

Figure 17.6 shows the distribution of leukocytes in the blood of the patient in this case. There is a prominent group of cells in the mid-right portion of the graph. The white blood cells are measured by the automated hematology analyzer as to their size and complexity. Eosinophils measure 11–16 μm in diameter and 70–130 fL in volume and have high complex granules. This scattergram reveals that the above noted group of cells in our patient corresponds to the location for eosinophils.

Figure 17.7 shows a normal distribution of white blood cells with only a few eosinophils for comparison. In normal adult patients neutrophils (N) account for 44–88%, lymphocytes (L) for 12–43%, monocytes for 2–11% (M), and eosinophils (E) for 0–5% of white blood cells.

A 22-year-old student with a lump on the side of his neck

CASE AND MCQS

Clinical history and presentation

A 22-year-old man presented with an enlarging mass on the left side of the neck. He stated that he had noticed this mass several months ago but it was much smaller in size. The patient denied any other symptoms including weight loss, fever, and night sweats. His past medical history was unremarkable. Physical examination revealed an alert, co-operative man in no distress. His temperature was 98.3°F (36.8°C), pulse rate was 80/min and regular, blood pressure was 120/85 mmHg, and his respiratory rate was 20/min. On the left anterior side of the neck a freely movable lymph node of rubbery consistency measuring about 2 cm in greatest dimension was palpable. No other lymphadenopathy was detected. The rest of the physical examination was unremarkable. The patient was scheduled for a lymph node biopsy.

Admission data

Table 18.1 Hematology

			SI Units	
WBC	12.1 H	(3.3–11.0 thou/µL)	12.1 H	(3.3–11.0 × 10⁹/L)
Neut	75	(44–88%)	75	(44–88%)
Band	0	(0–10%)	0	(0–10%)
Lymph	16	(12–43%)	16	(12–43%)
Mono	6	(2–11%)	6	(2–11%)
Eos	2	(0–5%)	2	(0–5%)
Baso	1	(0–2%)	1	(0–2%)
RBC	5.05	(3.9–5.5 mill/µL)	5.05	(3.9–5.0 × 10¹²/L)
HGB	15.3	(11.6–15.6 g/dL)	153	(116–156 g/L)
HCT	46.4	(37.0–47.0%)	0.464	(0.37–0.47)
MCV	91.9	(79.0–99.0 fL)	91.9	(79.0–99.0 fL)
MCH	30.3	(26.0–32.6 pg)	30.3	(26.0–32.6 pg)
MCHC	33.0	(31.0–36.0 g/dL)	330	(310–360 g/L)
Plts	262	(130–400 thou/µL)	262	(130–400 × 10⁹/L)

Table 18.2 Chemistry

			SI Units	
Glucose	103	(65–110 mg/dL)	5.71	(3.6–6.11 mmol/L)
Creatinine	0.9	(0.7–1.4 mg/dL)	80	(61.9–123.76 µmol/L)
BUN	13	(7–24 mg/dL)	4.6	(2.50–8.57 mmol/L)
Uric acid	5.6	(3.0–8.5 mg/dL)	0.33	(0.18–0.51 mmol/L)
Cholesterol	193	(150–200 mg/dL)	5.0	(3.88–5.17 mmol/L)
Calcium	9.9	(8.5–10.5 mg/dL)	2.48	(2.13–2.63 mmol/L)
Protein	7.3	(6–8 g/dL)	73	(60–80 g/L)
Albumin	4.5	(3.7–5.0 g/dL)	45	(37–50 g/L)
LDH	205	(100–250 U/L)	205	(100–250 U/L)
Alk Phos	75	(0–120 U/L)	75	(0–120 U/L)
AST	26	(0–55 U/L)	26	(0–55 U/L)
GGTP	25	(0–50 U/L)	25	(0–50 U/L)
Bilirubin	0.5	(0.0–1.5 mg/dL)	8.55	(0–25.7 µmol/L)
Bilirubin-direct	0.05	(0.02–0.18 mg/dL)	0.86	(0.34–3.08 µmol/L)
Amylase	34	(13–85 U/L)	0.58	(0.22–1.45 µkat/L

Table 18.3 Electrolytes

			SI Units	
Na	140	(134–143 mEq/L)	140	(134–143 mmol/L)
K	4.7	(3.5–4.9 mEq/L)	4.7	(3.5–4.9 mmol/L)
Cl	106	(95–108 mEq/L)	106	(95–108 mmol/L)
CO_2	28	(21–32 mEq/L)	28	(21–32 mmol/L)

Table 18.4 Coagulation

PT	11.4	(11–14 s)
aPTT	29.1	(22–32 s)
INR	0.94	

Table 18.5 Erythrocyte sedimentation rate (ESR)

ESR	10	(0–15 mm/hr)

Table 18.6 Urinalysis

Within normal limits

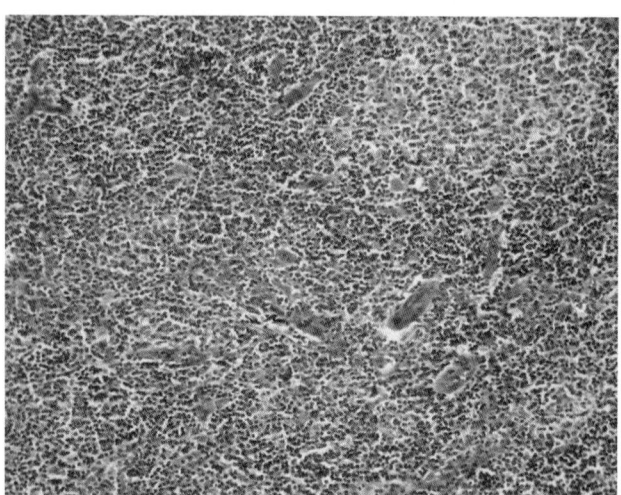

Figure 18.1 Left cervical lymph node biopsy (patient). Hematoxylin & eosin stain.

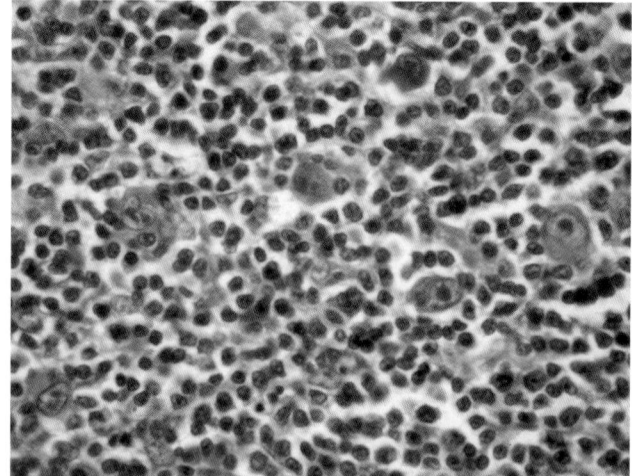

Figure 18.2 Left cervical lymph node biopsy (patient). Hematoxylin & eosin stain.

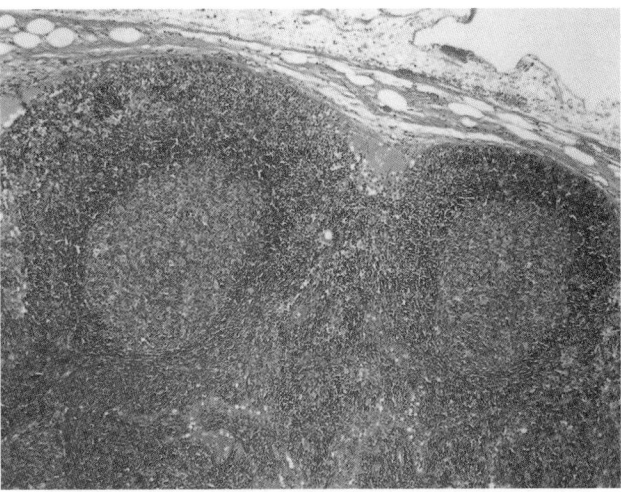

Figure 18.3 Lymph node biopsy (normal). Hematoxylin & eosin stain.

Questions

Based on the above information you can best conclude the following:

INTERMEDIATE

1. Lymph node biopsy images depicted in Figs 18.1 and 18.2 are consistent with:

   a. metastatic squamous cell carcinoma
   b. acute pyogenic lymphadenitis
   c. follicular hyperplasia
   d. granulomatous inflammation
   e. none of the above

INTERMEDIATE

2. Based on the information you have, your immediate action should be:

   a. to start intravenous antibiotic therapy
   b. to start antiviral therapy
   c. to start specific chemotherapy
   d. to ask the patient to come after 1 year for a follow-up visit
   e. none of the above

INTERMEDIATE

3. This patient's disease may be associated with:

   a. a T cell receptor (TCR) gene rearrangement
   b. an immunoglobulin gene rearrangement
   c. Epstein–Barr virus (EBV) infection
   d. all of the above
   e. none of the above

INTERMEDIATE

4. Which of the following factors is prognostically significant in this patient's disease?

   a. the patient's age at diagnosis
   b. the presence of systemic symptoms (fever, weight loss, and night sweats)
   c. the clinical stage of the disease
   d. all of the above
   e. none of the above

Clinical course

On his follow-up visit, the results of his lymph node biopsy, and the work-up required to stage his disease were discussed with the patient. He was admitted to the hospital for chest X-ray, chest, abdominal, and pelvic CT scan, and bone marrow biopsy. The patient underwent treatment, which he tolerated well. He was discharged and will be followed as an outpatient.

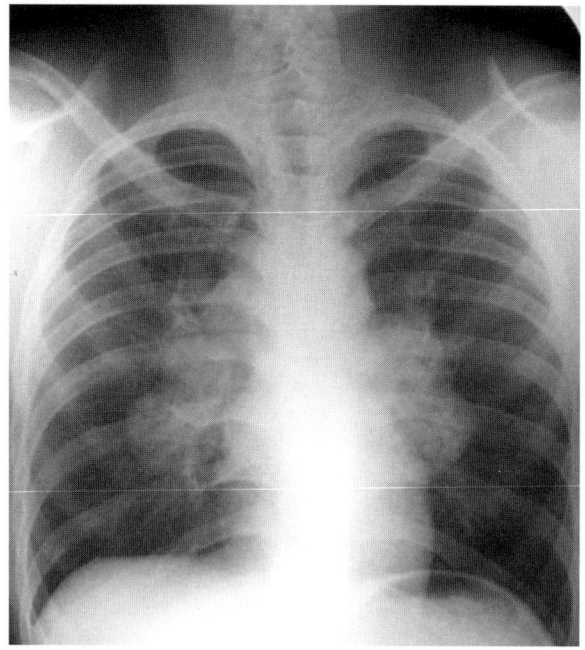

Figure 18.4 Chest X-ray, A-P view (patient).

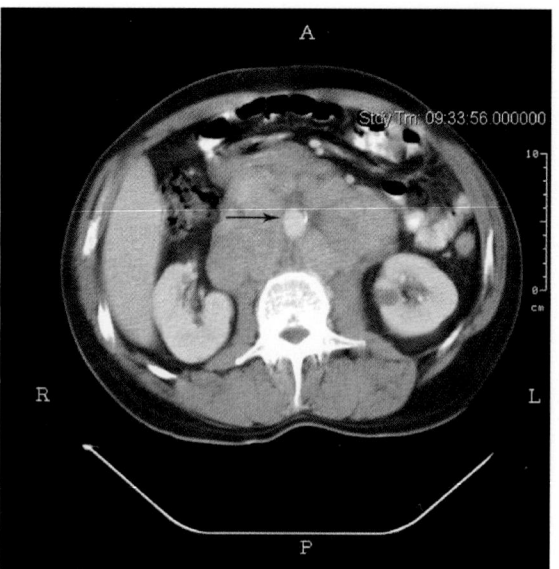

Figure 18.5 CT scan of abdomen (patient).

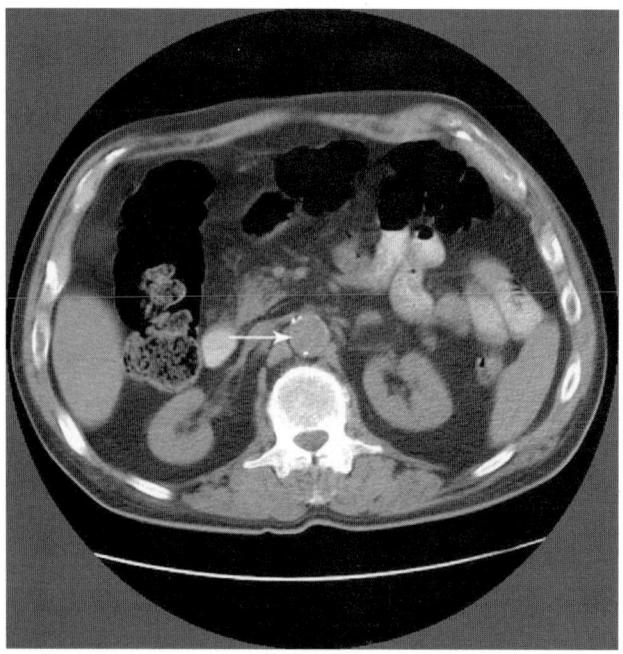

Figure 18.6 CT scan of abdomen (normal).

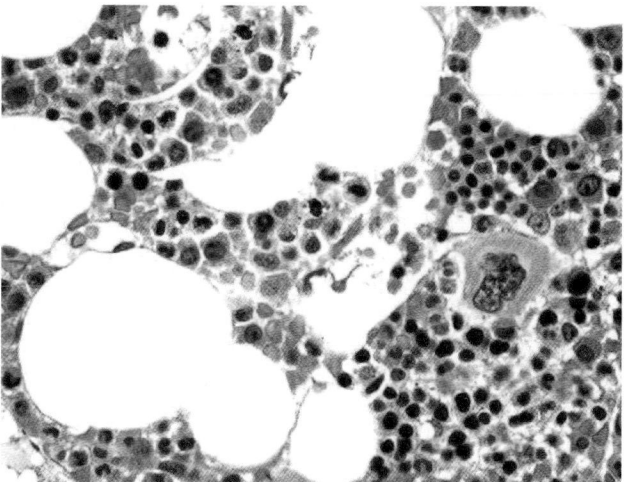

Figure 18.7 Bone marrow biopsy (patient). Hematoxylin & eosin stain.

Questions

INTERMEDIATE

5. This patient's chest X-ray (Fig. 18.4) shows:

    a. hilar lymphadenopathy
    b. cardiomegaly
    c. diffuse pulmonary infiltrate
    d. normal findings
    e. a solitary lung mass

INTERMEDIATE

6. Bone marrow biopsy (Fig. 18.7) in this patient:

    a. shows erythroid hyperplasia
    b. is normocellular
    c. shows marked fibrosis
    d. shows an increased number of abnormal plasma cells

INTERMEDIATE

7. Based on the above clinical, laboratory, and radiological findings, this patient's stage of the disease is:

    a. IA
    b. II
    c. IIA
    d. III$_{ES}$
    e. IIIA

INTERMEDIATE

8. Which of the following statements regarding this patient's disease is correct?

    a. it is caused by a transformation of a hematopoietic stem cell
    b. alcohol ingestion may induce pain
    c. hepato-splenomegaly is a frequent finding
    d. lymphoid tissue of Waldeyer's ring is usually involved
    e. extranodal involvement is common

INTERMEDIATE

9. Select the INCORRECT statement regarding a disease such as that of this patient:

    a. the erythrocyte sedimentation rate (ESR) is increased in active disease
    b. cell-mediated immunity is depressed
    c. hyperuricemia is a common finding in untreated patients
    d. anticonvulsants may produce histological changes resembling those seen in Fig. 18.1

INTERMEDIATE

10. In general, a disorder such as that of this patient is LEAST likely to be associated with:

    a. leukocytosis
    b. neutrophilia
    c. anemia
    d. eosinophilia
    e. lymphopenia

ANSWERS AND FURTHER INFORMATION

Figure descriptions

Figure 18.1 Left cervical lymph node biopsy (patient). Hematoxylin & eosin stain.
Hodgkin's disease, mixed cellularity: The lymph node architecture is effaced. This section shows a diffuse mixed cellular infiltrate of the lymph node. No lymphoid follicles or germinal centers are seen in this photomicrograph.

Figure 18.2 Left cervical lymph node biopsy (patient). Hematoxylin & eosin stain.
Hodgkin's disease, mixed cellularity: A higher magnification showing that the mixed cellular infiltrate is composed of small normal lymphocytes, scattered eosinophils, plasma cells, and histiocytes. There are many prominent larger cells with abundant eosinophilic cytoplasm and dense, sharply demarcated, eosinophilic nucleoli (mononuclear Hodgkin's cells). Two multilobed nuclei with prominent nucleoli (classical Reed–Sternberg cells) are also seen in this image. These morphological features are consistent with a diagnosis of Hodgkin's disease, mixed cellularity.

Figure 18.3 Lymph node biopsy (normal). Hematoxylin & eosin stain.
This is an image of a normal reactive lymph node with normal architecture, an open capsular space, and lymphoid follicles with prominent germinal centers.

Figure 18.4 Chest X-ray, A-P view (patient).
The chest X-ray shows a bilateral irregular widening of the hilus. This is most likely due to bilateral enlarged hilar lymph nodes.

Figure 18.5 CT scan of abdomen (patient).

Para-aortic lymphadenopathy: A bulky irregular mass of enlarged lymph nodes is seen surrounding the aorta (arrow). The kidneys and liver appear normal in this CT scan.

Figure 18.6 CT scan of abdomen (normal).

Normal CT scan of the abdomen at a slightly higher level than that of Fig. 18.5, showing a normal aorta (arrow), kidneys, liver, and spleen.

Figure 18.7 Bone marrow biopsy (patient). Hematoxylin & eosin stain.

The bone marrow is normocellular with trilineage hematopoiesis. No abnormal cellular infiltrate or Reed–Sternberg cells are noted in this image.

Answers

1. E. Figures 18.1 and 18.2 show a lymph node with a diffuse mixed infiltrate of eosinophils, plasma cells, histiocytes, and multiple binucleated large cells with prominent eosinophilic inclusion-like nucleoli (Reed–Sternberg cells). This pattern is consistent with Hodgkin's disease, mixed cellularity type. There are no morphologic features of follicular hyperplasia, metastatic squamous cell carcinoma, or of a granuloma. Pyogenic lymphadenitis would show a severe neutrophilic infiltrate and necrosis of the follicular centers, neither of which is evident in these photomicrographs.

2. E. The patient has Hodgkin's disease. A significantly large proportion of patients with Hodgkin's disease (HD) can be cured by radiotherapy, chemotherapy, or a combination of both. The appropriate choice of therapeutic plan for patients with HD is dependent on accurate staging of the disease. Accurate staging requires a complete history and physical examination, CBC (FBC), evaluation of renal and hepatic function, ESR, chest X-ray (AP and lateral views), abdominal and pelvic CT scan, bone marrow biopsy, and bipedal lymphograms. Under special circumstances staging laparotomy may be required. There is no role for antibiotic or antiviral therapy in the treatment of HD. To have a patient with HD wait for 1 year for staging of his or her disease would constitute malpractice.

3. D. In some patients with Hodgkin's disease the neoplastic cells show a T cell receptor (TCR) gene rearrangement, while others show an immunoglobulin gene rearrangement. In a large proportion (30–50%) of patients with Hodgkin's disease, EBV DNA can be identified in Reed–Sternberg cells. This association is more frequent in AIDS-related HD. Patients with a history of EBV infection are at a higher risk for HD than the normal population.

4. D. All listed factors (the patient's age at diagnosis, the presence of systemic symptoms, the clinical stage of the disease) and the histological type are well-documented prognostic factors in patients with Hodgkin's disease. A better prognosis has been observed in young patients (<40 years), in patients with clinical stage I of the disease, in the absence of systemic symptoms, and in patients with nodular sclerosis and lymphocyte predominance HD.

5. A. Chest X-ray shows mediastinal widening and bilateral hilar lymphadenopathy. There are no radiological features to suggest cardiomegaly, diffuse pulmonary infiltrate, or solitary lung mass (see Fig. 18.4 description).

6. B. Bone marrow biopsy (Fig. 18.7) shows normal hematopoietic cellularity for the patient's age (70%). There is no evidence of erythroid hyperplasia, marked fibrosis, or of increased number of abnormal plasma cells in this biopsy.

7. E. This patient was asymptomatic. His HD involved a cervical lymph node, hilar and paratracheal lymph nodes (Fig. 18.4), and retroperitoneal lymph nodes (Fig. 18.5). Involvement of lymph node regions on both sides of the diaphragm in the absence of systemic symptoms (weight loss, fever, and night sweats) is classified as stage IIIA.

8. B. The cell of origin in Hodgkin's disease (HD) is unknown; it is histologically heterogeneous. Alcohol-induced pain has been reported in some patients with Hodgkin's disease. It rarely involves lymphoid tissue of Waldeyer's ring and extranodal sites. Splenomegaly is present only in a small proportion of patients with Hodgkin's disease, and hepatomegaly is present in an even smaller proportion.

9. C. Hyperuricemia is an infrequent finding in patients with untreated Hodgkin's disease (HD); however, it is usually seen during therapy due to rapid tissue destruction. The active form of HD is associated with an abnormal ESR, serum copper level, and protein electrophoresis. The elevation of ESR correlates with constitutional symptoms. Cell-mediated immunity is depressed in patients with HD. Antibody production is minimally affected in untreated patients, but it is reduced following therapy. Some patients treated for epilepsy with anticonvulsants (diphenylhydantoin) may develop hypersensitivity reactions to the drug including lymphadenopathy, rash, eosinophilia, and fever. Histologically, lymph nodes from those patients show a mixed infiltrate of eosinophils, plasma cells, immunoblasts, and binuclear immunoblasts that closely resemble Reed–Sternberg cells. These histologic changes may pose a diagnostic challenge to distinguish them from those of HD and from non-Hodgkin lymphomas. These hypersensitivity reactions often disappear when use of the drug is stopped.

10. D. In Hodgkin's disease (HD), leukocytosis (mainly neutrophilia) may be observed. As with other malignant diseases normocytic normochromic anemia with low serum iron and normal or increased iron stores may be seen. Absolute lymphopenia is a frequent finding in patients with HD, especially in those with advanced disease. Eosinophilia, on the other hand, is rarely observed in HD. In general, neutrophilia, anemia, and lymphopenia are more common in patients with an advanced stage of Hodgkin's disease.

Final diagnosis and synopsis of the case

• Hodgkin's disease

A previously healthy young man presented with an enlarged cervical lymph node. Lymph node biopsy was diagnostic of Hodgkin's disease, mixed cellularity type. The patient had no systemic manifestations or signs of active disease. Staging radiological studies showed the involvement of the hilar, paratracheal, and para-aortic lymph nodes. His disease was classified as stage IIIA. Prognostic considerations, therapeutic options, and their possible complications were discussed with the patient.

Lab tips

World Health Organization/Revised European American Lymphoma (WHO/REAL) Classification of Hodgkin's disease

Type	Morphology	RS variants	%*	Comment
Nodular lymphocyte-predominant Hodgkin's lymphoma	• Nodular infiltrate of mature lymphocytes & histiocytes • L+H** cells (of B-cell lineage) • Eosinophils, plasma cells, neutrophils, and classic RS cells are rarely seen	L+H cells: a Reed–Sternberg (RS) cell variant with a large, lobulated nucleus (popcorn)	5%	• Young male • Excellent prognosis
Classical Hodgkin's lymphoma: nodular sclerosis	See Fig. 18.8	See Fig. 18.9	70	• More common in women • Usually involves lower cervical, supraclavicular, and mediastinal nodes • Early stage disease has excellent prognosis
Classical Hodgkin's lymphoma: mixed cellularity	See Fig. 18.10	See Fig. 18.11	23	• More common in males • Presents as a widespread disease • Most common form of HD AID
Classical Hodgkin's lymphoma: lymphocyte depletion	• Few lymphocytes and abundant RS cells or variants • Diffuse fibrosis subtype: hypocellular with fibrosis, atypical histiocytes and few RS cells • Reticular subtype: cellular with numerous pleomorphic atypical RS cells	Few classical RS cells or pleomorphic atypical RS cells	2	• A rare type of HD. When present it affects predominantly older males • Widespread, aggressive disease • Poor prognosis

* Frequency of the subtype of Hodgkin's disease. ** L+H = lymphocytic and histiocytic variants.

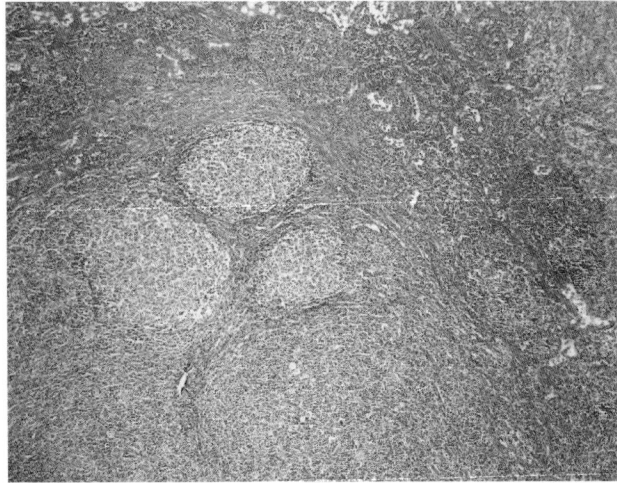

Figure 18.8 Nodular sclerosis HD.

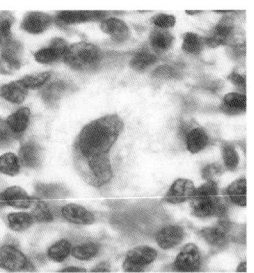

Figure 18.9 Lacunar cell.

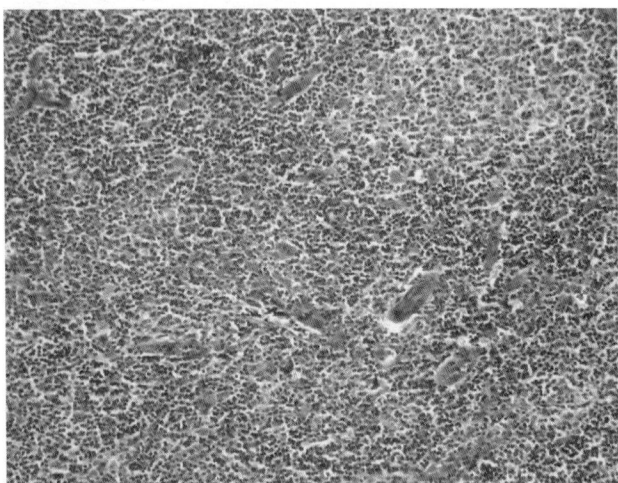

Figure 18.10 Mixed cellularity HD.

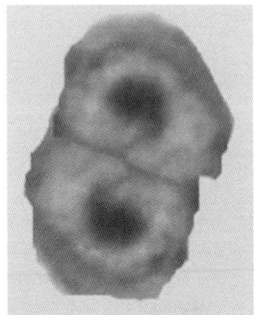

Figure 18.11 Classic RS.

Figure 18.8 Lymph node biopsy from another patient. Hematoxylin & eosin stain.

Classical Hodgkin's lymphoma, nodular sclerosis: The lymph node shows multiple irregular nodules separated by dense broad bands of collagen. The nodules contain a mixture of lymphocytes and many lacunar cells. In this type of Hodgkin's disease classic Reed–Sternberg cells are infrequent.

Figure 18.9 Lymph node biopsy from another patient. Hematoxylin & eosin stain.

Classical Hodgkin's lymphoma, nodular sclerosis: At this higher magnification the morphological features of a lacunar cell can be clearly seen, surrounded by many lymphocytes. Lacunar cells are variants of Reed–Sternberg cells and are only seen in tissue fixed with formalin (fixation artifact). They are mononuclear or multinuclear cells surrounded by clear spaces.

Figure 18.10 Lymph node biopsy (patient). Hematoxylin & eosin stain.

Hodgkin's disease, mixed cellularity: The lymph node architecture is effaced. This section shows a diffuse mixed cellular infiltrate of the lymph node. No lymphoid follicles or germinal centers are seen in this photomicrograph.

Figure 18.11 Lymph node biopsy from another patient. Hematoxylin & eosin stain.

Classical Hodgkin's lymphoma, mixed cellularity: At this higher magnification a binucleated Reed–Sternberg cell with prominent eosinophilic, inclusion-like nucleoli can be clearly seen.

A 70-year-old sailor with heartburn and crimson face

CASE AND MCQS

Clinical history and presentation

A 70-year-old man presented with epigastric pain and heartburn. He admitted to multiple similar episodes, which were occasionally associated with nausea and vomiting of dark, coffee-ground like material over the last 2 weeks. The patient stated that the pain often occurred at night and was somewhat relieved by food. He denied weight loss, cigarette smoking, and alcohol abuse. His past medical history included ischemic heart disease and hypertension. Physical examination showed an alert, co-operative man in mild

distress, with facial plethora. His temperature was 98.3°F (36.8°C), pulse rate was 86 beats/min and regular, blood pressure was 140/90 mmHg, and his respiratory rate was 18/min. Abdominal examination revealed a mild epigastric tenderness to palpation. The spleen was palpable. Rectal examination revealed mild prostatic enlargement and a guaiac-positive stool. The rest of the physical examination was unremarkable. An endoscopy was performed (Fig. 19.3).

Admission data

Table 19.1 Hematology

			SI Units	
WBC	21.59 H	(3.3–11.0 thou/μL)	21.59 H	(3.3–11.0 × 10⁹/L)
Neut	65	(44–88%)	65	(44–88%)
Band	10	(0–10%)	10	(0–10%)
Lymph	6 L	(12–43%)	6 L	(12–43%)
Mono	8	(2–11%)	8	(2–11%)
Eos	7 H	(0–5%)	7 H	(0–5%)
Baso	4 H	(0–2%)	4 H	(0–2%)
RBC	8.37 H	(3.9–5.0 mill/μL)	8.37 H	(3.9–5.0 × 10¹²/L)
HGB	21.2 H	(11.6–15.6 g/dL)	212 H	(116–156 g/L)
HCT	67.3 H	(37.0–47.0%)	0.673 H	(0.37–0.47)
MCV	80.4	(79.0–99.0 fL)	80.4	(79.0–99.0 fL)
MCH	25.4 L	(26.0–32.6 pg)	25.4 L	(26.0–32.6 pg)
MCHC	31.5	(31.0–36.0 g/dL)	315	(310–360 g/L)
Plts	948 H	(130–400 thou/μL)	948 H	(130–400 × 10⁹/L)

Table 19.2 Chemistry

			SI Units	
Glucose	100	(65–110 mg/dL)	5.55	(3.6–6.11 mmol/L)
Creatinine	1.1	(0.7–1.4 mg/dL)	97.2	(61.9–123.76 µmol/L)
BUN	16	(7–24 mg/dL)	5.7	(2.50–8.57 mmol/L)
Uric acid	9.3 H	(3.0–8.5 mg/dL)	0.55 H	(0.18–0.51 mmol/L)
Cholesterol	163	(150–200 mg/dL)	4.21	(3.88–5.17 mmol/L)
Calcium	9.0	(8.5–10.5 mg/dL)	2.25	(2.13–2.63 mmol/L)
Protein	7.4	(6–8 g/dL)	74	(60–80 g/L)
Albumin	4.2	(3.7–5.0 g/dL)	42	(37–50 g/L)
LDH	221	(100–250 U/L)	221	(100–250 U/L)
Alk Phos	74	(0–120 U/L)	74	(0–120 U/L)
AST	34	(0–55 U/L)	34	(0–55 U/L)
GGTP	14	(0–50 U/L)	14	(0–50 U/L)
Bilirubin	1.1	(0.0–1.5 mg/dL)	18.8	(0–25.7 µmol/L)
Bilirubin-direct	0.09	(0.02–0.18 mg/dL)	1.54	(0.34–3.08 µmol/L)
Amylase	20	(13–85 U/L)	0.34	(0.22–1.45 µkat/L)

Table 19.3 Electrolytes

			SI Units	
Na	138	(134–143 mEq/L)	138	(134–143 mmol/L)
K	4.4	(3.5–4.9 mEq/L)	4.4	(3.5–4.9 mmol/L)
Cl	100	(95–108 mEq/L)	100	(95–108 mmol/L)
CO_2	26	(21–32 mEq/L)	26	(21–32 mmol/L)

Table 19.4 Arterial blood gases

			SI Units	
pH	7.39	(7.35–7.45)	7.39	(7.35–7.45)
PCO_2	32	(32–46 mmHg)	4.27	(4.27–6.13 kPa)
PO_2	89	(74–108 mmHg)	11.9	(9.86–14.4 kPa)
HCO_3^-	25	(21–29 mEq/L)	25	(21–29 mmol/L)
O_2 saturation	97	(92–100%)	97	(92–100%)

Table 19.5 Erythrocyte sedimentation rate4

ESR	1		(0–15 mm/hr)

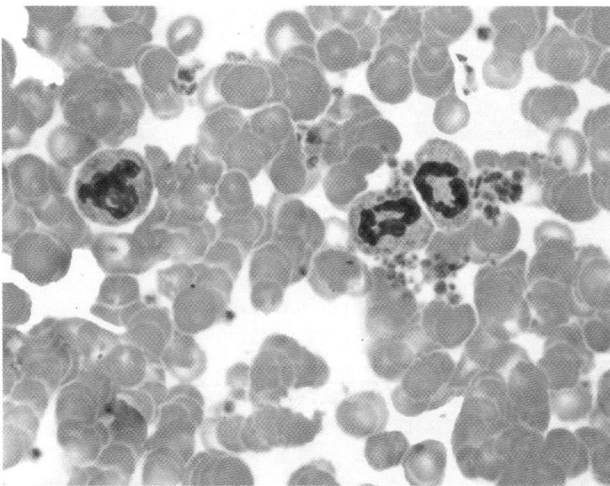

Figure 19.1 Peripheral blood smear (patient). Wright/Giemsa stain.

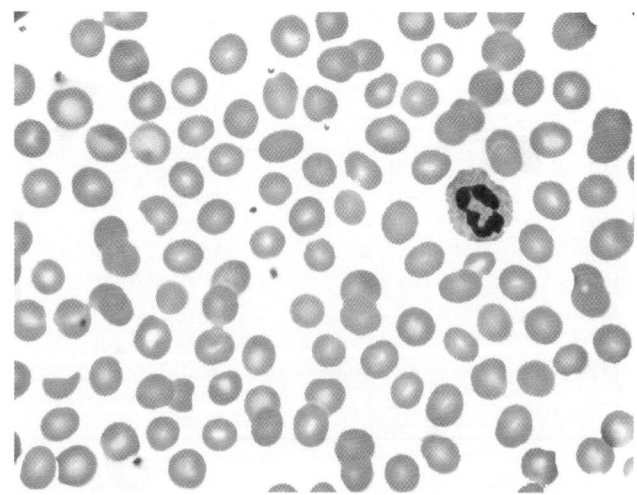

Figure 19.2 Peripheral blood smear (normal). Wright/Giemsa stain.

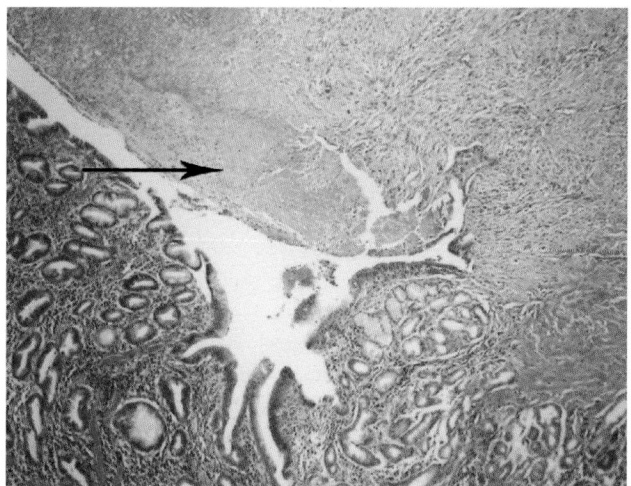

Figure 19.3 Duodenal biopsy (patient). Hematoxylin & eosin stain.

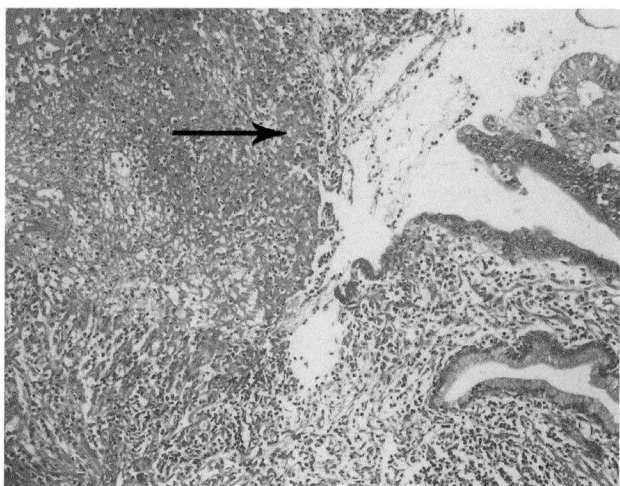

Figure 19.4 Duodenal biopsy (patient). Hematoxylin & eosin stain.

Questions

Based on the above information you can best conclude the following:

1. Peripheral blood smear (Fig. 19.1) and CBC (FBC) in this patient are consistent with:

   a. megaloblastic anemia
   b. increased numbers of lymphoblasts
   c. increased numbers of mature lymphocytes
   d. none of the above

2. The patient's duodenal biopsy depicted in Figs 19.3 and 19.4 is suggestive of:

   a. malignant ulcer
   b. hyperplastic polyp
   c. lymphoma
   d. peptic ulcer

3. This patient's erythrocytosis is most likely due to:

   a. hypoxia
   b. an obstructive lung disease
   c. a renal cell carcinoma
   d. a myeloproliferative disorder
   e. dehydration

4. This patient's increased level of serum uric acid can be best related to:

   a. liver cirrhosis
   b. increased cell turnover
   c. an acute renal failure
   d. a chronic renal disease
   e. splenomegaly

5. The most common cause of upper gastrointestinal bleeding in the Western hemisphere is:

   a. esophageal varices
   b. peptic ulcer
   c. gastric carcinoma
   d. esophageal squamous cell carcinoma

6. Which of the following factors may be implicated in the pathogenesis of the patient's lesion depicted in the duodenal biopsy (Figs 19.3 and 19.4)?

   a. increased numbers of basophils
   b. thrombosis
   c. *Helicobacter pylori* infection
   d. increased histamine levels
   e. all of the above

Clinical course

Abdominal ultrasound examination confirmed moderate splenomegaly, and showed mild hepatomegaly, and no other abnormalities. The patient was treated conservatively and his gastrointestinal symptoms improved. The results of additional laboratory tests aimed at investigating the patient's hematological abnormalities are shown below (Table 19.6 and Figs 19.5–19.7). A few days later he was discharged to be followed as an outpatient.

Table 19.6 Special hematology

Total blood volume	12 401 H	(adjusted to the patient's weight: 5025 mL)
Plasma volume	4055 H	(adjusted to the patient's weight: 3015 mL)
Red blood cell mass	8346 H	(adjusted to the patient's weight: 2010 mL)

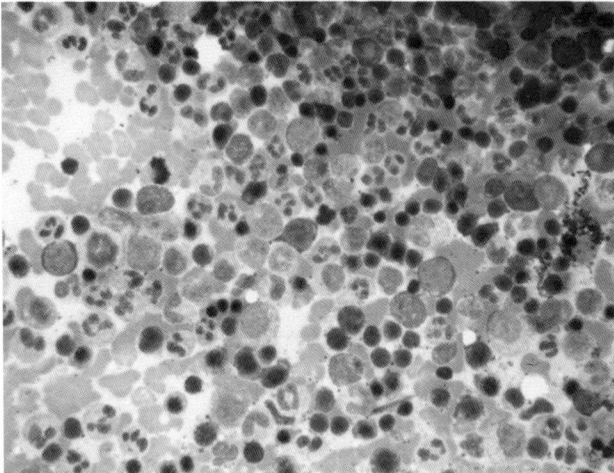

Figure 19.5 Bone marrow aspiration smear (patient). Wright/Giemsa stain.

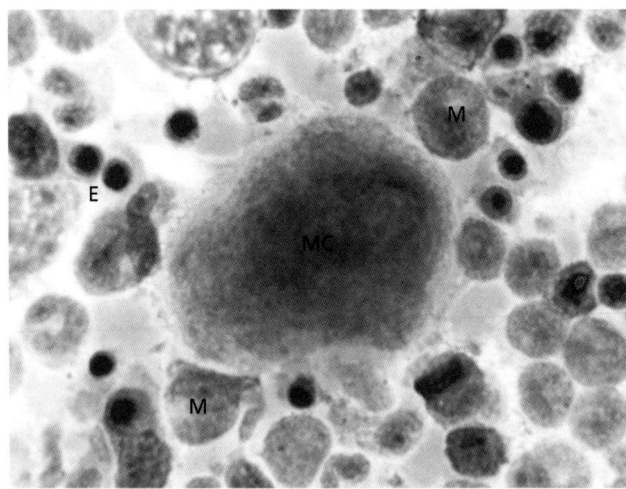

Figure 19.6 Bone marrow aspiration smear (patient). Wright/Giemsa stain.

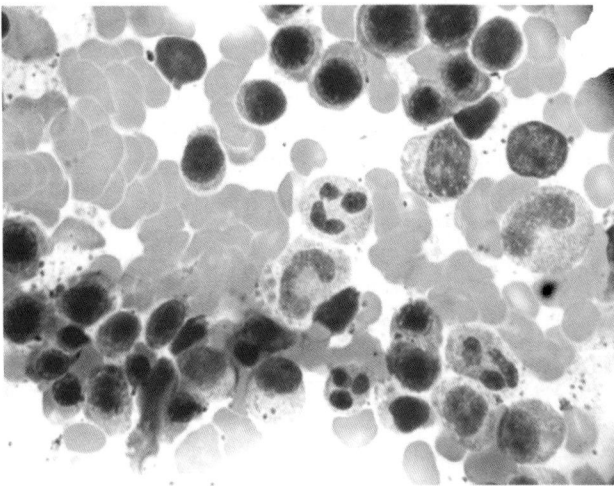

Figure 19.7 Bone marrow aspiration smear (patient). Wright/Giemsa stain.

Questions

7. All of the following statements regarding this patient's hematological problem are correct EXCEPT:

a. it is caused by a transformation of a hematopoietic stem cell

b. it is associated with an increased blood viscosity

c. morphological changes observed in the peripheral blood smear are in themselves diagnostic of his hematological problem

d. thrombotic episodes are the most common complication

ADVANCED

8. Bone marrow aspiration smear (Figs 19.5–19.7) in this patient:

a. shows erythroid hyperplasia

b. is hypocellular

c. shows a large cluster of atypical lymphocytes

d. shows an increased number of abnormal plasma cells

e. would show increased iron storage

INTERMEDIATE

9. Select the INCORRECT statement regarding the hematological condition affecting this patient:

a. reduction of this patient's hemoglobin content would decrease the spleen size

b. microscopic examination of the spleen would reveal extramedullary hematopoiesis

c. the microscopic examination of the bone marrow (Figs 19.5–19.7) shows atypical megakaryocytes

d. most untreated patients with this condition show no cytogenetic abnormalities

INTERMEDIATE

10. Select the INCORRECT general statement about the hematological condition of this patient:

a. it has a peak incidence in the sixth and seventh decades

b. the life span of the red blood cells is normal

c. it is a familial disease

d. it is frequently associated with intense itching after bathing

INTERMEDIATE

11. In general, the hematological disorder found in this patient:

a. is more common in woman

b. is usually associated with an increased level of vitamin B_{12}

c. is associated with a high serum level of erythropoietin

d. is not associated with cyanosis

ANSWERS AND FURTHER INFORMATION

Figure descriptions

Figure 19.1 Peripheral blood smear (patient). Wright/Giemsa stain.
This is an image of a well-spread peripheral blood smear with a large number of overlapping erythrocytes. There is also a marked increase in the number of platelets. Three neutrophils are noted in this field.

Figure 19.2 Peripheral blood smear (normal). Wright/Giemsa stain.
This normal peripheral blood smear shows normal red blood cells, an adequate number of platelets, and one neutrophil.

Figure 19.3 Duodenal biopsy (patient). Hematoxylin & eosin stain.
Duodenal ulcer: This image shows a duodenal ulcer (upper part of the image, arrow) with thick fibrinous exudate. On the left there is a portion of duodenal mucosa with intact mucosa and a marked inflammatory cell infiltrate.

Figure 19.4 Duodenal biopsy (patient). Hematoxylin & eosin stain.
Duodenal ulcer: At a higher magnification, the ulcer bed (arrow) shows denuded epithelium, mixed dense inflammatory cells, and fibrinous material.

Figure 19.5 Bone marrow aspiration smear (patient). Wright/ Giemsa stain.

Polycythemia rubra vera: This image shows a hypercellular bone marrow aspirate smear. There is a marked normoblastic hyperplasia. Numerous myeloid cells in different stages of maturation are also seen in this image. Elsewhere in this smear (not shown in this image), a megakaryocytic hyperplasia with atypical megakaryocytes was noted.

Figure 19.6 Bone marrow aspiration smear (patient). Wright/ Giemsa stain.

Polycythemia rubra vera: This photomicrograph shows an atypical mononuclear megakaryocyte (MC) and numerous myeloid (M) and erythroid (E) precursors.

Figure 19.7 Bone marrow aspiration smear (patient). Wright/ Giemsa stain.

Polycythemia rubra vera: This image of the patient's bone marrow aspiration smear shows normoblastic hyperplasia and a few myeloid precursors.

Answers

1. D. This patient's peripheral blood smear (Fig. 19.1) and CBC (FBC) show leukocytosis, thrombocytosis, and microcytic hypochromic erythrocytosis. Features of megaloblastic anemia include macrocytic hyperchromic anemia, hypersegmented neutrophils, numerous oval macrocytes, schistocytes, basophilic stippling, and Howell–Jolly bodies, none of which is present in this patient. There is also no lymphocytosis (the patient has 1290 lymphocytes/μL; lymphocytosis is defined as a lymphocyte count exceeding 4000 lymphocytes/μL).

2. D. Figure 19.3 shows a typical appearance of a peptic ulcer (see figure description). There are no morphologic changes to suggest malignant ulcer, hyperplastic polyp, or lymphoma.

3. D. The presence of facial plethora, pancytosis (erythrocytosis, leukocytosis, and thrombocytosis), normal O_2 saturation, and splenomegaly favor the diagnosis of polycythemia rubra vera (PRV) over secondary polycythemia. An increased number of circulating red blood cells in response to hypoxia, obstructive lung diseases with hypoxia, congenital heart disease or caused by inappropriate production of erythropoietin by tumor (renal cell carcinoma) is called secondary polycythemia. Dehydration, on the other hand, leads to a relative polycythemia, due to a decrease in the plasma volume.

4. B. The diagnosis of polycythemia rubra vera (PRV) was suspected because of the presence of facial plethora, pancytosis, normal O_2 saturation, and splenomegaly. In PRV, as in other myeloproliferative disorders, increased serum uric acid is related to increase in cell turnover (increase in nucleic acid breakdown) and to the production of an excess amount of free purine bases. This patient shows no signs or symptoms of acute or chronic renal disease. Liver cirrhosis and splenomegaly in themselves do not increase serum uric acid.

5. B. All listed conditions (esophageal varices, peptic ulcer, gastric carcinoma, and esophageal squamous cell carcinoma) lead to upper gastrointestinal bleeding. In the Western hemisphere the most common cause (40–50%) of upper gastrointestinal bleeding is peptic ulcer.

6. E. This patient has polycythemia rubra vera (PRV), which is associated with an increased prevalence of peptic ulcer (4 to 5 times normal). The pathogenesis of peptic ulcer in PRV patients is uncertain. Some investigators have suggested that peptic ulcer in patients with PRV is due to the action of digestive enzymes on necrotic areas produced by thrombosis in the vessels of the first part of the duodenum. Others have proposed that it is due to the increased release of histamine from the abnormally high number of basophils. In general, *Helicobacter pylori* infection appears to play an important role in the pathogenesis of peptic ulcer. The distribution of *Helicobacter pylori* is patchy, and its absence from a duodenal biopsy does not rule out the possibility of *Helicobacter pylori* infection as a contributing factor for this patient's peptic ulcer.

7. C. Polycythemia rubra vera (PRV) is due to a defect of a single hematopoietic stem cell, which leads to an increased production of all marrow elements. In PRV the blood viscosity is increased (5–8 times normal). The peripheral blood smear (Fig. 19.1) shows a large number of erythrocytes, and increased numbers of leukocytes and platelets, which in themselves are not diagnostic of PRV. Thrombotic episodes are the most common complication of PRV. Thrombotic complication of PRV may include hepatic vein thrombosis (Budd–Chiari syndrome), cerebrovascular accident, myocardial infarction, deep vein thrombosis, and pulmonary embolism.

8. A. Bone marrow aspiration smear (Figs 19.5–19.7) shows hyperplasia of all three hematopoietic cell lines (see figure descriptions), which by itself is not diagnostic of polycythemia rubra vera. There are no abnormal lymphocytes or plasma cells seen. In most patients with polycythemia rubra vera (PRV) serum iron concentration is low, and iron stores in the bone marrow are absent or low due to increased hematopoiesis and iron utilization.

9. A. Mild to moderate splenomegaly is seen in the majority of patients with polycythemia rubra vera (PRV). Reduction of the hemoglobin content by multiple phlebotomies does not lead to reduction of the size of the spleen. Microscopic examination of the spleen and the liver would show multiple foci of extramedullary hematopoiesis and congestion. The spleen in patients with PRV shows normal follicular architecture. Microscopic examination of the bone marrow (Fig. 19.6) shows atypical mononuclear megakaryocytes. Only 10–15% of patients with PRV have cytogenetic abnormalities (most frequently trisomy 9). In patients with PRV previously treated with radiation or chemotherapy, however, the incidence of cytogenetic abnormalities approaches 40%.

10. C. The majority of patients with polycythemia rubra vera (PRV) do not have a family history of the disease. PRV has a peak incidence in the sixth and seventh decades. The life span of the red blood cells is normal and the erythrocytosis is secondary to an increased production of RBCs. PRV is frequently associated with intense itching after bathing (aquagenic pruritus). The pathogenesis of pruritus is uncertain, but the increased number of cutaneous mast cells and the elevated histamine level present in these patients have been implicated. The pruritus tends to disappear after treatment.

11. B. In patients with polycythemia rubra vera (PRV) the level of vitamin B_{12} is usually increased due to the increased production of cobalophilin (transcobalamin I), also known as R-protein, by leukocytes. PRV is more common in men in their sixth and seventh decades. The serum level of erythropoietin in patients with PRV is low or absent. True cyanosis may be seen particularly in the distal portion of the extremities due to stagnation and deoxygenation of blood.

Final diagnosis and synopsis of the case

- Duodenal ulcer
- Polycythemia rubra vera

An elderly man presented with multiple episodes of epigastric pain, heartburn, nausea, vomiting, and hematemesis of 2 weeks' duration, which were diagnosed as being due to a duodenal ulcer. During routine laboratory testing he was found to have severe erythrocytosis, leukocytosis, and thrombocytosis. The presence of pancytosis, splenomegaly, normal O_2 saturation, and facial plethora favors the diagnosis of polycythemia rubra vera over secondary polycythemia. The diagnosis was confirmed by the presence of an elevated red blood cell mass. His duodenal ulcer is most likely a consequence of his polycythemia rubra vera (with increased release of histamine and/or a thrombotic complication). Multiple phlebotomies are the common initial treatment for most patients with PRV.

Lab tips

Laboratory investigations of polycythemia
Relative and absolute polycythemia can be distinguished by measurement of the red blood cell mass and plasma volume. This is an invasive procedure using radiolabeled red blood cells, and the test is useful when the cause of the polycythemia is clinically unclear. The test is not indicated when any of the following situations are present:

1. Hgb > 20 g/dL (200 g/L) or HCT >60% (0.60), reason: increased red blood cell mass assumed.
2. Decreased arterial PO_2, reason: absolute polycythemia is due to hypoxia.
3. Leukocytosis, thrombocytosis, and splenomegaly, reason: diagnosis is most likely polycythemia rubra vera.

The laboratory features of polycythemias

Laboratory test	Relative polycythemia	Absolute polycythemia	
		Secondary polycythemia	Polycythemia rubra vera
Red blood cell volume	Normal	Increased	Increased
Erythropoietin level	Normal	Usually normal (increased in inappropriate erythropoietin secretion by tumors)	Decreased
PO_2	Normal	Sometimes decreased	Normal
Carboxyhemoglobin	Increased (smokers)	Increased (smokers)	Normal
Leukocyte alkaline phosphatase	Usually normal	Usually normal	Increased
Serum ferritin	Normal	Normal	Decreased
Serum iron	Normal	Normal	Decreased
Serum uric acid	Normal	Normal	Increased
Serum vitamin B_{12}	Normal	Normal	Increased
Leukocytosis	May be present depending on disease	May be present depending on disease	Usually present
Thrombocytosis	May be present depending on disease	May be present depending on disease	Usually present
Bone marrow examination	Normal	May be abnormal (metastatic disease)	Abnormal (hematopoietically hypercellular)

A 62-year-old housekeeper with unusual gait

CASE AND MCQS

Clinical history and presentation

A 62-year-old woman complained of increasing fatigue, difficulty in walking, and of increasing weakness in her upper extremities over the last year. She described tingling sensations in all four extremities in a "stocking-and-glove distribution," which she first noticed at the tips of the toes 7 months ago. Recently, she has become irritable, forgetful, and has experienced mood swings. Her past medical history included multiple episodes of nausea, vomiting, and upper abdominal discomfort for which she underwent gastric biopsy 4 years ago (Figs 20.1 and 20.3). Physical examination reveals a pale woman with slightly icteric sclerae. Her temperature was 99.1°F (37.3°C), pulse rate was 94/min and regular, blood pressure was 125/85 mmHg. Her tongue appeared smooth and "beefy" red. Abdominal and chest examinations were unremarkable. Neurological examination revealed weakness and spasticity in the proximal muscles of all four extremities, hyperactive deep tendon reflexes, a positive Babinski's sign, and a loss of position and (high-frequency) vibration sense. There was no muscle fasciculation or significant muscle atrophy. Cranial nerve examination was normal.

Admission data

Table 20.1 Hematology

			SI Units	
WBC	2.8 L	(3.3–11.0 thou/µL)	2.8 L	(3.3–11.0 × 10⁹/L)
Neut	54	(44–88%)	54	(44–88%)
Band	0	(0–10%)	0	(0–10%)
Lymph	34	(12–43%)	34	(12–43%)
Mono	5	(2–11%)	5	(2–11%)
Eos	5	(0–5%)	5	(0–5%)
Baso	2	(0–2%)	2	(0–2%)
RBC	1.6 L	(3.9–5.0 mill/µL)	1.6 L	(3.9–5.0 × 10¹²/L)
HGB	6.7 L	(11.6–15.6 g/dL)	67 L	(116–156 g/L)
HCT	23 L	(37.0–47.0%)	0.23 L	(0.37–0.47)
MCV	144 H	(79.0–99.0 fL)	144 H	(79.0–99.0 fL)
MCH	41.9 H	(26.0–32.6 pg)	41.9 H	(26.0–32.6 pg)
MCHC	29.0 L	(31.0–36.0 g/dL)	290 L	(310–360 g/L)
Plts	161	(130–400 thou/µL)	161	(130–400 × 10⁹/L)
Retic	0.4	(0.1–2.0%)	0.4	(0.1–2.0%)

Table **20.2** Chemistry

			SI Units	
Glucose	100	(65–110 mg/dL)	5.56	(3.6–6.11 mmol/L)
Creatinine	1.1	(0.7–1.4 mg/dL)	97.2	(61.9–123.76 µmol/L)
BUN	17	(7–24 mg/dL)	6.07	(2.50–8.57 mmol/L)
Uric acid	5.6	(3.0–8.5 mg/dL)	0.33	(0.18–0.51 mmol/L)
Cholesterol	150	(150–200 mg/dL)	3.88	(3.88–5.17 mmol/L)
Calcium	9.2	(8.5–10.5 mg/dL)	2.3	(2.13–2.63 mmol/L)
Protein	7.1	(6–8 g/dL)	71	(60–80 g/L)
Albumin	4.3	(3.7–5.0 g/dL)	43	(37–50 g/L)
LDH	931 H	(100–250 U/L)	931 H	(100–250 U/L)
Alk Phos	74	(0–120 U/L)	74	(0–120 U/L)
AST	50	(0–55 U/L)	50	(0–55 U/L)
GGTP	14	(0–50 U/L)	14	(0–50 U/L)
Bilirubin	2.9 H	(0.0–1.5 mg/dL)	49.6 H	(0–25.7 µmol/L)
Bilirubin-direct	0.53 H	(0.02–0.18 mg/dL)	9.1 H	(0.34–3.08 µmol/L)
Amylase	24	(13–85 U/L)	0.41	(0.22–1.44 µkat/L)

Table **20.3** Electrolytes

			SI Units	
Na	138	(134–143 mEq/L)	138	(134–143 mmol/L)
K	4.4	(3.5–4.9 mEq/L)	4.4	(3.5–4.9 mmol/L)
Cl	100	(95–108 mEq/L)	100	(95–108 mmol/L)
CO_2	26	(21–32 mEq/L)	26	(21–32 mmol/L)

Table **20.4** Urinalysis

pH	6.5	(5.0–7.5)
Protein	Neg	(Neg)
Glucose	Neg	(Neg)
Ketone	Neg	(Neg)
Color	Yellow	(Yellow)
Clarity	Clear	(Clear)
Sp. grav.	1.021	(1.010–1.035)
WBC	2	(0–5/HPF)
RBC	1	(0–2/HPF)
Casts	Neg	(Neg)
Urobilinogen	2+ H	(Neg)

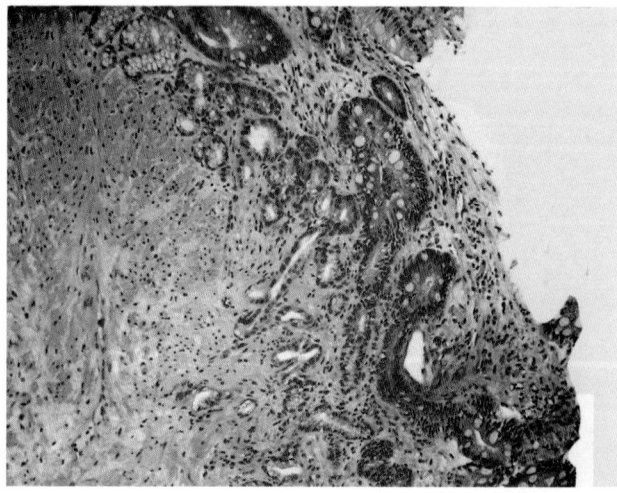

Figure 20.1 Gastric biopsy (patient). Hematoxylin & eosin stain.

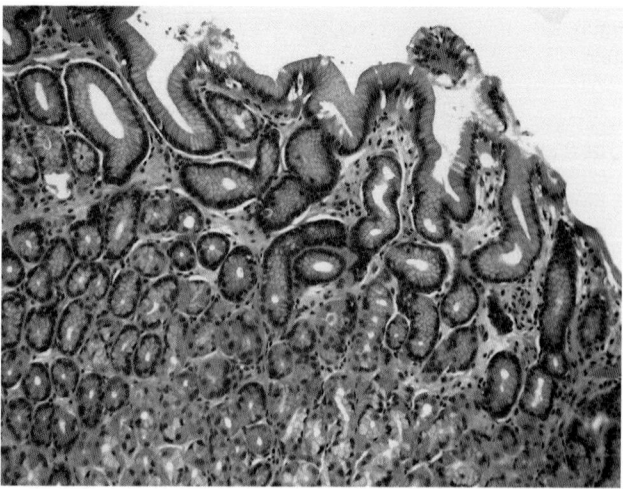

Figure 20.2 Gastric biopsy (normal). Hematoxylin & eosin stain.

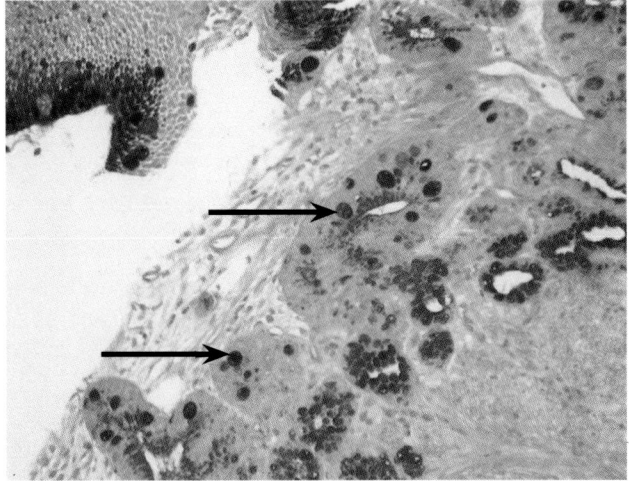

Figure 20.3 Gastric biopsy (patient). PAS/Alcian blue stain.

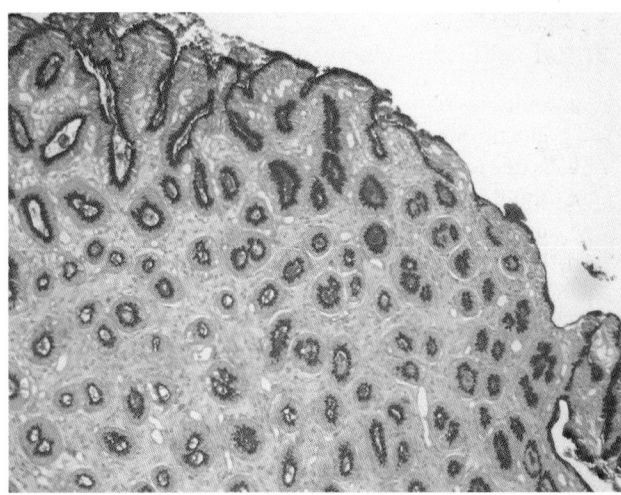

Figure 20.4 Gastric biopsy (normal). PAS/Alcian blue stain.

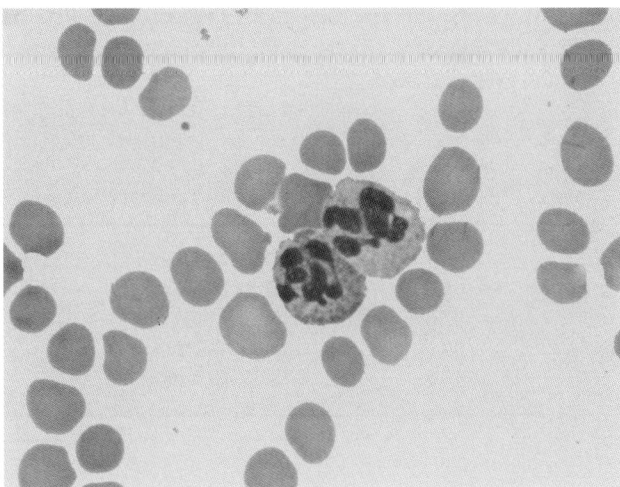

Figure 20.5 Peripheral blood smear (patient). Wright/Giemsa stain.

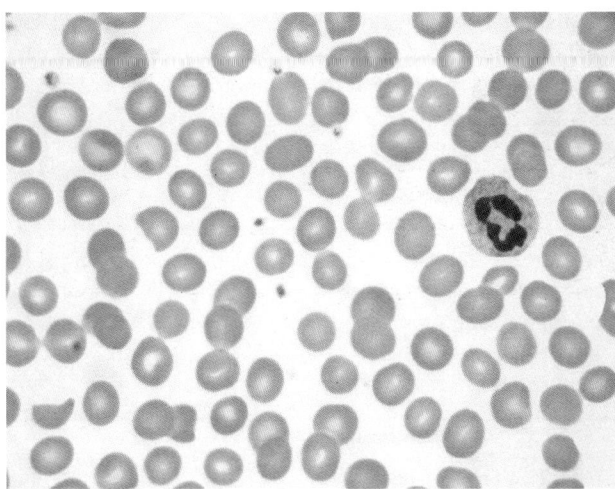

Figure 20.6 Peripheral blood smear (normal). Wright/Giemsa stain.

Questions

Based on the above information you can best conclude the following:

1. In general, the differential diagnosis of an anemia, such as that of this patient, should always include:

   a. alcohol abuse
   b. myelodysplastic syndromes
   c. liver disease
   d. all of the above
   e. none of the above

2. The patient's neurological signs and symptoms indicate involvement of:

   a. the dorsal columns of the spinal cord
   b. pyramidal tracts
   c. the lateral columns of the spinal cord
   d. all of the above
   e. none of the above

3. This patient's hyperbilirubinemia:

   a. indicates impaired canalicular transport of bilirubin glucuronides

   b. is due to increased RBC destruction

   c. should not be associated with an increased level of urine urobilinogen

   d. is predominantly composed of water-soluble bilirubin

   e. all of the above

4. This patient's gastric biopsy (Figs 20.1 and 20.3) is most consistent with:

   a. acute peptic ulcer

   b. adenocarcinoma

   c. lymphoma

   d. none of the above

5. This patient's gastric lesion (Figs 20.1 and 20.3) is usually associated with:

   a. an increased serum gastrin level

   b. intestinal metaplasia

   c. achlorhydria

   d. decreased numbers of parietal cells

   e. all of the above

Clinical course

Results of additional studies (Tables 20.5 and 20.6 and Fig. 20.7) evaluating this patient's anemia, including bone marrow examination, are seen below. Several days after the initiation of specific therapy the patient's hematological status significantly improved (Table 20.7); her neurological symptoms, however, persisted.

Table 20.5 Special hematology (Day 2)

			SI Units	
Iron	179 H	(42–135 µg/dL)	32.1 H	(7.5–24.2 µmol/L)
TIBC	310	(280–400 µg/dL)	55.5	(50.1–71.6 µmol/L)
Transferrin saturation	58 H	(15–50%)	0.58 H	(0.15–0.50)
Serum B_{12}	90 L	(225–1000 pg/dL)	90 L	(225–1000 pmol/L)
Serum folate	8.6	(1.7–12.6 ng/dL)	19.5	(3.85–28.5 mmol/L)

Table 20.6 Schilling test (Day 2)

Schilling I	6.9 L	(10–40%)
Schilling II	18.9	(10–40%)

Table 20.7 Hematology (8 days post therapy)

			SI Units	
WBC	6.8	(3.3–11.0 thou/µL)	6.8 H	(3.3–11.0 × 10^9/L)
RBC	4.1	(3.9–5.0 mill/µL)	4.1	(3.9–5.0 × 10^{12}/L)
HGB	11.7	(11.6–15.6 g/dL)	117	(116–156 g/L)
HCT	33 L	(37.0–47.0%)	0.33 L	(0.37–0.47)
Plts	200	(130–400 thou/µL)	200	(130–400 × 10^9/L)
Retic	5.4 H	(0.1–2.0%)	5.4 H	(0.1–2.0%)

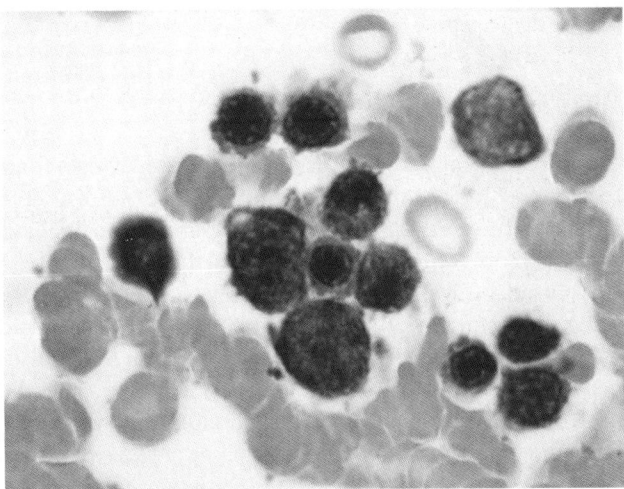

Figure 20.7 Bone marrow aspiration smear (patient). Wright/Giemsa stain.

Questions

6. The LEAST likely feature of this patient's anemia is:

    a. a decreased level of haptoglobin
    b. increased neutrophil myeloperoxidase
    c. morphological changes of RBCs and neutrophils
    d. an increased total leukocyte count
    e. anisocytosis and poikilocytosis

7. Bone marrow aspiration smear (Fig. 20.7) in this patient:

    a. shows erythroid hypoplasia
    b. would show decreased iron storage
    c. shows evidence of nuclear-cytoplasmic dissociation
    d. shows all of the above
    e. shows none of the above

8. This patient's elevated serum LDH level:

    a. is mainly due to an increase in LDH_1 and LDH_2 isoenzymes
    b. is due to ineffective erythropoiesis
    c. would return to normal within 2 weeks of therapy
    d. all of the above

9. The patient's increased reticulocyte count after 8 days of therapy (Table 20.7):

    a. is a favorable sign
    b. indicates an ongoing RBC hemolysis
    c. reflects impaired RBC production
    d. none of the above

10. Which of the following features of this patient's condition is not going to be corrected or improved by therapy?

    a. atrophic gastritis
    b. leukopenia
    c. hemolytic tendency
    d. increased serum iron level

11. Select the INCORRECT general statement about the hematological disease diagnosed in this patient:

    a. neurological abnormalities observed in patients with such a disease are due to impaired DNA synthesis in neurons
    b. a smooth beefy tongue may be seen in the absence of anemia
    c. epithelial cells of the buccal and vaginal mucosae may show morphological alteration
    d. muscle biopsy (Fig. 20.6) shows features consistent with an upper motor neuron lesion
    e. the Schilling test confirms the diagnosis

ANSWERS AND FURTHER INFORMATION

Figure descriptions

Figure 20.1 Gastric biopsy (patient). Hematoxylin & eosin stain.
Chronic atrophic gastritis: This image shows decreased numbers of gastric glands, mild to moderate gastric atrophy, mild cellular infiltrate of the lamina propria, the absence of parietal cells, focal intestinal metaplasia, and focal mucosal fibrosis, consistent with chronic atrophic gastritis.

Figure 20.2 Gastric biopsy (normal). Hematoxylin & eosin stain.
Normal gastric mucosa: This image shows a normal gastric mucosa. There is no significant inflammatory cell infiltrate in the lamina propria or hemorrhage. Gastric glands are intact. The surface epithelial cells are mucus-secreting cells.

Figure 20.3 Gastric biopsy (patient). PAS/Alcian blue stain.
Chronic atrophic gastritis: This section is stained with PAS/Alcian blue stain for mucopolysaccharides. It shows multiple blue-staining goblet cells (arrows), indicating focal intestinal metaplasia.

Figure 20.4 Gastric biopsy (normal). PAS/Alcian blue stain.
Normal gastric mucosa: No intestinal metaplasia is noted in this image.

Figure 20.5 Peripheral blood smear (patient). Wright/Giemsa stain.
Macrocytic anemia: This peripheral blood smear shows aniso-poikilocytosis, large oval red blood cells, and two hypersegmented neutrophils.

Figure 20.6 Peripheral blood smear (normal). Wright/Giemsa stain.
Normal blood smear: The red blood cells appear uniform and are normocytic. A neutrophil and platelets are seen in this image.

Figure 20.7 Bone marrow aspiration smear (patient). Wright/Giemsa stain.
Erythroid precursors with megaloblastic features: The patient's bone marrow aspiration smear is hypercellular. This image shows a cluster of erythroid precursors with dyserythropoiesis and nuclear-cytoplasmic dissociation. The peripheral blood smear and bone marrow findings are consistent with a megaloblastic anemia.

Answers

1. D. This patient has a macrocytic anemia, as is evident from the peripheral blood smear (Fig. 20.1) and RBC indices (Table 20.1). Macrocytosis can be detected by examination of blood smear or more accurately by determining the mean corpuscular volume (MCV). Macrocytes have MCV exceeding 100 fL. The most common cause of macrocytosis is megaloblastic anemia, which is most commonly due to vitamin B_{12} or folate deficiency. Alcoholism, hepatic diseases, hemolytic anemia, post-hemorrhagic anemia, post-splenectomy status, myelodysplastic syndromes, and aplastic anemia are known causes of non-megaloblastic, macrocytic anemia.

2. D. This patient's neurological manifestations indicate the involvement of the dorsal column of the spinal cord (loss of vibration and position senses), and involvement of the lateral columns of the spinal cord (pyramidal tracts). Pyramidal tract involvement is manifested by weakness and spasticity in the proximal muscles of all four extremities, hyperactive deep tendon reflexes, a positive Babinski's sign, and by the absence of fasciculation and significant muscle atrophy.

3. B. This patient's hyperbilirubinemia is mainly due to an elevated level of unconjugated bilirubin (conjugated bilirubin is less than 20% of total bilirubin). Unconjugated bilirubin is highly insoluble in aqueous media. Predominantly unconjugated hyperbilirubinemia is usually caused by RBC hemolysis and by rare hereditary diseases associated with defects in bilirubin conjugation or transport in the liver. Impaired canalicular transport of bilirubin glucuronides, on the other hand, would lead to predominantly conjugated hyperbilirubinemia and is the underlying mechanism for Dubin–Johnson and Rotor's syndromes. Urobilinogens are bacterial degradation products of bilirubin in the bowel, mainly excreted in the feces. About 20% of urobilinogen is reabsorbed and returned to the liver to be excreted into bile (enterohepatic circulation). A small proportion of urobilinogen escapes the enterohepatic circulation and is excreted in urine. In patients with increased bilirubin overload (increased RBC destruction), the urine urobilinogen level is increased.

4. D. This patient's gastric biopsy (Figs 20.1 and 20.3) shows mild to moderate gastric atrophy, mild cellular infiltrate of the lamina propria, focal intestinal metaplasia, and focal mucosal fibrosis, consistent with chronic atrophic gastritis. There is no evidence to suggest the diagnosis of an acute peptic ulcer, adenocarcinoma, or lymphoma.

5. E. The most likely diagnosis of gastric mucosal atrophy with only minimal inflammatory cellular infiltrate (seen in Figs 20.1 and 20.3) in a patient with severe macrocytic anemia, neurological symptoms, and glossitis is that of immunologic (autoimmune) chronic gastritis. In autoimmune gastritis the volume of gastric acid secretion, hydrogen ion secretion in response to histamine stimulation, and the secretion of intrinsic factor are markedly reduced or absent owing to autoimmune destruction of parietal cells. The serum gastrin level is usually increased in response to the decreased gastric acidity.

6. D. The patient has a severe macrocytic anemia. The presence of chronic atrophic gastritis (autoimmune gastritis), of a low level of serum vitamin B_{12}, and of an abnormal Schilling test (stage I) and a normal Schilling test (stage II) confirmed the diagnosis of pernicious anemia (PA), due to a gastropathy leading to deficient intrinsic factor secretion and cobalamin deficiency. In patients with PA the peripheral blood smear shows hypersegmented neutrophils, ovalomacrocytes, anisocytosis, and poikilocytosis. The total leukocyte count is reduced or normal and there is an increased neutrophil myeloperoxidase. In PA there is increased intramedullary hemolysis (decreased RBC life span), which leads to a decreased serum level of haptoglobin.

7. C. Bone marrow aspiration smear (Fig. 20.7) shows erythroid hyperplasia (increased numbers of erythroid precursors), multiple megaloblasts, with abundant mature (pink) cytoplasm and an immature (delicate nuclear chromatin) nucleus (i.e. nuclear-cytoplasmic dissociation). Bone marrow biopsy in patients with pernicious anemia would show increased bone marrow iron storage and sideroblasts.

8. D. This patient has pernicious anemia. In the majority of patients with pernicious anemia the serum LDH level is increased (due to ineffective erythropoiesis in the bone marrow and RBC destruction). This increase reflects increased levels of LDH_1 and LDH_2 isoenzymes. LDH_1 increase is greater than that of LDH_2. The LDH level usually returns to normal within 2 weeks of the onset of therapy.

9. A. The patient was started on parenteral cyanocobalamin therapy for her pernicious anemia. The response to this therapy is usually brisk and the presence of reticulocytosis is a favorable sign, which indicates effective erythropoiesis rather than ongoing RBC hemolysis.

10. A. In pernicious anemia the gastric changes are primary and are believed to result from immunologically mediated destruction of gastric mucosa, which leads to vitamin B_{12} deficiency. Since these changes are not the effect of vitamin B_{12} deficiency, the parenteral administration of cyanocobalamin (vitamin B_{12}) will not correct the gastric atrophy or achlorhydria. Leukopenia and a hemolytic tendency are direct consequences of vitamin B_{12} deficiency and, therefore, will be corrected by therapy. The increased iron level is expected to fall after therapy, due to marked utilization of previously unused iron and due to correction of the hemolytic tendency.

11. A. Neurological abnormalities observed in patients with pernicious anemia (PA) are due to lack of tissue S-adenosylmethionine (SAM), which is produced by cobalamin-dependent reactions. SAM is required for some transmethylation reactions essential for synthesis and maintenance of myelin. Since neurons do not divide, impaired DNA synthesis plays no role in the pathogenesis of the neurologic abnormalities observed in patients with PA. Glossitis (smooth "beefy" red tongue) may be seen in patients with PA in the absence of hematologic abnormalities. Epithelial cells of the buccal and vaginal mucosae in patients with PA may show morphologic alterations similar to those seen in the bone marrow and red blood cell precursors (enlarged nuclei and nuclear-cytoplasmic dissociation). The presence of an abnormal Schilling I and a normal Schilling II test indicate that vitamin B_{12} deficiency is due to intrinsic factor deficiency and confirms the diagnosis of PA.

Final diagnosis and synopsis of the case

- Subacute combined degeneration of spinal cord
- Chronic atrophic gastritis
- Pernicious anemia

An elderly woman, who was diagnosed 4 years previously as having chronic atrophic gastritis, presented with symptoms suggesting subacute combined degeneration of the spinal cord (fatigue, difficulty in walking, weakness of the upper extremities, forgetfulness, tingling sensations in all four extremities, and mood swings), with atrophic glossitis, and with a severe macrocytic anemia. The work-up of her anemia revealed a reduced level of serum vitamin B_{12} and megaloblas-tic changes in her peripheral blood smear and bone marrow. The diagnosis of pernicious anemia (PA) was confirmed by an abnormal Schilling test. All the findings in this patient were related to her atrophic gastritis, which leads to vitamin B_{12} deficiency. Vitamin B_{12} deficiency leads to nuclear-cytoplasmic dissociation in all proliferating cells (e.g. RBC megaloblastic changes), degeneration of the posterior and lateral columns of the spinal cord (neurologic manifestations), ineffective erythropoiesis, and a hemolytic tendency (hyperbilirubinemia, increased LDH level, increased serum iron level). The patient's hematologic abnormalities promptly responded to parenteral therapy with cyanocobalamin (vitamin B_{12}).

Lab tips

Schilling test

Schilling test examines cobalamin (vitamin B_{12}) absorption. It is performed in two stages.
- Stage I: ^{57}Co-cyanocobalamin is given orally and subsequently the 24-hour urinary excretion of the radioactive cyanocobalamin is measured. If this stage is abnormal (i.e. abnormal absorption of cobalamin), proceed to stage II.
- Stage II: the test is repeated with the concomitant administration of intrinsic factor.

If the absorption of cyanocobalamin improves after the administration of intrinsic factor (normal Schilling II), the patient's vitamin B_{12} malabsorption is most likely to be due to deficient intrinsic factor secretion (pernicious anemia). Decreased hydrochloric acid secretion (achlorhydria) affects the absorption of the protein-bound vitamin B_{12} (in food), which could lead to vitamin B_{12} deficiency. This deficiency, however, is not associated with an abnormal Schilling test since the absorption of free cyanocobalamin (such as measured in Schilling test) does not depend on the presence of hydrochloric acid. For this reason, in patients with a simple achlorhydria, Schilling test stages I and II are normal.

A 72-year-old librarian with diabetes

CASE AND MCQS

Clinical history and presentation

A 72-year-old woman was seen at her physician's office for a routine check-up. Her medical history included non-insulin dependent diabetes mellitus of 12 years' duration. She had a myocardial infarction 2 years ago, and she has well-controlled congestive heart failure. Her hyperglycemia was controlled by an oral medication. She continued to smoke at least a pack of cigarettes a day, against the advice of her physician. Physical examination revealed an obese, elderly female, oriented, and in no acute distress. She was afebrile. Her blood pressure was 170/80 mmHg, pulse rate 74/min and regular, and respirations 16/min. The lungs were clear to auscultation, there was edema of both legs and there were prominent varicose veins. The abdomen was soft but a pulsatile mass was palpated.

Admission data

Table 21.1 Hematology

			SI Units	
WBC	9.2	(3.3–11.0 thou/μL)	9.2	(3.3–11.0 × 10^9/L)
Neut	80	(44–88%)	80	(44–88%)
Band	0	(0–10%)	0	(0–10%)
Lymph	12	(12–43%)	12	(12–43%)
Mono	5	(2–11%)	5	(2–11%)
Eos	1	(0–5%)	1	(0–5%)
Baso	2	(0–2%)	2	(0–2%)
RBC	4.7	(3.9–5.0 mill/μL)	4.7	(3.9–5.0 × 10^{12}/L)
HGB	14.4	(11.6–15.6 g/dL)	144	(116–156 g/L)
HCT	43.0	(37.0–47.0%)	0.43	(0.37–0.47)
MCV	91.6	(79.0–99.0 fL)	91.6	(79.0–99.0 fL)
MCH	30.6	(26.0–32.6 pg)	30.6	(26.0–32.6 pg)
MCHC	33.4	(31.0–36.0 g/dL)	334	(310–360 g/L)
Plts	255	(130–400 thou/μL)	255	(130–400 × 10^9/L)

Table 21.2 Chemistry

			SI Units	
Glucose	118 H	(65–110 mg/dL)	6.55 H	(3.6–6.11 mmol/L)
Creatinine	1.2	(0.7–1.4 mg/dL)	106	(61.9–123.8 µmol/L)
BUN	20	(7–24 mg/dL)	7.14	(2.50–8.57 mmol/L)
Uric acid	7.0	(3.0–8.5 mg/dL)	0.42	(0.18–0.51 mmol/L)
Cholesterol	290 H	(150–200 mg/dL)	7.50 H	(3.88–5.17 mmol/L)
Calcium	9.1	(8.5–10.5 mg/dL)	2.28	(2.13–2.63 mmol/L)
Protein	7.4	(6–8 g/dL)	74	(60–80 g/L)
Albumin	3.9	(3.7–5.0 g/dL)	39	(37–50 g/L)
LDH	180	(100–250 U/L)	180	(100–250 U/L)
Alk Phos	110	(0–120 U/L)	110	(0–120 U/L)
AST	40	(0–55 U/L)	40	(0–55 U/L)
GGTP	41	(0–50 U/L)	41	(0–50 U/L)
Bilirubin	0.7	(0.0–1.5 mg/dL)	12	(0–25.7 µmol/L)
Bilirubin-direct	0.15	(0.02–0.18 mg/dL)	2.6	(0.34–3.08 µmol/L)
BNP (B-type natriuretic peptide)	130 H	(<100 pg/mL)	130 H	(<100 ng/L)

Table 21.3 Electrolytes

			SI Units	
Na	136	(134–143 mEq/L)	136	(134–143 mmol/L)
K	4.6	(3.5–4.9 mEq/L)	4.6	(3.5–4.9 mmol/L)
Cl	97	(95–108 mEq/L)	97	(95–108 mmol/L)
CO_2	24	(21–32 mEq/L)	24	(21–32 mmol/L)

Table 21.4 Urinalysis

pH	6	(5.0–7.5)
Protein	Neg	(Neg)
Glucose	Neg	(Neg)
Ketone	Neg	(Neg)
Color	Yellow	(Yellow)
Clarity	Clear	(Clear)
Sp. grav.	1.017	(1.010–1.035)
WBC	4	(0–5/HPF)
RBC	0	(0–2/HPF)
Casts	Neg	(Neg)
Bacteria	Neg	(Neg)

Questions

Based on the above information you can best conclude the following:

1. Which of the following problems would you NOT expect in the type of diabetes such as this patient has?

   a. a reduced responsiveness of peripheral tissues to insulin
   b. impaired insulin secretion by β-cells
   c. increased susceptibility to infection
   d. ketoacidosis upon decompensation
   e. a vascular involvement by the disease

2. Complications resulting from this type of diabetes include all of the following EXCEPT:

   a. varicose veins of the leg
   b. accelerated atherosclerosis
   c. microangiopathy
   d. nephropathy
   e. neuropathy

3. Which of the following tests would give you the best information about this patient's control of blood glucose over an extended period of time?

   a. random testing of urine
   b. the total amount of glucose in a 24-hour collection of urine
   c. a random morning blood glucose level
   d. random testing for ketones in blood
   e. the measurement of glycosylated hemoglobin "HbA$_{1c}$"

4. This patient has coronary artery disease. Which of the following factors in this patient is considered to be a risk for atherosclerosis-related disease?

   a. diabetes mellitus
   b. hypertension
   c. high serum cholesterol
   d. age
   e. all of the above

5. Which of the following vascular lesions is more common in a diabetic than in a non-diabetic population in the same age group?

   a. atherosclerosis
   b. hyaline arteriolosclerosis of afferent and efferent glomerular arterioles
   c. severe atherosclerosis of the aorta
   d. diffuse thickening of the capillary basement membrane
   e. all of the above

Clinical course

An ultrasound examination of the abdomen was performed to evaluate the patient's abdominal mass (Fig. 21.1). The findings were discussed with the patient and she underwent a surgical procedure. She tolerated the procedure well and her recovery was uneventful. Figures 21.3–21.6 show the appearance of the abdominal lesion's content.

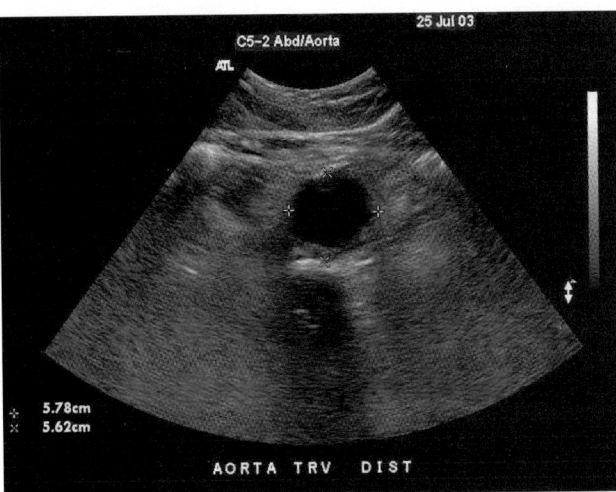

Figure 21.1 Ultrasound examination of the abdominal lesion (patient).

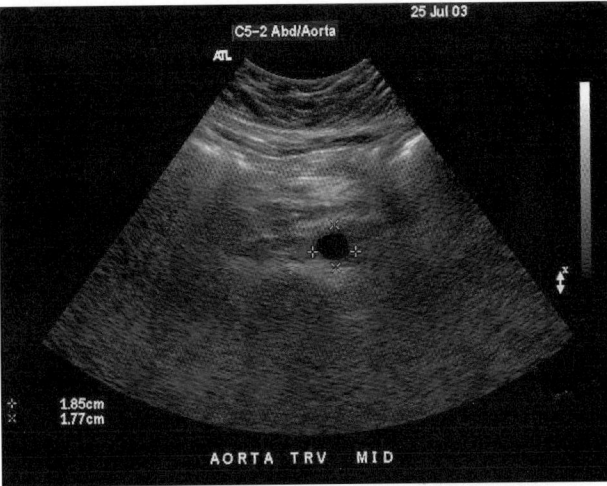

Figure 21.2 Ultrasound examination of an area proximal to the abdominal lesion (patient).

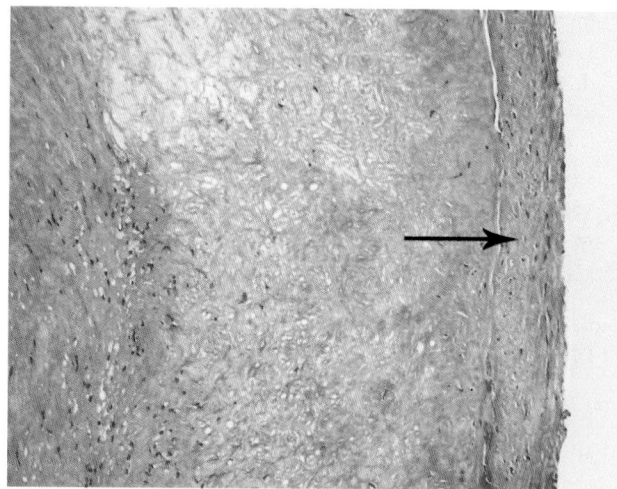

Figure 21.3 Material from the abdominal lesion (patient). H&E stain.

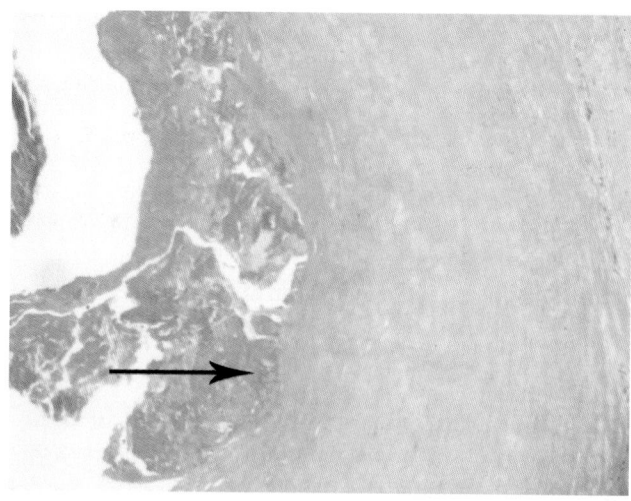

Figure 21.4 Material from the abdominal lesion (patient). H&E stain.

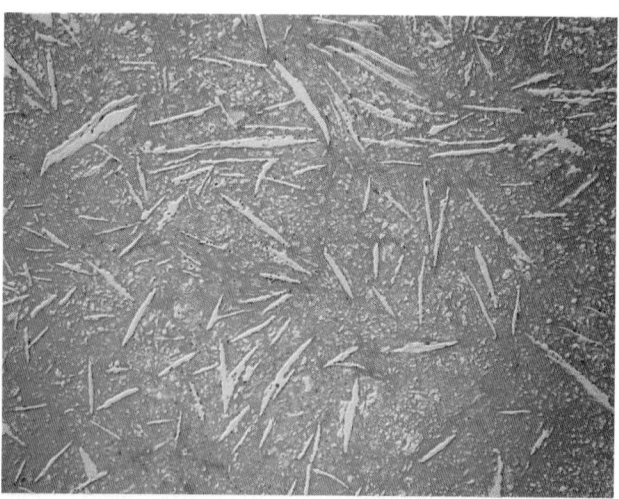

Figure 21.5 Material from the abdominal lesion (patient). H&E stain.

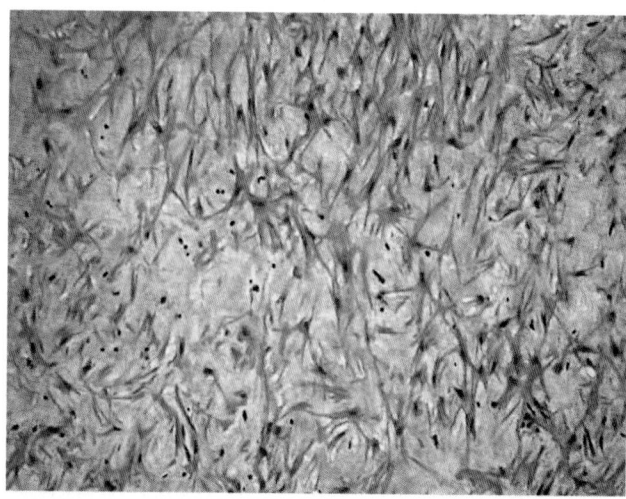

Figure 21.6 Material from the abdominal lesion (patient). H&E stain.

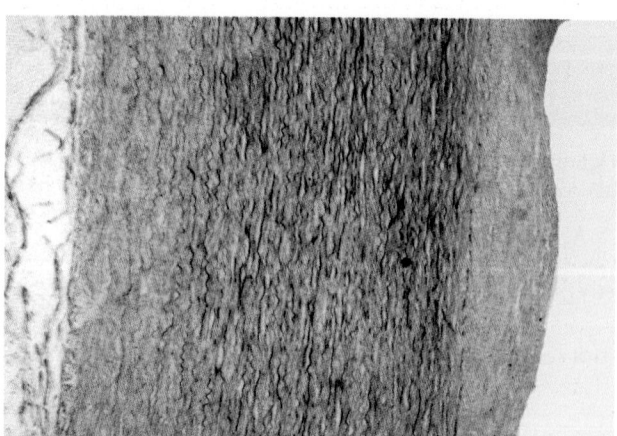

Figure 21.7 Abdominal aorta (normal). Elastic stain.

Questions

INTERMEDIATE

6. Identify the correct statement about this surgically removed lesion:

    a. the location of this patient's lesion is not typical for such a lesion of atherosclerotic origin

    b. such a lesion is more common in women

    c. such a lesion may be a cause of pulmonary embolism and infarction

    d. all of the above

    e. none of the above

INTERMEDIATE

7. The microscopic appearance of the material from the abdominal lesion (Figs. 21.3–21.6) depicts all of the following EXCEPT:

    a. dissection of the wall by blood

    b. fibrin deposition

    c. an area of necrosis

    d. cholesterol crystals

    e. lipid-laden macrophages

INTERMEDIATE

8. The patient has isolated systolic hypertension. In general, the most likely cause of this type of hypertension is:

    a. pheochromocytoma

    b. decreased aortic and arterial compliance

    c. narrowing of the renal artery

    d. chronic renal disease

    e. none of the above

ANSWERS AND FURTHER INFORMATION

Figure descriptions

Figure 21.1 Ultrasound examination of the abdominal lesion (patient).
Aortic aneurysm: This transverse ultrasound image shows an infrarenal aortic aneurysm measuring 5.78 × 5.62 cm. Surgical repair is not a surgical emergency when the aortic aneurysm is less than 5 cm in diameter.

Figure 21.2 Ultrasound examination of an area proximal to the abdominal lesion (patient).
A transverse ultrasound image of an area proximal to the aortic aneurysm shows the normal non-aneurysmal caliber of the vessel, with a diameter of 1.85 cm, for comparison.

Figure 21.3 Material from the abdominal lesion (patient). Hematoxylin & eosin stain.
Material from the aortic aneurysm removed during surgery, showing a thinned portion of the tunica media on the right (arrow). The intima is thickened, loose, and contains an atheromatous plaque.

Figure 21.4 Material from the abdominal lesion (patient). Hematoxylin & eosin stain.
This image exhibits a portion of the atheromatous plaque showing fibrin deposition, necrotic debris, and microcalcification (arrow).

Figure 21.5 Material from the abdominal lesion (patient). Hematoxylin & eosin stain.
This photomicrograph shows a portion of the atheromatous plaque showing cholesterol crystal clefts.

Figure 21.6 Material from the abdominal lesion (patient). Hematoxylin & eosin stain.
Portion of the atheromatous plaque showing smooth muscle proliferation and a few foamy macrophages in this photomicrograph.

Figure 21.7 Abdominal aorta (normal). Elastic stain.
This is a section from a normal adult aorta. A normal tunica intima is seen on the right side of this image. The tunica media is thick and contains smooth muscle and elastic fibers (black staining). The tunica adventitia is seen on the left side of the image.

Answers

1. D. The patient has type II diabetes mellitus, which is characterized by two major metabolic defects: derangement of insulin secretion by β-cells and a reduced responsiveness of peripheral tissues to insulin. Both defects lead to hyperglycemia and eventual β-cell exhaustion. In both type I and type II diabetes there is an increased susceptibility to infection.

The disease process affects large and small vessels' basement membrane, kidney, nerves, retina, and other tissues. Upon decompensation, however, patients with type I diabetes develop ketoacidosis (due to severe insulin deficiency and an absolute or relative increase of glucagon). Patients with type II diabetes usually do not suffer from severe deficiency of insulin and do not develop ketoacidosis. They could develop (due to hyperglycemic diuresis) severe dehydration and so called hyperosmotic non-ketotic coma, but not ketoacidosis.

2. A. Type II diabetes mellitus leads to all the listed complications (accelerated atherosclerosis, microangiopathy, nephropathy, and neuropathy) except varicose veins of the leg. These are formed in response to intraluminal venous pressure and there is a familial tendency for their development.

3. E. The measurement of glycosylated (glycated) hemoglobin (HbA$_{1c}$) level in the blood provides the best information about the control of glycemia over the past several weeks. Glycosylated hemoglobin is produced by non-enzymatic attachment of the glucose molecules with free amino groups on the globin component of hemoglobin. The glycohemoglobin circulates within red blood cells up to 120 days and therefore provides information about the level of glycemia during that period. The higher the glycemia, the higher will be the level of glycohemoglobin. Random laboratory tests mentioned (of blood or urine) do not provide information about the control of hyperglycemia over an extended period of time.

4. E. The major risk factors for the development of atherosclerosis-related diseases include all factors listed: diabetes mellitus, hypertension, hypercholesterolemia, and increasing age.

5. E. Diabetes leads to a variety of morphologic changes in the vascular system. Atherosclerosis of large arteries (aorta and renal artery) occurs in diabetics at earlier age and is of greater severity than in non-diabetics. A microangiopathy, diffuse thickening of the capillary basement membrane, is also seen in elderly non-diabetics, but not to the extent seen in long-standing diabetics. Hyaline arteriolosclerosis of afferent and efferent glomerular arterioles is almost exclusively seen in diabetics.

6. E. The surgery was done to correct and repair a large abdominal aortic aneurysm. Atherosclerosis is the most common cause of aneurysm and such aneurysms most frequently occur in the abdominal portion of the aorta. Abdominal aortic aneurysm is more common in men than women. While it is true that embolism from the atheroma or mural thrombus occurs, it affects the arterial system; pulmonary embolisms originate from the venous system, most often from deep calf veins.

7. A. Figures 21.3–21.6 show the histological appearance of the aortic aneurysm material, removed during surgery. Figure 21.3 shows thickened intima with an atheromatous plaque. Figures 21.4 and 21.5 show fibrin material and cholesterol crystal (cleft), respectively. A portion of thinned media is seen in Fig. 21.3. There is no morphologic evidence of dissection noted in Figs 21.3–21.6.

8. B. The patient has isolated systolic hypertension (an increased systolic blood pressure with a normal diastolic pressure). Such a finding accounts for more than 50% of hypertension in people over 60 years of age. This kind of hypertension is caused by decreased aortic and arterial compliance and is not as benign as previously thought. It should be treated. The other causes of hypertension (pheochromocytoma, renal artery stenosis, and chronic renal disease) lead to increase in both systolic and diastolic blood pressure.

Final diagnosis and synopsis of the case

- Type II diabetes mellitus
- Isolated systolic hypertension
- Abdominal aortic aneurysm

The patient is a 72-year-old woman with a 12-year history of diabetes mellitus and ischemic heart disease. On routine check-up, a large pulsating abdominal mass was discovered.

Abdominal CT scan showed an abdominal aortic aneurysm, which was surgically treated. She tolerated the procedure well and there were no post-operative complications. She will continue to take her oral hypoglycemic medication and will be seen by her cardiologist to re-evaluate her hypertension therapy.

SI units conversion table

	Conventional units	Conversion factor	SI units
ACTH, serum (adrenocorticotrophic hormone)	pg/mL	0.22	pmol/L
ALT (alanine aminotransferase)	U/L	1	U/L
APTT (activated partial thromboplastin time)	seconds	1	seconds
AST (aspartate aminotransferase)	U/L	1	U/L
Acetaminophen (paracetamol)	µg/mL	6.62	µmol/L
Albumin	g/dL	10	g/L
Albumin, cerebrospinal fluid	mg/dL	10	mg/L
Aldosterone, serum	ng/dL	0.0277	nmol/L
Alkaline phosphatase	U/L	1	U/L
Amylase, serum (Dupont aca)	U/L	0.017	µkat/L
Amylase, urinary (Dupont aca)	U/hr.	1	U/hr.
Angiotensin-1-converting enzyme	U/L	0.017	uKat/L
Apoprotein A-1 (apolipoprotein A-1)	mg/dL	0.01	g/L
Apoprotein B100 (apolipoprotein B)	mg/dL	0.01	g/L
BUN (blood urea nitrogen)	mg/dL	0.357	mmol/L
Bands, blood (band neutrophils)	%	0.01	fraction
Base, excess	mEq/L	1	mmol/L
Bilirubin, direct	mg/dL	17.1	µmol/L
Bilirubin, total	mg/dL	17.1	µmol/L
B-type natriuretic peptide (BNP)	pg/mL	1	ng/L
CA-125 (cancer antigen 125)	AU/mL	1	kAU/L
CEA (carcinoembryonic antigen)	µg/L	1	µg/L
CK (creatine kinase)	U/L	1	U/L
CO_2, venous whole blood (carbon dioxide)	mEq/L	1	mmol/L
CPK MB (creatine kinase MB isoenzyme)	%	0.01	fraction
CPK MM (creatine kinase MM isoenzyme)	%	0.01	fraction
Calcium, total	mg/dL	0.2500	mmol/L
Cholesterol	mg/dL	0.025 86	mmol/L
Cl (chloride)	mEq/L	1	mmol/L
Creatinine	mg/dL	88.40	µmol/L
Eos, blood (eosinophils)	%	0.01	fraction
Ferritin	ng/mL	1	µg/L
Fibrin degradation products (FDP)	µg/mL	1	mg/L
Fibrinogen	mg/dL	0.01	g/L
Folate	ng/mL	2.265	nmol/L
GGTP (gamma glutamyl transferase)	U/L	1	U/L
Glucose, blood	mg/dL	0.055 51	mmol/L
Glycosylated hemoglobin	%	0.01	fraction
HCO_3^-, arterial whole blood (carbon dioxide content)	mEq/L	1	mmol/L
HDL (high-density lipoprotein cholesterol)	mg/dL	0.0259	mmol/L

Continued

	Conventional units	Conversion factor	SI units
Haptoglobin	mg/dL	10	mg/L
HCT (hematocrit)	%	0.01	fraction
Hgb (hemoglobin)	g/dL	10	g/L
Iron, total	µg/dL	0.1791	µmol/L
Iron-binding capacity, total	µg/dL	0.1791	µmol/L
K (potassium)	mEq/L	1	mmol/L
LDH (lactate dehydrogenase)	U/L	1	U/L
LDH_1, LDH_2, LDH_3, LDH_4, LDH_5	%	0.01	fraction
LDL (low-density lipoprotein cholesterol)	mg/dL	0.0259	mmol/L
Lipase, serum	U/L	0.017	µkat/L
MCH (mean corpuscular hemoglobin)	pg	1	pg
MCHC (mean corpuscular hemoglobin concentration)	g/dL	0.01	fraction
MCV (mean corpuscular volume)	fL	1	fL
Monos, blood (monocytes)	%	0.01	fraction
Na (sodium)	mEq/L	1	mmol/L
O_2 saturation, arterial whole blood	%	0.01	fraction
PCO_2, arterial whole blood (carbon dioxide partial pressure)	mmHg	0.1333	kPa
PO_2, arterial whole blood (oxygen partial pressure)	mmHg	0.1333	kPa
PT (prothrombin time)	seconds	1	seconds
Plt (platelets)	thou/µL	1000 000	$\times 10^9$/L
Prostate-specific antigen (PSA)	ng/mL	1	µg/L
Prostatic acid phosphatase (PAP)	ng/mL	1	µg/L
Protein, total	g/dL	10	g/L
RBC, blood (red cell count)	mill/µL	1000 000	$\times 10^{12}$/L
RF (rheumatoid factor)	U/mL	1	kU/L
Reticulocytes	%	0.01	fraction
Transferrin saturation	%	0.01	fraction
Triglycerides	mg/dL	0.011 29	mmol/L
Uric acid	mg/dL	0.059 48	mmol/L
Vitamin B_{12}	pg/mL	0.7378	pmol/L
WBC, blood (total white cell count)	thou/µL	1000 000	$\times 10^9$/L
WBC, synovial fluid (total white cell count)	cells/µL	1000 000	cells/L

Topics explored

A. Pathology topics

Pathology topics	Chapters
Abscess	10
Acute appendicitis	7
Acute lymphoblastic leukemia	2
Acute pyelonephritis	6
Adynamic ileus	15
Anemia of chronic disease	1, 3, 4, 13
Anemia, hemolytic	11, 13
Anemia, macrocytic	3, 13
Anemia, megaloblastic	3, 13, 19, 20
Anemia, microcytic	3, 4, 13
Anemia, pernicious	20
Aortic aneurysm	21
Atherosclerosis	15, 21
Bacteremia	7, 11
Beta thalassemia	13
B-lymphocyte antigens	2, 16
Carcinoma of colon	3
Carcinoma of endometrium	15
Carcinoma of lung	9
Carcinoma of oral cavity	5
Carcinoma of prostate	12
Chronic blood loss	3
Chronic granulomatous disease	10
Chronic idiopathic cold agglutinin immune hemolytic anemia	11
Congestive heart failure	3
Diabetes mellitus	9, 21
Eosinophilia	17
Erythema multiforme	17
Erythromelalgia	14

Pathology topics	Chapters
Essential thrombocythemia	14
Gastritis, acute	14
Gastritis, atrophic	20
Gastritis, chronic active	4
Gastroenteritis	13
Gilbert syndrome	13
Granuloma	1
Hodgkin's disease	18
Immune hemolytic anemia	11
Inflammation, acute	1
Inflammation, chronic	1
Jaundice	13, 20
Malnutrition	10
Multiple myeloma	7
Mycosis fungoides	16
Osteomyelitis	10
Oxygen-dependent killing of microorganisms	10
Pathological bone fractures	7, 9
Peptic ulcer	19
Pneumonia	1, 17
Polyclonal hypergammaglobulinemia	17
Polycythemia rubra vera	19
Premalignant lesions of oral cavity	5
Sarcoidosis	1
Sinusitis	14
Skin lesions	16, 17
Systolic hypertension	21
T lymphocyte antigens	2, 16
Urinary tract infection	6, 11, 13
Vaginal bleeding	15

B. Laboratory medicine topics

Laboratory medicine topics	Chapters	Laboratory medicine topics	Chapters
Arterial blood gases	1, 3, 10	Hypercalcemia	7
Azotemia	3, 9, 11	Hyperglycemia	9, 21
B lymphocyte antigens	2, 16	Hypoalbuminemia	9, 17
Bacteriuria	6, 11	Hypocalcemia and hypoalbuminemia	9
Bence-Jones proteins	7	Hypocalcemia	9
Bilirubin	11, 13	Hypokalemia	10
Blood cultures	1	Immunofixation of serum protein	7
Bone marrow composition	2	Iron studies	4
BUN (blood urea nitrogen)	6, 9, 10, 13	LDH (lactate dehydrogenase)	15
Carcinoembryonic antigen (CEA)	3	Leukocytosis	2, 6, 8, 13
Casts in urine	6	Lymphocytosis	2, 6, 8, 12
Cold agglutinins	11, 17	NBT (nitroblue tetrazolium test)	10
Coombs' test	2	Platelets	14, 15
Eosinophils	17	Prostate-specific antigen (PSA)	12
Erythrocyte sedimentation rate (ESR)	2	Prostatic specific acid phosphatase (PSAP)	12
Ferritin	1	Proteinuria	6
Flow cytometric analysis	2, 16	RDW (red cell distribution width)	4, 13
GGTP (gamma glutamyl transferase)	4	Reticulocytosis	10, 11
Glycosylated hemoglobin	21	Schilling test	20
Guaiac test for occult blood	3, 14	Serum protein electrophoresis	7, 10, 17
Haptoglobin	2, 11	Sputum analysis	1
Helicobacter pylori	4	T lymphocyte antigens	2, 16
Hematuria	6, 11, 12	Urinalysis	6, 11
Hemolysis	11	Urinary protein electrophoresis	7

Lab tips

Final diagnoses

Final diagnoses	Chapters
Abdominal aortic aneurysm	21
Acute appendicitis	8
Acute bacterial pneumonia	1
Acute bacterial sinusitis	14
Acute gastritis	14
Acute lymphoblastic leukemia of mixed lineage	2
Acute pyelonephritis	6
Acute urinary tract infection (*Proteus mirabilis*)	13
Adenocarcinoma of the prostate	12
Anemia	2
Anemia of chronic disease	1, 10
Bone pain due to infiltration by leukemic cells	2
Bowel obstruction	15
Bronchopneumonia	10
Carcinomatosis	15
Chronic atrophic gastritis	20
Chronic blood loss	4
Chronic granulomatous disease	10
Chronic idiopathic cold agglutinin immune hemolytic anemia	11
Colonic adenocarcinoma	3
Congestive heart failure (CHF)	3
Duodenal ulcer	19
Eosinophilia	17
Erythema multiforme	17
Erythromelalgia	14
Escherichia coli bacteremia	8, 11

Final diagnoses	Chapters
Essential thrombocytosis (thrombocythemia)	14
Gastritis; *Helicobacter pylori* infection	4
Gilbert's syndrome	13
Hodgkin's disease	18
Iron deficiency anemia	4
Isolated systolic hypertension	21
Lower urinary tract infection	11
Malnutrition	10
Metabolic alkalosis	10
Microcytic hypochromic anemia	3
Multiple abscesses (*Enterobacter aerogenes*)	10
Multiple myeloma	7
Mycosis fungoides	16
Non-small-cell carcinoma of the lung	9
Oral squamous cell carcinoma involving the mandible	5
Osteomyelitis (*Enterobacter aerogenes*)	10
Papillary serous adenocarcinoma of the endometrium	15
Pathologic bone fracture	7, 9
Pernicious anemia	20
Pneumonia	17
Polyclonal hypergammaglobulinemia	17
Polycythemia rubra vera	19
Sarcoidosis	1
Subacute combined degeneration of spinal cord	20
Type II diabetes mellitus	21

Index

Page range references covering several pages, e.g. 70–8, indicate the major topics explored (Appendix 2) and final diagnoses (Appendix 3). References with parentheses, e.g. 4(7), indicate a question and its answer.